INTERVIEWING CHILDREN AND ADOLESCENTS

ALSO BY JAMES MORRISON

Diagnosis Made Easier, Second Edition:
Principles and Techniques for Mental Health Clinicians

DSM-5 Made Easy: The Clinician's Guide to Diagnosis

The First Interview, Fourth Edition

When Psychological Problems Mask Medical Disorders, Second Edition:
A Guide for Psychotherapists

Interviewing

Children

and Adolescents

SECOND EDITION

**SKILLS AND STRATEGIES
FOR EFFECTIVE DSM-5® DIAGNOSIS**

James Morrison
Kathryn Flegel

THE GUILFORD PRESS
New York   London

Copyright © 2016 The Guilford Press
A Division of Guilford Publications, Inc.
370 Seventh Avenue, Suite 1200, New York, NY 10001
www.guilford.com

Paperback edition 2018

Printed in the United States of America

This book is printed on acid-free paper.

Last digit is print number: 9   8   7   6   5   4   3   2

The authors have checked with sources believed to be reliable in their efforts to provide formation that is complete and generally in accord with the standards of practice that are accepted at the time of publication. However, in view of the possibility of human error or changes in behavioral, mental health, or medical sciences, neither the authors, nor the editor and publisher, nor any other party who has been involved in the preparation or publication of this work warrants that the information contained herein is in every respect accurate or complete, and they are not responsible for any errors or omissions or the results obtained from the use of such information. Readers are encouraged to confirm the information contained in this book with other sources.

Library of Congress Cataloging-in-Publication Data

Names: Morrison, James R., 1940- author. | Flegel, Kathryn, author.
Title: Interviewing children and adolescents : skills and strategies for effective DSM-5 diagnosis / James Morrison and Kathryn Flegel.
Description: Second edition. | New York, NY : The Guilford Press, [2016] | Includes bibliographical references and index.
Identifiers: LCCN 2016023930 | ISBN 9781462526932 (hardback : acid-free paper); 9781462533794 (paperback : acid-free paper)
Subjects: LCSH: Interviewing in child psychiatry. | Interviewing in adolescent psychiatry. | Mental illness--Diagnosis. | BISAC: PSYCHOLOGY / Psychotherapy / Child & Adolescent. | MEDICAL / Psychiatry / Child & Adolescent. | SOCIAL SCIENCE / Social Work. | PSYCHOLOGY / Psychopathology / General.
Classification: LCC RJ503.6 .M67 2016 | DDC 618.92/89075--dc23
LC record available at https://lccn.loc.gov/2016023930

The "Essential Features" boxes; Tables 16.1, 24.1, 25.1a, 25.1b, and 27.1; and the sidebar on page 331 are all reprinted or adapted from *DSM-5® Made Easy: The Clinician's Guide to Diagnosis* by James Morrison, copyright © 2014 The Guilford Press.

DSM-5 is a registered trademark of the American Psychiatric Association. The APA has not participated in the preparation of this book.

For the children and adolescents in my life:
Emily, Jasper, Lucia, Maia, Nikolas, Rebecca, and Soren
—J. M.

For my family: Nicki, Joe, and Katie
—K. F.

About the Authors

James Morrison, MD, is Affiliate Professor of Psychiatry at Oregon Health and Science University (OHSU) in Portland. He has extensive experience in both the private and public sectors. With his acclaimed practical books—including *DSM-5 Made Easy*; *Diagnosis Made Easier, Second Edition*; *The First Interview, Fourth Edition*; and *When Psychological Problems Mask Medical Disorders, Second Edition*—Dr. Morrison has guided hundreds of thousands of mental health professionals and students through the complexities of clinical evaluation and diagnosis.

Kathryn Flegel, MD, is Assistant Professor of Child and Adolescent Psychiatry at OHSU. Dr. Flegel was a primary care doctor for 16 years before becoming a psychiatrist. She completed her psychiatry residency and child psychiatry fellowship at OHSU and currently provides inpatient and outpatient care to children, adults, and families. Dr. Flegel is a Fellow of the American Psychiatric Association.

Acknowledgments

We are grateful to Mary Morrison, who provided valuable criticism at various stages throughout the project. Our editor, Kitty Moore, and copyeditor, Marie Sprayberry, have given their usual all. We also acknowledge the assistance of Anna Brackett, Martin Coleman, David Mitchell, and the many others at The Guilford Press whose efforts made this book possible. Patricia Casey and William Lenderking provided invaluable help as well. Above all, we express our thanks to Thomas F. Anders, MD, the child psychiatrist who provided much of the material and guidance for the first edition of this book.

List of Abbreviations

Several of these abbreviations denote more than one term; which one is meant should be clear from the context. With the exception of ADHD, most abbreviations for disorders are used only in the Part II chapters where the disorders are primarily discussed.

AD	adjustment disorder
ADHD	attention-deficit/hyperactivity disorder
AMC	another medical condition
AN	anorexia nervosa
ARFID	avoidant/restrictive food intake disorder
ASD	autism spectrum disorder, acute stress disorder
ASPD	antisocial personality disorder
BDD	body dysmorphic disorder
BED	binge-eating disorder
BMI	body mass index
BN	bulimia nervosa
CBT	cognitive-behavioral therapy
CD	conduct disorder, conversion disorder
CGAS	Children's Global Assessment Scale
CM	cytomegalovirus
CT	computerized tomography ("CAT scan")
DA	dissociative amnesia
DCD	developmental coordination disorder
DDD	depersonalization/derealization disorder
DID	dissociative identity disorder
DMDD	disruptive mood dysregulation disorder
DQ	developmental quotient
DSED	disinhibited social engagement disorder
DSM	*Diagnostic and Statistical Manual of Mental Disorders*
EEG	electroencephalogram

EMG	electromyogram
FDIA	factitious disorder imposed on another
FDIS	factitious disorder imposed on self
GAD	generalized anxiety disorder
GAF	Global Assessment of Functioning
GD	gender dysphoria
HD	hoarding disorder
HIV	human immunovirus
HMO	health maintenance organization
HPI	history of the present illness
ICD	*International Classification of Diseases*
ICSD	*International Classification of Sleep Disorders*
ID	intellectual disability
IQ	intelligence quotient
LD	language disorder
LPE	with limited prosocial emotions (specifier for conduct disorder)
LSD	lysergic acid diethylamide
MDD	major depressive disorder
MDMA	methylenedioxymethamphetamine ("ecstasy")
MRI	magnetic resonance imaging
MSE	mental status examination
NCD	neurocognitive disorder
OAD	overanxious disorder of childhood (DSM-III-R only)
OCD	obsessive–compulsive disorder
ODD	oppositional defiant disorder
OSAH	obstructive sleep apnea hypopnea
PANS	pediatric acute-onset neuropsychiatric syndrome
PCP	phencyclidine
PMDD	premenstrual dysphoric disorder
PTSD	posttraumatic stress disorder
RAD	reactive attachment disorder
REM	rapid eye movement
SAD	separation anxiety disorder
SCD	social communication disorder
SLD	specific learning disorder
SM	selective mutism
SMD	stereotypic movement disorder
SOC	social anxiety disorder
SSD	speech sound disorder, somatic symptom disorder
SSDPP	somatic symptom disorder with predominant pain
TD	Tourette's disorder
WISC	Wechsler Intelligence Scale for Children

Contents

PART II

DSM–5 DIAGNOSES APPLICABLE TO CHILDREN AND ADOLESCENTS

APPENDICES

Purchasers of this book can download and print a larger version of Appendix 3, "A Questionnaire for Parents," at *www.guilford.com/morrison7-forms* for personal use or use with individual clients (see copyright page for details).

INTERVIEWING CHILDREN AND ADOLESCENTS

Introduction

A few months ago, a dog bit 3-year-old Melissa on her face. Her history and presentation stimulated a case conference discussion that ranged far wider than the immediate cause for referral.

Melissa's maternal grandmother had related that she had always been a "squirmy" child who couldn't sit still during story time. She would fuss when required to stop watching TV or go to bed, or even when told they couldn't visit the cereal aisle every time they shopped at the Safeway. Initially, she would just yell and flap her hands. Lately, when frustrated, she would hit, kick, and bite—one tantrum lasted nearly half an hour. "Sometimes she needs a bear hug until she winds down," her grandmother said.

In a brief video recording made on the day of her evaluation, Melissa appeared healthy and well nourished. She quickly hugged and kissed her grandmother before she readily skipped along with the interviewer, with whom she engaged in a lively discussion about kittens, Cookie Monster, and her own bedroom. Speech patterns, vocabulary, and motor activity appeared developmentally appropriate.

Melissa's mother, who has intellectual disability, had conceived her while living in a group home. Ever since the normal prenatal care and uncomplicated delivery, Melissa had lived with her mother and grandparents. Lately, she had started wetting the bed once or twice a week. At nursery school, she would shove any other child who stepped ahead of her in line. Teachers had worried that her vocabulary was limited for her age.

The brisk discussion of diagnostic possibilities included attention-deficit/hyperactivity disorder, oppositional defiant disorder, disinhibited social engagement disorder, intellectual disability, and enuresis. A specialist in autism suggested, yes, autism spectrum disorder. By the time all the gathered material had been presented, mood and anxiety issues had been added to the differential diagnosis—along with the reaction to the trauma from the dog bite.

This brief presentation of Melissa illustrates the two principal aspects of evaluating any patient—information gathering and diagnosis—that constitute the focus of this book. Interview technique and mental diagnosis for children and adolescents are so mutually interdependent that we find it hard to write about one without covering the other. That's why we have presented them together in a single volume. In the first part, we discuss the mental health interview as it applies to young people and their families; in the second, we address the science (and art) of diagnosis.

Obtaining clinical information from young people, especially children under the age of 12, requires special technical skills and clinical experience in interviewing that are different from those necessary for interviewing adults.

1. Children's vocabularies are relatively limited, and their perspectives are more closely circumscribed than are those of adults. Younger children have not yet begun to think in abstract terms; their thought processes tend to be concrete. Interviewers must be sensitive to all children's need for developmentally appropriate terms that are understandable without sounding condescending.

2. There is a danger that any patient may withhold necessary diagnostic information, but a child patient especially may not realize the importance of forthright communication in a clinical evaluation.

3. Even a child who can be made to understand the importance of full disclosure may not realize what information is necessary to achieve it.

4. The stages of human development add complexity (and interest) to interviewing and the diagnostic process. A fundamental knowledge of development is essential for clinicians working with juveniles.

5. Sometimes concern about a child's behavior serves as an entry when the real problem lies elsewhere—parental couple conflicts or personal mental disorder, for example. Although parental and couple/family disorders lie beyond the scope of this book, a mental health professional who treats children and adolescents must be alert to all possible causes of a patient's troubles.

6. Flexibility and a youthful spirit are especially important capacities for mental health professionals who work with children and adolescents.

Talking with young people needs to be distinguished from talking to and about them. Parents* and teachers talk to young people—to teach, sometimes to admonish them. Parents talk with mental health professionals or teachers about their children. But most adults need to learn how to talk with children and adolescents in a way that encourages two-way communication. That is what we focus on in this book—methods of talking with kids to

---

*Throughout this book, we intend the term *parents* to include biological and adoptive parents, legal guardians, and "significant others"—in short, anyone who acts as a primary caregiver to a child or adolescent. In parallel fashion, we use *teachers* to stand for all educational personnel, including principals, counselors, and librarians.

elicit clinically relevant information. These methods necessarily vary according to the age and developmental stage of each young patient.

By some estimates, just over 20% of all children and adolescents in the United States (more than 16 million) have a diagnosable mental disorder. Many of these are serious; that is, they cause significant distress or interfere with a child's or adolescent's ability to study or to relate to family or friends. Although some young people referred for mental health evaluation do not require treatment, hardly any referral we can imagine should be regarded as trivial. Pretty much every referred child or adolescent will have worried someone, sometime. This thought underscores the importance of obtaining all the information relevant to the accurate diagnosis of each young patient who comes to a mental health professional. At present there are far too few well-trained mental health professionals to evaluate more than a small fraction of all these potential patients.

PART I. INTERVIEWING CHILDREN AND ADOLESCENTS

Especially in the field of child and adolescent mental health, we need to gather our information from multiple sources whenever possible, including parents, teachers, and other health care providers. Grandparents and other relatives may provide additional useful information. We clinicians must become adept at balancing all views and sources of information, and at using clinical and developmental judgment to establish a diagnosis that is in the best interest of a young person.

Teachers can be particularly valuable resources, in part because their broad experience and training provide them the opportunity to make comparisons between referred children and other children their age. Another advantage is that because teachers' self-esteem is usually not at stake when referred children are being evaluated, they can often report certain childhood skills and behaviors more objectively than parents can. Bear in mind, however, that teachers also tend to be personally uninvolved with young people; are sometimes burdened by large class size and inadequate support; and may overgeneralize, using labels to facilitate the removal of boisterous children or obstreperous adolescents from the classroom. Some teachers may recommend medication to control behavior when a child's or adolescent's disruptiveness is actually a response to stresses that originate within the classroom.

Certain general principles do seem universal to all successful interviews. They include listening carefully with an open mind, directing and following conversation, establishing rapport, and following up on important clues. Interviewers should focus not just on problems, but also on a child's and family's strengths and supports. We must also pay special attention to the family's values and cultural beliefs. The most scholarly presentation of these principles has been that of Cox and colleagues, who in the 1980s published a series of studies based on interviews with parents whose children had been brought for evaluation. The principles they derived apply to nearly every patient, relative, friend, or other informant encountered by a mental health professional. (See Appendix 1 for a reference to Cox et al.'s work.)

Although Part I of this book is not intended as a textbook on interviewing, we do present some of the methods commonly used to obtain diagnostic information from patients and informants. Chapter 1 reviews material pertinent to any mental health interview. Chapter 2 discusses the steps needed to establish a relationship with a young mental health patient. Chapter 3 presents developmental information relevant to the initial interview, as well as a table of developmental milestones.

To demonstrate principles of interviewing, the remainder of Part I comprises edited transcriptions of actual interviews. In Chapter 4, we present something that has become much discussed and used in recent years—an "infant/toddler interview," which is actually an interview with a mother while the clinician interacts with the child. Chapters 5–7 contain interviews that demonstrate a variety of techniques useful for school-age children: toys, drawing, and dolls. As you will note, clinicians often use all three modalities in a single interview. Chapter 8, containing an interview with a teenager, demonstrates many of the same interview techniques that apply to an adult patient. Chapter 9 presents the basics of family interviewing in an annotated initial encounter with a boy and his mother.

Because we believe that learning occurs best when it is illustrated by concrete examples, we rely throughout on modified transcriptions of actual patient interviews. These we have annotated with discussions of our impressions of the interviewers' goals, methods, and effectiveness, as well as with descriptions of other material that might be sought (or at least considered) in similar interviewing circumstances. We have not attempted to cover both sexes at every age. Although young patients of varying ages and developmental stages will inevitably require modifications and adaptations, the basic techniques remain much the same. Throughout this book, names and other identifying data in case material have been changed to preserve anonymity.

Finally, in Chapter 10, we discuss the written report. We cover formulation, in which we show how all the information gathered from records, informants, and the patient is brought together to create a clear statement of the problem; a list of most likely diagnoses (the differential diagnosis); and a working plan for further evaluation and treatment.

PART II. DSM–5 DIAGNOSES APPLIED TO CHILDREN AND ADOLESCENTS

The second part of this volume presents mental diagnoses that are usually first made during childhood or adolescence, plus diagnoses from other sections of the American Psychiatric Association's *Diagnostic and Statistical Manual of Mental Disorders*, fifth edition (DSM-5) that are often applied to young persons. We cover this material in several ways:

- We begin most Part II chapters with a Quick Guide that contains the necessary information for a rapid scan of possible diagnoses, including those in other DSM-5 chapters.

- Then we present some of the basic information that mental health professionals need to know about the presentation, demographics, and possible causes.

- In some cases (such as the substance-related disorders), we have condensed descriptive material about several disorders into tables that readers can consult at a glance, rather than flipping back and forth between sections.

- Rather than copying down the DSM-5 criteria, which—to be candid—tend to be a bit ponderous, we've used what we call Essential Features. These are usually the same as (or only slightly revised from) those in James Morrison's *DSM-5 Made Easy*. Sometimes called *prototypes*, they reflect the way experienced clinicians actually make diagnoses. Yet, in some studies (of mood and anxiety disorders), they have performed at least as well as the official criteria. And beginning clinicians find them easier to use.

- We often illustrate the symptoms of a diagnosis with a clinical vignette.

- For each vignette, we use both the DSM-5 criteria and the Essential Features as discussion points for a differential diagnosis. Each patient's final diagnosis includes code numbers from the *International Classification of Diseases*, 10th revision (ICD-10)—the version of ICD that became standard for clinical use in the United States as of October 2015.*

- For each major diagnostic category, a special section addresses the techniques of interviewing for the specific diagnoses. To help integrate the material from Parts I and II, we discuss age-specific interviewing skills and developmentally relevant diagnostic information.

- Whenever possible, we include material on differences in presentation that can be expected at various developmental stages. But note that the ages mentioned here are not set in stone; children can progress and mature at vastly different rates and still be normal.

- Throughout the book, we've attempted to write in clear, jargon-free prose. We believe that understanding is improved when the material is shorn of cant and legalistic boilerplate.

---

*Technically, the version of ICD-10 we're using here is called ICD-10-CM (the CM stands for Clinical Modification)—but we're referring just to ICD-10 throughout, for simplicity's sake.

Using the Essential Features

Most children and adolescents referred for evaluation will have at least one diagnosis, and some will have two or more. Sometimes these diagnoses will be more or less independent; at other times they will interact with one another. DSM-5 insists that the main diagnosis for a hospitalized patient is termed the *principal diagnosis*, whereas one for an outpatient should be termed the *reason for visit*. We don't know anyone who actually adheres to this convention; for all patients, we'll use something on the order of *main diagnosis* (or *best diagnosis*), which is the one listed first.

Each Essential Features begins with a prototype description. In this brief statement—sometimes just a single sentence—we've tried to capture the essence of what the DSM-5 criteria say about a patient's symptoms. The prototype distills the meaning of the actual criteria into a few words that clinicians can use as the basis for pattern matching, which is the way clinical diagnoses tend to be made in actual practice.

Besides the prototype descriptions, the Essential Features employs a variety of boiler-plate statements for further defining the population addressed. These are included in the Fine Print, which mostly comprises what we refer to as *the D's*, as well as *coding notes*:

- *Duration.* How long have the symptoms lasted—6 months (as in oppositional defiant disorder)? One month (pica)?

- *Demographics.* Some disorders are restricted to certain ages, such as intellectual disability, which must begin in early childhood. Antisocial personality disorder cannot be diagnosed until a patient is at least 18.

- *Distress or disability.* Examples: A condition hinders educational or occupational achievement or social functioning (as in stuttering, among many others); a condition causes distress (as in enuresis). Note, however, that stress or suffering by itself is never synonymous with mental disorder.

- *Differential diagnosis.* Here we gather together all of the conditions that should be ruled out when a patient is being considered for the diagnosis. This list includes other mental disorders, physical illnesses, and substance use disorders.

- *Coding notes.* In many instances, specific code numbers are included here, along with symptom specifiers and indicators of severity and remission. Mutually exclusive choices for specifiers are indicated in curly braces (usually, {with}{without} . . .).

We recommend that you (mentally, at least) assign a number that indicates how closely your patient fits the ideal of any diagnoses you are considering. Here's the accepted convention: 1 = little or no match; 2 = some match (the patient has a few features of the disorder); 3 = moderate match (there are significant, important features of the disorder); 4 = good match (the patient meets the standard; the diagnosis applies); 5 = excellent match (a classic case). Of course, we've written our vignettes to match at the 4 or 5 level.

Psychosocial and Environmental Problems

DSM-IV had an entire axis (diagnostic section) devoted to environmental or psychosocial stressors that might affect diagnosis or management. DSM-5 has done away with this axis (in fact, with the entire axial system) and uses ICD-10 numbering to indicate these conditions, as well as the non-mental-disorder conditions that used to be called the *V-codes* in DSM-IV. In Chapter 27, we've described the codes of these types that are most commonly used with children. Any information that doesn't fit neatly into one of these categories should be mentioned in the body of the evaluation.

Assessments of Functioning

DSM-5 has also abandoned the Global Assessment of Functioning (GAF) and the Children's Global Assessment Scale (CGAS), used for many years to assess overall impairment on a 100-point continuum. However, we believe that an overall assessment of function, even though subjective, is a valuable part of the evaluation of any patient. We rely principally on the CGAS, although for patients who are 18 or over, we refer to the GAF. (Both are reprinted in some of James Morrison's earlier books, and both are widely available online.) They are structurally analogous, so their scores should be essentially the same.

Pointers for Making a Diagnosis

Here are some pointers to keep in mind when evaluating patients for diagnosis.

1. Have you obtained all the data?
    - History of the present illness
    - Personal, family, and social background
    - Sensitive subjects (substance use, suicide ideas/attempts, violence/delinquency, physical/sexual abuse)
    - Medical history with review of systems
    - Physical exam (as relevant)
    - Family history (especially mental disorders)
    - Mental status examination
    - Testing

2. Select all possible areas of diagnosis:

Likely in younger children

Adjustment disorder
Anxiety disorders (including separation anxiety disorder)
Attachment disorders (reactive attachment disorder and disinhibited social engagement disorder)
Attention-deficit/hyperactivity disorder
Autism spectrum disorder
Conduct disorder
Elimination disorders
Intellectual disability
Learning disorders
Stereotypic movement disorder
Tics and Tourette's disorder

Likely in older children and adolescents

Cognitive disorders*
Eating disorders
Gender identity disorder
Mood disorders*
Posttraumatic stress disorder
Psychotic disorders
Somatization disorder*
Substance-related disorders

3. For diagnostic possibilities (differential diagnosis), consult the introductory sections of DSM-5 or the Quick Guides at the beginnings of Chapters 11–25 in this book.

4. In using the Essential Features, don't limit yourself to the prototype; also consider the Fine Print. For each possible diagnosis, ask:

- Are inclusion criteria met?

- Are exclusion criteria met?

- Have you considered the D's (described above)?

5. What further information do you need—additional history or background material from informants? More interviews with the patient? Time for observation? Testing?

6. Is a definitive diagnosis even possible? Consider the possible ways of saying, "I'm not sure," expressed here for a patient with depressive symptoms and listed in decreasing order of certainty:

F32.0   Major depressive disorder, single episode, mild (provisional)
F32.8   Other specified depressive disorder**
F32.9   Unspecified depressive disorder

*Cognitive disorders, mood disorders, and somatization disorder represent three instances where we prefer to retain DSM-IV terminology. DSM-5 now refers to cognitive disorders as neurocognitive disorders, and has divided the DSM-IV chapter on the mood disorders into separate chapters for depressive and bipolar disorders. We describe our reservations about DSM-5 somatic symptom disorder, which has superseded DSM-IV somatization disorder, in Chapter 18.

**The *other specified* designation is for a disorder that doesn't fully meet diagnostic criteria, and you specify the reason(s) (duration too brief, criteria too few, or others). With the *unspecified* designation, you do not give the reasons.

F48.9   Unspecified nonpsychotic mental disorder
F99   Other specified mental disorder
F99   Unspecified mental disorder

7. Is it possible that a child or adolescent should have no diagnosis at all? If that's the decision after an evaluation, you'd use Z03.89 (briefly, no mental disorder).

DSM-5 as It Applies to Children and Adolescents

Much that we accept today about mental disorders in children and adolescents has been extrapolated from studies of adults—an assumption fraught with risk. Furthermore, many DSM-5 definitions are based on research that was done with criteria sets that are no longer current. As a result, the reliability of diagnoses in childhood and adolescence lags somewhat behind that for adults. This is not to say that we believe the criteria we have today are useless—only that some are based on information less solid than that used for the adult mental disorders. The mere fact of having clearly stated (if not always validated) diagnoses provides a starting point for future studies that will eventually produce more reliable criteria.

Here are some additional thoughts about using DSM-5 with children and adolescents:

- Its structure and content make DSM-5 a snapshot in time. Many disorders, and nearly all criteria sets, have been changed from those in the previous editions of DSM. This suggests that further evolution in how the mental disorders of young people are defined awaits us in DSM-6 and beyond.

- Validating data may be sparse. An example is the newly defined disruptive mood dysregulation disorder, where clinical study is, so to speak, in its infancy.

- Psychopathology in infants and toddlers, rarely fixed, often depends on context. Symptoms and prevalence rates change with age.

- Symptoms can cut across diagnostic boundaries. For example, inattentiveness can be found in alcohol (and other substance) intoxication, attention-deficit/hyperactivity disorder, delirium, generalized anxiety disorder, major depressive episode, and manic episode.

- Many children and adolescents turn out to have more than one diagnosis. Comorbidity is especially common in young people with intellectual disability, anxiety disorders, learning disorders, and disorders of conduct and attentiveness. Intellectual disability may also be diagnosed in children or adolescents who have autism spectrum disorder.

- When children do have illnesses typically diagnosed in adults, the symptoms may be different. For example, a child with posttraumatic stress disorder is likely to relive the event through repetitive play, rather than through flashbacks, dreams of specific content, or other adult manifestations. The gender dysphoria criteria for children differ in several respects from those used for adults.

■ There is a danger that unfamiliar diagnoses will be missed or made on incorrect or insufficient grounds. Of course, this caveat might be applied to any patient; however, it is especially true for children and adolescents, in whom symptoms may be normal developmental variants whose symptomatic time course may not match DSM-5 criteria.

■ We acknowledge that some clinicians won't have much need for certain diagnostic categories (a specialist in early childhood is unlikely to encounter bipolar disorder or schizophrenia). But to promote wide differential diagnoses, as well as to encourage referrals, every clinician should be aware of each diagnosis.

■ Although it is used the world over, DSM-5 is a distinctly American document that reflects U.S. experiences and tastes. European clinicians are much less likely to diagnose, for example, attention-deficit/hyperactivity disorder or anorexia nervosa. The prevalence of these conditions will be very different in series reported from abroad.

■ Similarly, even within the United States, children of different cultural origins may present with different intensities or patterns of symptoms that nevertheless meet DSM-5 criteria. Because they often affect compliance, family values and cultural beliefs are especially important to consider when treatment is prescribed.

Appendix 1

Appendix 1 presents general references for further reading, as well as descriptions of various structured and semistructured interviews that can be used to guide clinicians and researchers in the quest for standardized assessments of children and adolescents.

Appendix 2

Appendix 2 lists the principal DSM-5 diagnoses with their appropriate ICD-10 code numbers, the approximate age at which each disorder begins, and the age range in which they are commonly found.

Appendix 3

In Appendix 3, we provide a questionnaire designed to help clinicians obtain relevant information about a child and family in conjunction with the initial interview. Using this questionnaire can help jog parents' memories and allow clinicians to focus the interview efficiently on the problem at hand. Readers are invited to photocopy these pages for use with patients.

PART I
INTERVIEWING CHILDREN
AND ADOLESCENTS

A Background
for Evaluating Children
and Adolescents

CHAPTER 1

Interviewing Informants

The Basics

To be sure, every part of the workup of a child or adolescent with mental or behavioral problems is important. But if we had to assign some order of importance to the various steps in the process, obtaining reliable information from multiple informants would appear at the top of our list. With every patient, but especially a young one, observers tend to have diverse viewpoints. Certainly teachers and parents often differ in their assessments. Even two parents may offer diverging opinions as to the nature and seriousness of their child's problems. Without the multiple perspectives of those who know your patient well, at best you will have a difficult time arriving at a correct diagnosis and appropriate treatment; at worst you might never get there.

A number of studies can guide us as we set about interviewing informants. For much of this discussion, we rely upon work that was done in Great Britain by Cox and colleagues. In a series of articles published in the early 1980s, these authors determined which interview techniques were most likely to succeed in obtaining different sorts of historical information. Their findings apply equally well to all types of informants—young patients themselves (especially older children and adolescents), parents, relatives, and others. There's a reference to Cox et al.'s work in Appendix 1. Although there are more contemporary writers about interview style, the work of Cox and colleagues stands the test of time, and the data they generated remain uniquely relevant.

TWO STYLES OF INTERVIEWING

Two fundamental styles of interviewing have been described: *directive* and *nondirective*. As a rule, young children usually respond best to simple, direct, structured questions. Children who are preadolescent or younger don't usually respond well to nondirective, open-ended questioning, but usually do respond to play. But both of the basic interviewing styles are useful in obtaining information from informants *about* children or adolescents.

Nondirective Interviewing

Nondirective interviewing allows the respondent maximum control over the course of the conversation. A nondirective style doesn't ask for "yes" or "no" answers; it doesn't present a multiple-choice format. Instead, open-ended questions give respondents the freedom to speak at length, perhaps bringing in a variety of facts. It encourages people to think deeply, talk freely, and share personal feelings and intimate ideas about their families and themselves. When you use nondirective interviewing, you accomplish several important goals:

1. Because you haven't constrained the answer with requests for specific types of information, you increase the range of possible answers—some of which may surprise you.

2. You increase the accuracy of the answers. This is logical: When people respond at length and choose their own words, they tend to express their ideas better than if they must limit their answers to a word or two.

3. Nondirective interviews promote rapport. A greater sense of relaxation, and the opportunity to reveal something spontaneously about themselves, help informants feel that you are interested in them and in the young people you are discussing.

Throughout this chapter, we illustrate some of the principles discussed here with examples—some good, others not so good—from a session conducted largely by an inexperienced interviewer. The patient is 17-year-old Kevin, who has been brought to an adolescent inpatient unit.

Kevin's examiner begins well enough:

EXAMINER: Good morning. What brought you to the hospital?

KEVIN: I started thinking about killing myself. I tried to stab myself. My voices started to kick in.

Here are some other nondirective beginnings: "Why did you bring Sheila for counseling?" "What sort of difficulty has Jeremy had in school?"

Directive Interviewing

A directive style, which confines the patient to a narrow focus of the examiner's choosing, helps focus the respondent's attention on aspects of the problem that the interviewer finds especially important, and it increases the amount of information obtained. The minute or so of interview following the examiner's opening question (above) is given below in its entirety. Notice that each of the examiner's questions serves to direct Kevin's subsequent narrative.

EXAMINER: Tell me about those thoughts.

KEVIN: I don't remember, exactly. First I went over to my cousin's house and talked to him, and told him I wanted to see a therapist.

EXAMINER: What made you want to see a therapist?

KEVIN: I'm tired of thinking about killing myself.

EXAMINER: You've been thinking about killing yourself. How long has that been going on?

KEVIN: Four or five years. And then the voices.

Using directive requests, the examiner in this sequence follows up each of Kevin's key words or phrases: "killing" and "therapist." As is typical for an adolescent, Kevin responds in short phrases that don't add much detail to the examiner's knowledge base.

Open- and Closed-Ended Questions

Many of the questions interviewers use to obtain information from patients and others are *open-ended*; that is, they allow informants maximum latitude to respond as they see fit. "Tell me more about that." "Tell me about your son's illness." "What happened next?" But *closed-ended* questions—those that can be answered in a word or two without elaboration—also have their place in mental health interviews. They are useful as probes of important areas already uncovered during an earlier, nondirective portion of the interview. And requests for yes–no (or sometimes multiple-choice) answers can help to rein in patients whose verbosity slows down an interview. The last question asked by the examiner in the excerpt above is a closed-ended one that yields a specific answer—and, as we shall see, an opportunity. The proportion of open-ended to closed-ended questions you employ will usually be determined by your respondent's strengths (such as staying on theme and degree of insight) and limitations (such as vagueness or circumstantial speech).

Conducting the Interview: Blending the Two Styles

From our discussion so far, it should be clear that each of the two basic interviewing styles is important in any initial interview. In general, a nondirective, open-ended style of questioning is important during the early stages, when you want to give the respondent greatest leeway to volunteer important observations concerning the child's or adolescent's behavior and emotional life. A bit later, as you come to understand the scope of your respondent's concerns, you can use questions that require short answers to increase the depth of your knowledge.

To elicit the informant's *chief complaint* (the reason the child or adolescent was brought for treatment), your first question should be directive yet open-ended. It will sound something like "Please tell me why you brought Jason for this evaluation." You'll probably hear a pretty specific response, such as "He's seemed very depressed," or "He can't sit still in class." You can then reply with an open-ended encouragement, such as "Please tell me some more about that," and your interview will be off and running.

Occasionally your request for a chief complaint will yield a reply that tells you the informant doesn't really have much information about the circumstances of referral: "His mother made the appointment; he's only been staying with me for 4 days," or "His teacher said I should." Then you may have to guide the informant's responses with specific questions about growth, development, emotions, scholastic achievement, moods, or social relationships.

After you hit upon a fruitful topic, give the informant maximum leeway to discuss it fully. Remember that during the early part of the interview, you want to pick up the broadest range of information about the child or adolescent, as well as about family, friends, and the environment at home and at school. You also want to build a trusting relationship with the informant. Be respectful, listen carefully, and try to suggest acceptance and understanding with your body language—for example, nodding assent, leaning toward the informant, and smiling. With children and younger adolescents, keep the questions simple, give examples illustrating what you want to learn, and use praise when indicated ("I know this is hard to talk about, but you're doing fine"). Always be alert to hints of problems in the following major clinical areas:

- Difficulty thinking (cognitive disorders)

- Substance use

- Psychosis

- Mood disturbance (depression or mania)

- Anxiety, avoidance behavior, and arousal

- Physical complaints

- Developmental delay

- Socialization problems at school or at home

- Personality problems

Make a note about any of these areas that will require further investigation later in the interview. But for now, strive to keep out of the way and let your informant speak.

ENCOURAGEMENTS AND CLARIFICATIONS

Anything you say could distract your respondent, so as long as you are obtaining material that is relevant to the patient's condition, you should just listen. But sooner or later your interviewee will run out of steam, take a wrong turn, or simply look at you for guidance. Then a verbal or nonverbal encouragement from you can help shape the course of the interview for maximum efficiency and productivity.

The least intrusive encouragements you can make are nonverbal ones. A smile or nod of the head may be enough to indicate that the interview is going well and that you want to hear more. One clinician we know manages to do all this just by blinking his eyes! And of course, maintaining eye contact can help establish a bond of sympathy and intimacy. By simply leaning forward, some clinicians subtly indicate support for someone who is recounting information that is particularly stressful. If it seems indicated, you can show sympathy and support by offering a box of tissues, without interrupting the flow of information.

Let's return to the interview with Kevin. The interviewer seizes the opportunity Kevin offered in his previous answer and branches out in another direction.

EXAMINER: The voices?

KEVIN: For about 3 years.

EXAMINER: Ah.

KEVIN: He [Kevin's cousin] was telling me the names of psychiatrists and everything, and he gave me the number, and I lost it. Then we went over to his homeboy's house and people started drinking. Then things got out of hand.

Notice from the sample above that a nearly nonverbal response leads to more material. Here the examiner gets considerable good from a very few words. Sometimes a syllable or two—"I see" or "Uh-huh"—is all that's needed. At other points, especially when the interview seems to be stuck, you will need to be more articulate. Here are some suggestions:

1. Directly request information, as Kevin's examiner does next:

    EXAMINER: What got out of hand?

    KEVIN: My voices started telling me to kill myself. I got a knife and tried to stab myself.

    Another way of putting this question might be "Please tell me some more about what got out of hand." Similar questions in other cases might be "I'd like to hear more about Brad's drinking," or "Can you describe Tiffany's problems in school?"

2. If you don't understand an answer (or if your informant has mistakenly answered the wrong question), don't hesitate to ask your question again. You can make it seem less like an interrogation by saying something like "I still don't understand" before re-asking your question.

3. To ensure that you understand the broad outline of what your informant has been trying to say, you can occasionally offer a brief summary. This will be no more than a sentence or two, and will generally begin with "Do you mean that . . . " or "So you feel that . . . "

EXAMINER: Do you mean that you tried to kill yourself?

TRANSITIONS

Your interview will work better if it flows naturally from one subject to the next, like a real conversation. To that end, you can provide *transitions,* or bridges from one topic to another. Wherever possible, try to follow the informant's lead. Such a process allows respondents to feel that they are full participants in the evaluation, encouraged to convey all important facts.

As the interview shifts from the initial "free-form" phase, you will need to become more directive in the techniques you employ. Several of them can help you move comfortably from one topic to another.

First, notice the *lack* of adequate transition in this exchange:

EXAMINER: Whom do you live with?

KEVIN: My mom and my grandma.

EXAMINER: Where's your dad?

KEVIN: Dead.

EXAMINER: So you were born in 1981. Did you start school when you were 6?

The abrupt shift of topic suggests that the examiner is uncomfortable with Kevin's stark, second response: "Dead." You can reduce the abruptness of transitions by picking up on the last couple of words (or any recent thought) of your informant. In the next example, notice how the interviewer uses Kevin's own words to encourage more detail:

EXAMINER: Earlier, you mentioned hearing voices . . .

To smooth out the flow of conversation, you can move from one topic to another by using any factor the topics may have in common, such as place, time, activities, or family relationships:

KEVIN: There are four voices. They're always telling me to do things. Right now they're just screaming, "Go to hell!"

EXAMINER: And what about the rest of your family—have they ever experienced anything like those screaming voices?

If you find that you need to make an abrupt change, say something that tells the informant that you realize you are changing gears. If your informant seems to have more to say on the first topic, you can offer to return to it later, when there's more time. Here is one way of doing this with Kevin:

EXAMINER: I think I understand about the problems with the voices. Now I'd like to hear about your problem with drinking alcohol.

PROBING FOR INFORMATION

After a few minutes of listening to the respondent's free-form reasons for the evaluation, you will reach a point of diminishing returns. To ensure that the main concerns have at least been touched upon, ask whether there are any other *major* problem areas (see the earlier list of such areas) that have not been covered. If not, you can begin to examine more closely the areas you have already identified.

Of course, any symptom has its own unique characteristics that require exploration. But common to all symptoms and behaviors are certain features you must probe to obtain more accurate detail. Consider, for example, how these questions would apply to a child who has been showing aggressive behavior:

- Type—physical or verbal?
- Severity—scuffles or all-out fist fights?
- Frequency—daily, weekly, or only once or twice?
- Duration—how long ago did the behavior begin?
- Context—spontaneous or provoked, as by taunts or abuse?

You can elicit and record similar descriptors for virtually every problem area identified.

As you begin to seek specific details, you will need greater control over the responses you obtain. Here are some of the techniques you can use:

1. Make your requests with closed-ended questions: "Did Matthew ever wet the bed?" "How old was he when he stopped?"

2. When you get a response that is brief and to the point, show your approval with smiles or nods.

3. Explicitly state what you need: "Now I'm going to ask you some questions that call for short answers."

However, when you want to assess feelings (concerning the patient, the informant, other family members, a situation), research shows that open-ended questions provide the most accurate, complete information about emotions.

OTHER INTERVIEWING TIPS

Be careful not to let the way you phrase a question suggest the answer. Here's an obvious example: "Russell hasn't been using drugs, has he?" The question itself makes it easy for the informant to give an answer that is negative, and not necessarily accurate.

Keep questions short. A complicated syntax that includes a lot of explanation is confusing and wastes time.

Don't try to economize by asking double questions; they will be confusing. If you ask, "Has Jessica ever run away from home or ditched school?", your respondent could focus on only half the question. Neither of you may realize that the part you'd really like to know about has been lost. Here's an unfortunate example from the interview with Kevin:

EXAMINER: How old were you when you and your mom moved in with Grandma?

KEVIN: Two or three.

EXAMINER: Does Grandma have any problems? And you've lived there ever since?

Encourage precision. If you are offered a vague description, ask for dates, time intervals, and numbers, as in the more productive line of questioning that follows. It is often helpful to draw a time line with anchor points, such as a birthday, a grade in school, or a holiday.

EXAMINER: Do you have any legal problems?

KEVIN: Not really.

EXAMINER: What do you mean?

KEVIN: I was never really arrested.

EXAMINER: Well, what kind of legal problems do you have?

KEVIN: Carjacking, robberies.

EXAMINER: So you've committed crimes that you've never been caught for?

KEVIN: Right.

EXAMINER: What sort were they?

KEVIN: Robbery.

EXAMINER: Like armed robbery?

KEVIN: Couple of times.

EXAMINER: Two armed robberies. Like a mugging?

KEVIN: No. Store robberies.

EXAMINER: Store robberies. For money?

KEVIN: Just to do it. To get the thrill of it.

EXAMINER: What else?

KEVIN: Shootings. Stabbings.

EXAMINER: How many people have you shot?

KEVIN: Maybe five or six.

EXAMINER: Have you ever killed anybody?

KEVIN: I'm not sure.

EXAMINER: So you don't know if any of these people died?

KEVIN: No.

EXAMINER: How is it that you've shot people, but never got arrested?

KEVIN: I throw the gun away or sell it.

EXAMINER: How many people have you stabbed?

KEVIN: About three people.

EXAMINER: Do you know any of the people that you shot or stabbed?

KEVIN: Some of them.

> *Despite the strongly positive history of antisocial and violent behavior obtained from this series of specific, quantitative questions, Kevin's veracity is difficult to determine. There's a real possibility of exaggeration and grandiosity to impress the examiner. For diagnostic purposes, this information needs corroboration from court records or statements from Kevin's mother or teachers.*

PARTS OF THE INITIAL INTERVIEW

The diagnostic mental health interview is traditionally divided into a number of discrete parts, the exact titles and content of which vary with the interviewer (and patient). However, the overall effect is always the same: to obtain the most complete account possible of the patient's life, problems, and potential. In the remainder of this chapter, we discuss these aspects under the following headings: "The Present Illness," "Personal, Familial, and Social Background," "Sensitive Subjects," "Medical History," "Family History," and "Mental Status Examination." Table 1.1 provides a more complete outline of the initial interview.

The Present Illness

For each of the problem areas identified during the information-gathering process, you should pursue the following lines of inquiry with both the patient and with a parent or other informant:

What kind of stressors might have preceded the onset of symptoms? Try to understand what circumstances or precipitating events preceded the onset.

Changes in sleep and appetite ("vegetative symptoms") may be encountered even in young patients, especially those who have mood disorders.

For disorders that occur episodically (again, especially mood disorders), when did they start? Are the symptoms the same each time? Do they appear in a specific order? What is the first sign of disorder? What comes next? Do the symptoms resolve completely between episodes? Here you may need to distinguish between episodes of the present illness; of course, onset can sometimes be quite gradual, with no clearly definable beginning.

Almost regardless of the duration of symptoms, you will want to know about previous treatment. Was medication used? If so, what effects did it have, wanted as well as unwanted (side effects)? How well did the patient and parents comply with the treatment regimen? If individual or family counseling was pursued, what was the focus of the therapy, and what was gained? What issues remained unresolved?

What have been the consequences of the illness for school attendance or grades, relationships with siblings, and the patient's ability to make and maintain friendships? Have there been any legal consequences? Have there been any changes in interests (including hobbies, reading, TV watching)?

In this excerpt, Kevin's examiner pursues details of the hallucinations:

EXAMINER: You said that about 3 years ago, you started to hear voices.

KEVIN: I think it was junior high. It was in the summer, I know.

EXAMINER: And how old were you then?

KEVIN: I don't . . . I can't even tell you. About 13 or 14.

TABLE 1.1. Outline of the Initial Mental Health Interview for a Child or Adolescent

Chief complaint

History of the present illness

Precipitating stressors? Onset? Symptoms?

Any previous episodes? If so, course and treatment (medication, hospitalization, counseling)?

Effects on patient, family, others?

Personal, familial, and social background

Patient's birthplace, number of siblings, sibship position?

Present family constellation? Patient's present residence?

Developmental history (milestones, possible traumatic events)?

Family ethnic background, religious preferences, cultural values?

Parents' relationship: Length/stability of marriage? Separation or divorce? Remarriages? Relationships within reconstituted families?

Physical/verbal violence or substance misuse in home?

Is patient adopted? If so, intra- or extrafamilially? At what age? Facts (if known) about natural parents? What does patient know?

Extended family involvement in caregiving? Foster care? Other alternative care?

Degree of family closeness?

Social supports for family?

Patient's age at puberty (if adolescent)? Dating and sexual history? Sexual orientation?

Education: Current or most recent grade? Scholastic problems? School refusal? Behavioral problems? Truancy? Suspensions/expulsions?

Hobbies/interests? Participation in sports/other physical activities? TV, phone/internet/social media use? Any changes due to illness?

Friends? Strengths, positive qualities/outcomes? Sources of satisfaction? Self-esteem?

Sensitive subjects

Substance use by patient: Type of substance? Duration of use? Quantity? Effects? Consequences (medical, personal/interpersonal, school/job, legal, financial)?

Suicide ideas/attempts: Seriousness? Methods? Drug- or alcohol-associated? Consequences? Was it disclosed or discovered?

Violence/delinquency: Nature? History? Legal system involvement (arrests, incarcerations)? Illegal behaviors for which patient was not apprehended?

Physical or sexual abuse: Exact nature of events? Perpetrator? Legal system involvement? Effects on patient and family? Witness to domestic violence?

Medical history

Mother's health during pregnancy? Any problems at birth?

Physical health since birth: Major illnesses? Operations? Hospitalizations? Allergies (environmental, food, medication)? Medications (mental or physical) and their side effects? Physical impairments?

Review of relevant systems: Disorders of appetite (anorexia/bulimia nervosa, binge-eating disorder)? Weight (obesity)? Sleep (regularity, disruptions)? Head injury? Seizures? Chronic pain? Unconsciousness? Premenstrual syndrome (for adolescents)? Possible somatization disorder?

Family history

Describe parents and other close relatives.

Any history of mental disorder in relatives? Medical family history?

Mental status examination (make age-appropriate)

Appearance: Apparent age? Race? Posture? Nutrition? Hygiene? Hairstyle? Body ornamentation? Clothing (style, cleanliness, neatness)?

Behavior: Activity level? Tremors? Tics? Mannerisms? Smiles? Eye contact?

Mood: Type? Lability? Appropriateness? Relation to examiner?

Flow of thought: Word associations? Rate and rhythm of speech?

Content of thought: Fantasies? Fears? Phobias? Anxiety? Worries? Obsessions, compulsions? Thoughts of suicide? Delusions? Hallucinations? Self-esteem?

Language: Comprehension? Fluency? Naming? Repetitions? Reading? Writing? Speech articulation?

Orientation: Person? Place? Time?

Memory: Immediate? Recent? Remote?

Attention and concentration: Simple math? Count backward by 1's?

Cultural information?

Abstract thinking: Similarities, differences?

Insight and judgment?

Personality characteristics

Response to limit setting?

Impulsiveness?

Distractibility?

Frustration tolerance?

EXAMINER: What were they like?

KEVIN: First I heard soft mumbling. Then as I started getting older, they started getting stronger and stronger and became constant for longer periods of time.

EXAMINER: Where do they come from?

KEVIN: Just in the back of my mind.

EXAMINER: They don't call you from outside?

KEVIN: No, not at all.

EXAMINER: And they tell you to do what?

KEVIN: To rob people. To hurt other people, watch them suffer. Things like that.

EXAMINER: And what can you do to make them go away?

KEVIN: Sometimes I just try to go to sleep or smoke weed or drink.

EXAMINER: Can you describe the voices some more for me?

KEVIN: There are four voices, screaming.

EXAMINER: Do they talk about you among themselves?

KEVIN: Yeah, they think I'm a fag. And they're constantly telling me to do things.

EXAMINER: What kind of things?

KEVIN: Right now they're telling me to just grab you and start strangling you, because you want to lock me up.

A directive interviewing technique has revealed a great deal about these hallucinations—their type (auditory), location, intensity, number (of voices), content, when they occur, and Kevin's age when they first began. Kevin's are command hallucinations—they tell him what to do. This requires further investigation.

EXAMINER: So they're screaming at you right now?

KEVIN: Yes.

EXAMINER: And they're telling you to grab me?

KEVIN: Grab you and try to get out of here.

EXAMINER: Are you able to control them right now?

KEVIN: I'm able to control them right now.

EXAMINER: Will you tell me if you're not?

KEVIN: Yes.

Although the nature of these voices seems exaggerated, as Kevin's description of his antisocial behavior has seemed, the examiner is sensitive to the possibility that Kevin may pose a danger. Asking whether a patient intends to hurt an examiner is important. If the answer is "yes," then of course the examiner should seek help or terminate the interview. With a "no" answer, the examiner can proceed, though still exercising due caution.

EXAMINER: Do you do what they say sometimes?

KEVIN: Sometimes.

EXAMINER: What kinds of things have they told you to do?

KEVIN: To rob people. Or when people come up and start saying something, start talking shit to them, or sometimes I'll black out.

EXAMINER: How many times have you blacked out?

KEVIN: Countless times.

EXAMINER: How long does it last?

KEVIN: Sometimes for hours, sometimes for a day.

EXAMINER: When did that start?

Blackouts may signal an organic or toxic etiology, so the interviewer veers off on a new tack to pursue possible causes. However, Kevin may barely perceive this change in course.

KEVIN: Two or three years ago.

EXAMINER: Same time as the voices?

KEVIN: Probably before, or a little after.

EXAMINER: Ever lost consciousness for any reason?

KEVIN: No.

EXAMINER: Have you ever had a head injury?

KEVIN: No.

EXAMINER: Ever been in an accident?

KEVIN: No.

The examiner has asked a number of closed-ended questions to pursue the specifics of a possible seizure disorder. Asking about head injuries and accidents may seem redundant, but the interviewer evidently hopes that the repetition will jog Kevin's memory.

Personal, Familial, and Social Background

You will obtain much material about the patient's personal, familial, and social background as you pursue the details of the present illness. Many of these important details can be learned only from a parent or other close relative.

Of course, it's important to ask about the patient's birthplace, number of siblings, and position in the sibship (oldest, middle child, youngest). Was this a planned pregnancy? (If there are siblings, were the other pregnancies planned?)

Try to learn about the developmental history. Focus on developmental milestones and possible traumatic events, such as moves, deaths, and other losses. As an infant, at what age did the patient sit, walk, and speak words and sentences? If any of these were delayed, did the parents seek advice? Did they learn anything about the cause?

What can you learn about the ethnic background, religious preferences, and cultural values of the family?

Learn how well the parents get along. Have there been separations or a divorce? In the absence of a two-parent family, describe any remarriages, relationships with stepparents, and time spent with the noncustodial parent. Also, how is the patient disciplined? Is there violence at home, either physical or verbal? Are alcohol or drugs abused in the house?

If the patient was adopted, what were the circumstances? Was the adoption intra- or extrafamilial? At what age did the adoption take place? What, if anything, is known about the natural parents? What does the patient know of these matters? What has been the role of the extended family in the patient's rearing? Has the patient had any history of foster care or other alternative caregivers?

What does the family do for fun? What is dinnertime like? Who eats together? How often? What is the routine at bedtime?

For an adolescent, determine the age at which puberty occurred (voice change, first menses). If dating has begun, at what age did it start? How much sexual experience does the adolescent have? "Do you have a girlfriend . . . or boyfriend?" (Or ask, "Do you have a romantic interest?" This can give a patient the opportunity to convey sexual orientation without implying assumptions.) Does a patient who is sexually active use protection regularly?

How far has the patient gone in school? Has there been any history of school refusal? Scholastic problems? Behavior problems in school? Truancy? Suspensions or expulsions? (What collateral information is available from teachers and counselors at school?) What kinds of friends does the patient have? Does the patient participate in sleepovers, in sports, in summer camps? Ask about strengths and positive outcomes as well. Is the patient popular? In what areas is the patient successful? What gives the patient pleasure and a sense of satisfaction? How is the patient's self-esteem?

Sensitive Subjects

Right from the beginning of any evaluation, the ground rules of confidentiality need to be made explicit. Here's an example: "Everything you say here is confidential except for two conditions: If you are going to hurt someone else, or if you are going to hurt yourself, I would have to share that information with your parents. If someone might be hurting you, we'd need to discuss it with others to keep you safe." Otherwise, make it clear to children, family members, and other informants that "What's said here is confidential."

Several sensitive subjects must be broached even when you are inquiring about young children. Admittedly, parents and other adults may not know everything that even latency-age children have been up to, but it is vital to avoid missing important information for want of asking. Even knowledgeable parents may feel reluctant to volunteer information about these subjects, which are probably far more common factors in the histories of child and adolescent mental health patients than they are generally acknowledged to be. Be mindful of the possibility that parents feel responsibility or guilt for their child's problems and that they may need some supportive encouragement to disclose information. You can use statements such as "I can see how difficult it has sometimes been to parent your child," or "There is rarely one single cause of a child's difficulties; this sensitive information is just one piece of a large and complex puzzle."

Use of Drugs and Alcohol

To the informant's knowledge, has the patient used any substances? Ask specifically about alcohol, marijuana, cocaine, opioids, sedatives, hallucinogens, inhalants (especially popular with younger adolescents), and central nervous system stimulants. For any positive answer, try to ascertain amounts, age at which use has occurred, duration of use, effects, consequences (medical, loss of control, personal and interpersonal, school or job, legal, financial), and attempts at treatment.

> EXAMINER: Do you take PCP, LSD, heroin, cocaine, speed?
>
> KEVIN: No.
>
> EXAMINER: Not this year? Last year? Any year? Never tried it?
>
> KEVIN: [Shakes his head in response to each question.] I tried crank [methamphetamine] before.
>
> EXAMINER: How many times?
>
> KEVIN: Once.
>
> EXAMINER: When was that?
>
> KEVIN: About a year ago.
>
> EXAMINER: And just one time?
>
> KEVIN: Just one time.
>
> EXAMINER: Did it cause any problems, like medical?

Suicide Ideas and Attempts

Has this patient ever shown evidence of thoughts about self-harm? Most obvious is an actual attempt, but more likely are wishes for death or relief from mental or physical pain. If there have been only ideas, were plans ever made? If attempts, what were the methods? How serious were the consequences? Did others know about it, and how did they find out?

Especially in very young children, even a history of accident-proneness could provide a clue. Any such behavior or statement is especially likely in a patient who has been depressed, abused, rejected, or involved with drugs or alcohol. Statements such as "Nobody cares about me," or "I want my friend Joe to have my dog," or "A friend told me that he almost got run over by a car" sometimes provide indirect clues to the suicidal ideation of a young child.

Even today, some clinicians may hesitate to ask about self-harm in the mistaken impression that such inquiry could "put new ideas into young heads." Although we have always dismissed such concerns as unlikely, actual evidence from a 2005 study demonstrated that screening for suicide ideas did not increase subsequent suicidal ideation. In fact, in this randomized controlled study of over 2,300 high school students, screening was associated with a significant *reduction* in stress for those who reported previous depressive symptoms or suicide attempts. Nevertheless, addressing such concerns can be tricky; words and phrasing could initially raise anxiety for patient and clinician alike. Ask about stresses that an older child or adolescent may be experiencing at home, in school, or with friends. "How laid back are you?" "How mellow . . . ?" "How stressed out . . . ?" are phrases that may help you across this patch of ice.

Violence and Delinquency

Especially for an older child or adolescent, inquire about any history of violence, such as fighting, destruction of property, or cruelty to animals. Also ask about any involvement with the legal system, including truancy, running away, theft, and other behaviors. What were the offenses and outcomes? Do the informants know of any other illegal activities for which the patient was not apprehended?

Sexual and Physical Abuse

Because of its exquisite sensitivity, abuse is an uncomfortable topic to tackle. Yet it is distressingly common, affecting children of all ages, of both genders, and at all socioeconomic levels. A gentle but direct approach may produce the least resistance from informants.

In the case of sexual abuse, you might ask, "Is there any possibility of sexual activity?" or "To your knowledge, has [the patient] ever been approached for sex by a peer or by an adult?" A positive answer must be explored carefully for details: What actually happened? Was there physical contact? How many times did it happen? At what ages? Who was the perpetrator? Was this a blood relative? How did the patient react? How did the parents find out? How did they react? How have these incidents affected the patient and family since? Has the abuse, even suspected abuse, been reported to authorities? What happened then?

In the case of physical abuse, you might start out by asking what punishment is typically used. Then you could ask, "Do you ever feel you get [spanked, whipped] too hard?" Once again, you will need to follow up all the pertinent details.

Legislatures and parliaments in many parts of the world have mandated the reporting of child abuse. Clinicians everywhere must acquaint themselves with the mandatory reporting requirements that pertain to them. However, what must be reported, to whom, and within what time frame all vary, depending on the jurisdiction. Even where law is lacking or unclear, medical and mental health professionals (as well as teachers, caseworkers, the clergy, and even laypeople) have an ethical duty to protect children from physical and mental harm.

Some clinicians inform all clients about requirements of reporting abuse; others mention it only if the suspicion of abuse arises. We favor being as open and honest as possible, using statements such as this: "If I find out this kind of information, I am required by law to report it. Reporting does not imply guilt; it does allow for an assessment of safety for the child."

Leisure Time and Use of Technology

For both children and parents, it is important to ask questions and make behavioral observations that are appropriate to each child's developmental stage and the economic circumstances, cultural values, and social context of the entire family. In the past few years, child-oriented marketing has promoted proficiency with cell phones, computers, texting, social networking, and video gaming. Although experts don't agree about the effects of these activities on child development and psychopathology, a comprehensive mental health evaluation should include questions about technologies associated with the Internet and the cyber world.

For example, the American Academy of Pediatrics recommends that infants up to the age of 2 years should not be exposed to television programming. So you might include questions to learn whether the TV is used as a "minder" to occupy very young infants. If so, for how much time on average, each day, are toddlers and preschool children exposed to TV? What is the content of the TV and video gaming in which children participate?

Here are some other questions with a similar focus: Which Internet sites do children and teens visit? Do they get sufficient sleep at night, or do they text and telephone until late? What content do children and teenagers upload to their social networking sites? Are there specific concerns about a child's or adolescent's use of social media?

Pursued in moderation and with parental awareness, technology-based activities probably will not harm a child's development or the family's sense of well-being. However, these are activities that can lead to interference with schoolwork, preoccupation with violence, and confusion about sexually explicit material—or even to conduct disorder, early use of alcohol or drugs, cyberbullying, and access to predatory adults. It is important to learn whether parents are aware of areas of potential controversy and discuss them with their children.

Medical History

What were the facts about the mother's pregnancy with this child? How was her health during pregnancy? Was the delivery vaginal or cesarean? Did the baby breathe right away? Was there jaundice? If so, why—was this an Rh-positive baby? Was a transfusion required? Did mother and child go home together?

Have the informant describe the patient's physical health since birth, including traumatic brain injury, seizures, asthma, operations, hospitalizations, and allergies. Is there a weight problem (underweight, overweight, frank obesity)? Is sleep irregular? Ask about current and past medications for mental and physical conditions. For each medication, what is (or was) the dose and frequency?

Family History

In terms of family involvement and personal characteristics, how would you describe the parents? (If your only information about one of them is from the other, be aware that it may be colored by the feelings surrounding partner strife or divorce.) And does a parent or any other relative have a history of mental disorder? To learn of any mental health difficulties in family members, you may have to bend your rule about asking long questions (although it is far better to ask short, single-answer questions about each of the difficulties):

> "Has anyone related by blood had nervousness, nervous breakdown, psychosis or schizophrenia, depression, problems from drug or alcohol abuse, suicide or suicide attempts, delinquency, arrests or other trouble with the police, a lot of physical complaints or doctor visits, mental hospitalization, or treatment for mental disease? By *relative*, I mean to include parents, brothers, sisters, grandparents, uncles, aunts, cousins, nieces, or nephews."

> "Has anyone in your family had thyroid problems, seizures, diabetes, high blood pressure, cardiac problems, or sudden death?"

Depending on the informant's level of sophistication, you may need to define some of these terms.

Mental Status Examination

The mental status examinations of children and adults have much in common. However, there are a number of distinguishing factors:

- Because young patients vary in age and developmental stage, the examiner must be familiar with the spectrum of normal behaviors at all ages (see Table 3.1).

- The examiner must have materials available for eliciting age-appropriate behaviors.

- The evaluation of a young child is usually carried out in part with other family members present, in part with the child alone.

- Depending on the child's age, toys of varying complexity or other age-appropriate projective material can be used to facilitate the communication.

At the conclusion of the evaluation, the clinician organizes the interactions and observations of behavior with the child and family into a coherent mental status report. The categories of the mental status examination usually include appearance, speech and language, motor activity, sensory capacities, affect and mood, thinking, intelligence, attention, orientation, and relationship with the examiner and with other significant participants.

CHAPTER 2

Structuring the First Interview
with the Young Patient

An adult who appears for a mental health evaluation usually knows more or less what to expect: The clinician invites the patient into the office; both patient and clinician get comfortable in their chairs; and they begin to converse. The patient describes a set of symptoms or problems to the clinician, who listens to content, observes behavior, and evaluates mood and affect. All of this is done in the service of establishing rapport and trust, and thus of obtaining reliable information that can be integrated into a diagnostic formulation with a differential diagnosis and a plan for further evaluation and/or treatment.

Clinicians who evaluate juvenile patients have the same ends in mind, but they must use methods carefully tailored to each individual child or adolescent. After all, their patients may be unable either to understand the purpose of the evaluation or to convey adequately in speech many subtleties of meaning. Diagnostic impressions often must be inferred. How rapid, how thorough, how abstract the interview can be will depend on a patient's chronological age, developmental stage, and cognitive capacities—as well as on the complexity of the story. Of course, rapport is just is every bit as important with a young patient as with an adult.

SETTING UP THE FIRST INTERVIEW

Although adults usually understand why they have been referred for a mental health evaluation, this is not the case for most children and for some adolescents. Because parents or teachers may regard the behavior under review as "being bad," young children especially may experience the evaluation as a form of punishment. Or, when told they are "going to the doctor," young children may expect a physical examination or an injection. Many children receive no information at all about the visit and arrive totally unprepared. And though parents may understand the reason for the evaluation, too often they have misguided expectations of what will take place or what will happen as a result.

Inadequate preparation makes the initial contact more difficult. Helping young patients and their parents understand what to expect—and to have the same expectations—can greatly facilitate the gathering of information. Usually this means that the clinician educates parents and gives them instructions about what to pass along to their child.

All family members involved should know that this appointment will be different from a visit to other health care professionals—that the emphasis will be on feelings and behavior, not physical well-being, and that as a clinician, you will need to understand the nature of these problems so as to be able to help. Parents should be instructed that you will talk with them and their child both together and separately. If possible, discourage families from bringing other children. If that is not possible, request that a minder for the other children also come along.

Depending upon the age of the child being interviewed, specifics of the evaluation should be reviewed in advance. For example, young children should be made aware beforehand of planned formal psychological testing, play techniques, family interviewing, or separation from their parents. They need to know that the initial visit should take a certain length of time, that they are not being punished, and that they will be returning home after the visit (unless the evaluation is for inpatient or residential care). Young children should also be reassured that the professional will not hurt them; if a physical examination is a possibility, this too should be made clear.

Communicating these difficult concepts is an immediate, practical task. Parents should be helped to select language and phrases that are appropriate to the child's age, level of development, and level of cognitive comprehension. In an initial phone interview, a parent can be asked what words and phrases a young child uses, and then can be encouraged to convey the description of the evaluation in the child's own language. It is often useful in opening the session to ascertain a young patient's understanding of and expectations for the evaluation ("What have you been told about this visit?"). This question can be followed up with one about what the patient knows about the problems that are of concern.

THE FIRST CONTACT

A youngster may be reluctant to talk directly about symptoms or problems, and may be frightened by a strange professional and unfamiliar surroundings. Like some adults, children can become anxious in a doctor's office. So a typical concrete response by a young child to the more adult-appropriate question "What brought you here today?" is "My mother." Similarly, "How are you feeling [doing] today?" is usually answered, "Fine."

What type of first interview should you use? Clinicians disagree, perhaps in part because young people and their situations can differ so greatly. Controlled studies do not help in choosing one mode over the other, so you should choose an initial interview style that is based on what you already know about a patient from the referral source, the patient's age, and your own interviewing experiences and preferences. Sometimes the structure of the initial evaluation will derive from external circumstances, such as an insurance plan's number of authorized visits. Don't try to follow a rigid plan; it is more important to establish a positive therapeutic alliance with the patient and family from the first moment of contact. Structured and semistructured interviews—which pursue a schedule of questions, sometimes with branching questions, even "twigs" and "leaves"—may assure coverage of all aspects of mental health, but they are less successful in eliciting emotions and unusual historical material.

The adults who schedule the interview may be able to help determine how the first interview should be structured. (Some clinicians prefer to interview the parents of a young child first and without the child present.) Do they feel that they can speak freely in the young patient's presence? Will the child's behavior be too distracting? At the time of the initial referral call, emphasize that both parents should attend the first session if at all possible. However, if only one parent shows up (as is often the case), request to meet later with the other parent or other family members involved in the care of the child.

A parent should usually be present for a part of the initial interview with the child, so you can observe the parent–child interaction. A good rule of thumb for a young child is to divide the first interview so you see the parent and child together for the first part, and then ask the parent to leave while you continue to interview the child alone. If a young child will permit a brief separation from the parent, you can observe how the child tolerates separation and then reunites with the parent in the session. This can provide important information about the attachment styles of both child and parent(s). For an adolescent, meeting first with the patient often works well.

Sometimes when a child or adolescent is brought for evaluation, you recognize that the problem extends beyond the identified patient. For example, the young person may be reacting with symptomatic behavior to a parental separation, death of a relative, or some other problem that began elsewhere in the family. Because it sometimes happens that no one openly acknowledges the other problems, you will need to observe sensitively, using your own clinical judgment to evaluate the multiple sources of stress and dysfunction.

ESTABLISHING RAPPORT

An initial evaluation has three components that proceed simultaneously: establishing a positive therapeutic alliance, gathering information, and (to a lesser extent) intervening therapeutically. Your first task is to establish a working relationship with the young patient and the family. This takes flexibility, a good working knowledge of children's capacities at different developmental stages, and lots of patience and good will. More than one session may be necessary. With a young child, you will often use toys or play materials to break the ice (see "The Play Interview," below, and see Chapters 5 and 6 for examples).

You may need to begin with a conversation that isn't at all related to the reason for referral—what with an adult we'd call "small talk." Topics that are interesting to a child or adolescent help develop rapport and will be viewed as nonthreatening. To draw young patients into participation, you might try questions about familiar TV programs, movies, sports events, computer games, or other relevant, age-appropriate activities that capture their interest. Your ability to make a young patient feel comfortable and relaxed, avoiding condescension or manipulation, is crucial to building a trusting relationship.

INTERVIEW STYLE

The memories of young children can be easily influenced by circumstance. In their desire to please an adult, children may give answers they think an interviewer would like to hear. You should therefore strive for candor with questions that encourage spontaneous recall. Keep questions simple and relevant, and rephrase questions from slightly different perspectives to see how concordant the answers are. Pay close attention to nonverbal cues, such as signs of anxiety, withdrawal, and mood shifts, as well as to emerging negativism and sudden shifts of topic. (See the material on nondirective interviewing in Chapter 1.)

Whereas adolescents are often able and willing to answer questions directly and to elaborate on feelings, preadolescent children are more likely to express feelings and portray conflict through themes that emerge in play. You will also need to observe how the interview develops over time. For example, does a shy, recalcitrant child warm up and engage during the course of the session? Does an anxious, scattered, hyperactive child settle down as the interview proceeds?

CONFIDENTIALITY AND SAFETY

In every case, the participants need to be assured about confidentiality. Of course, you must explain to child and adolescent patients that you will have to share with the appropriate responsible adults any information about situations potentially harmful to the patients' health or well-being. The issue of confidentiality should be discussed with all children older than about 7 years. You might tell an adolescent,

> "What we talk about alone will stay confidential with me. I won't tell your parents or anyone else. The only exception would be if I am worried that you are doing something that is dangerous to yourself or others. Then I'd have to tell your parents. But I won't do that without telling you first. And, if at all possible, I will talk about you only when you are in the room."

With a younger child, you might have this to say:

> "What we talk about in here is only for us. Once in a while, I may want your mom and dad to come into the room with you so we can all talk together. But unless you're there, I won't talk about what we do in this room. When your mom has some worries about you, I will want her to tell me when you're present, so you can hear them, too."

In the presence of the child or adolescent, you might tell a parent,

> "Whatever I learn in our sessions, I will keep confidential unless I am worried about [the patient's] safety or well-being. Then I will ask you to join us, and we can discuss what worries me. Similarly, I will keep to myself what you tell me in confidence about yourself or your family."

Although you will usually want to watch a young patient interact with at least one parent, you must first protect the patient from information that is potentially harmful—parental love affairs, an impending divorce or lawsuit, or the possibility of a parent's job loss. Any of these may eventually become known to the patient, but if so, this should occur at a time and place better suited for it than the first interview. Some parents will report just about everything while their children sit listening; others seem reluctant to mention anything potentially anxiety-provoking in the presence of their children. Either extreme suggests patterns of family interaction that are important to understand. Over time, experience will indicate what information you should impart to young patients, based on its nature, the parents' observed sensitivity, and the patients' developmental stage.

At what age should you begin to interview children alone? Of course, it will depend greatly upon a child's maturity, the focus of the interview, and the cooperation of the parent(s). But a rule of thumb might be this: Encourage a parent to remain with a child who is up to 10 years of age, but devote part of the evaluation with an older child to a private session. We usually prefer to interview adolescents first, before their parents, to emphasize to the patients that this evaluation is for them, as well as about them. For younger children and those who are developmentally less advanced, it is usually beneficial first to ask parents to outline the presenting problems and issues.

THE PLAY INTERVIEW

Rationale and Materials

Why do clinicians so often use play? Young children frequently tell a story through play as they make believe that events happen to dolls or imaginary human figures. In a play interview, the interviewer is a participant-observer, following the child's lead in choosing the direction of play. Play provides the child with the safety of distance from the emotions created by the problem. It also serves as a natural bridge for communication between the child and the adult. Because children are familiar with play at home and with their peers, it helps decrease their anxiety in strange surroundings. Play can also reflect situations and behavior a child experiences in real life, and can provide an opportunity to experience mastery of various physical and intellectual tasks.

Play materials should allow for fantasy production. Human and animal figures that can be constructed into family constellations are popular, as are materials with which to draw or build. We especially like *transformers*—that is, colorful action toys that a child can manipulate to create a variety of forms. Remember that the more structured the games and toys, the less personalized they are. Board games such as checkers and Candy Land, and card games such as Old Maid or Black Jack, may elicit interest and cooperation from the child, but they rarely yield much clinically useful information. At best, they indicate whether a child can understand and follow the principles of rule-bound games. (Most adolescents prefer to talk about their problems, but some find it easier to talk while working on a jigsaw puzzle or playing with pipe cleaners.) During the preparatory phone call, you might ask the parent which play materials might be most suitable for this particular child.

Clinical experience demonstrates that an adult professional who gets down on the floor at the same level as a child who is seated on the floor, or lower than a child who is seated in a chair, is less intimidating and often more successful in eliciting engagement. If a parent and child enter an interview room that provides an appropriate selection of play materials, it is often helpful for the clinician to sit at the level of the child, either on the floor or at a play table. The parent, who is familiar and nonthreatening, can sit in a comfortable chair.

Conducting the Play Interview

Invite the child to explore the play materials. As the child begins to verbalize action or ideas related to the play materials, ask for elaboration: "What shall we call this guy?" "Is he a good guy or a bad guy?" "What are we going to do with him next?" As the theme develops, it will often reflect the child's concerns. Through make-believe, as noted above, children can distance themselves from powerful emotions they may be experiencing.

Sometimes resistance may appear in the form of play disruption. The play seems to be going smoothly, and the child appears intensely involved; suddenly the child shifts the focus of interest to another game or breaks up a previous construction. Such play disruptions should be noted, but, like themes of conflict, their interpretation should be saved for a time when you have become better acquainted with child and family.

Although play will usually involve only you and a child, in the first several sessions it is sometimes useful to allow a parent's presence in the room, or even to involve the parent in the play. The parent's response as a participant in or interpreter of the play may provide useful additional information about the parent–child relationship.

Interactional Engagement Strategies

A skillful interviewer employs a number of interactional engagement strategies in play interviews. In the chapters that follow, we present examples of these strategies, many of which are also applicable outside the play context.

Engagement refers to a clinician's strategies for building a respectful, interactive relationship. Some of these have been previously mentioned. Examples include letting the child set the pace of the interview; sitting at the child's level; keeping the child informed of what will be happening; and listening to and following in play, rather than directing it.

Exploration attempts to elicit information about both positive and negative aspects of the lives of the child and family. Getting the child and parent to relate their separate versions of events; asking the child to elaborate on a play theme with questions that maintain the "imaginary" mask of distance ("How do you suppose Jack [a doll] should handle this?"); and using an interactive style that puts the child at ease are examples of this strategy. It is usually more productive to ask children what they understand about an event or topic ("What happened when you got home that day?") than to ask them to explain it.

Continuity/deepening allows the clinician to expand a child's thematic play or dialogue to elicit additional information related to a particular problem behavior. Commenting on the child's drawings, or whatever the child is playing with, works better than asking the child to discuss a particular topic or to elaborate on feelings in the abstract.

Remembering-in-play (interpretation) acknowledges reenactments of behaviors of which the child has been unaware, possibly because they occurred at a developmental stage prior to the onset of verbal language. Such interpretations should be few in number and brief in presentation, and they should usually occur later rather than earlier in therapy. As a rule, they are generally not appropriate in an initial evaluation.

Limit setting requires a clinician's intervention to maintain boundaries. A basic rule in interviewing children is to set the fewest limits and controls possible. However, hurting the therapist or another person, or intentionally destroying play materials or office equipment, must be prohibited early and consistently. Each interviewer must define a personal comfort zone of acceptable behavior. Averting temptation is far better than repeatedly telling a child not to use something because it makes a mess; arranging the office or playroom before a session in a way that will minimize the need for limit setting may be the key. Obviously, an office that contains a scattering of fine lamps and small art objects is not the place to evaluate a child who has been described as "hyperactive and impulsive." Clay, paints, or sand and water should not be provided as play materials if it is important to keep the office neat. When specific play materials (Play-Doh figures, paintings) are used, be sure to save them from one session to the next.

SPECIAL ISSUES

There is no formula that will make every interview simple and successful. If a child or adolescent is going to receive treatment from you after the initial evaluation, then establishing rapport and gaining compliance are much more important goals of early meetings than obtaining reliable or valid information; information can always be gathered from additional sources. Clinical experience, an appreciation of the young patient's developmental stage, and an empathic approach to the patient's problems within the context of family, friends, and school should facilitate the establishment of rapport. Nevertheless, because they have experienced significant trauma and disappointments, many children and adolescents referred to mental health professionals have a limited capacity for trust. Only a safe, accepting, and consistent therapeutic milieu can rebuild their ability to harbor nurturing relationships. In the remainder of this chapter, we consider questions that may arise in the course of interviewing such patients.

How should I deal with strong negative emotions, such as "I hate my father"?

Children and adolescents often express powerful negative emotions, such as hatred for a parent or the wish to kill a sibling. Recognizing that these can be projections of self-hatred or suicidal feelings, a therapist needs to tolerate such negative emotions. Sometimes, however, these feelings reflect the reality that a young patient is being abused; in such a case, the patient must be protected. Whatever their meaning, the clinician must accept such expressions of negative affect and attempt to understand them.

At the same time, we all have a duty as clinicians to protect others, even those with whom they may not be acquainted. This means that we must take affirmative action to warn intended victims if a patient threatens to kill someone specific or take a weapon to school.

How can I respond to a child or adolescent who habitually resists communicating, as with "I don't know"?

Of course, if a young patient genuinely doesn't comprehend, rephrasing questions is appropriate. Sometimes, however, "I don't know" means a fear of answering; perhaps the child has been warned by a parent not to reveal certain information. Assurances of confidentiality may succeed with older children or adolescents, but clinicians must guard against making promises they cannot keep. For example, an admission of physical or sexual abuse may not, by law, be held confidential by a therapist.

A clinician may suspect abuse or harsh treatment from the themes expressed in play. A child who persistently examines the genitals of a doll, causes animal figures to mount one another, or hits at a doll and calls it "bad" may be demonstrating a possible clue to the problem. Observing such play and making comments, such as "Why is the dog being hit all the time? I think he is trying to be a good dog," will probably elicit further information. For example, a child may reply, "No, he's being bad. He's always messing up the house." The interviewer can then respond, "I bet he tries to be good, but the daddy dog doesn't believe him."

In working with a young patient, a clinician must constantly balance the adult, neutral, professional self who is observing the patient with the self who is engaging the patient in interaction. The participating self—the clinician's "inner child"—can react in a benevolent way to the patient's expressions of negative affect, whereas the adult, observing self can note the interactions and the progressive deepening of their meanings.

When is it permissible to touch a young patient? When not?

The same general rules that apply to touching adult patients apply to children and adolescents. For some young patients, even a touch might seem to represent a potential sexual advance or physical assault. For others, it could seem a sign of undeserved familiarity or being treated like "a baby." A clinician must walk the line between social appropriateness (a handshake, a congratulatory pat on the back) and condescension or overfamiliarity. Every situation merits individual therapeutic scrutiny. Transference and countertransference issues are important in the treatment of children and adolescents, just as they are for adults.

That said, sometimes young patients—especially younger children—may need physical restraint if they are becoming out of control and destructive. Because restraint can trigger trauma or worsen unwanted behavior, it's a good idea to discuss ahead of time how parents manage out-of-control behavior at home. Some young children express extreme anxiety in certain situations. It is perfectly acceptable for a clinician to ask a child if a hug would help. If the answer is "yes," the clinician should sit beside the child and use a "side hug," explaining that this is how hugs work in the office. The side hug provides a gesture of comfort without violating physical boundaries; we discourage allowing a child to sit on a clinician's lap. Again, whenever possible, the clinician should discuss these measures with the parent ahead of time and gain parental consent.

How should I respond to a child or adolescent who lies?

Whereas children and adolescents are often evasive, withholding, or vague ("I don't know," "I don't remember," "Maybe, maybe not"), it is unusual in the course of an interview for a young patient to tell a flat lie. Of course, to escape the consequences of their behavior, some patients (usually older children or adolescents who have engaged in delinquent activities) will say, "I didn't do it"—and perhaps accuse someone else. Although assurances of confidentiality may yield the truth, they can also backfire, as when a clinician must warn parents of life-endangering activities. A direct confrontation early in the course of a relationship with a child or adolescent will usually engender only ill will; the best approach is prevention.

One strategy is to explain how confusing lies can be to clinicians and how they can get in the way of what young patients want (for example, release from the hospital). Then offer an alternative: "If you don't want to talk about something, it's better to say, 'I don't want to talk about that.'" Early in the therapeutic relationship, *not* seeking every detail of an event or behavior can sometimes reduce the likelihood of a lie. Of course, if the information seems critical to an accurate diagnosis or an appropriate treatment plan, questions should be asked. However, if it is something that can be obtained from other sources or is not immediately necessary, delaying until more trust is established will reduce the necessity to lie.

A special challenge is an angry child who accuses a parent of abuse. Sometimes such an accusation may reflect reality, but there are other instances in which, for various reasons, the move is a manipulation to involve the parent with police. If you are in doubt, report your suspicions to child protective services personnel. It is their job to assess safety for the child.

How can I engage a child who neither talks nor plays?

Some children may completely refuse to talk, play, or interact with a clinician. In such cases, neurological disorders, intellectual disability, and autism spectrum disorder must of course be ruled out, but children with selective mutism may also refuse to engage. Usually the history from other sources is helpful in differentiating these diagnoses. Such behavior that emerges in a child who has previously interacted may signify new trauma or a change in attitude about the clinician or the therapy. In such a case, it's important to speak with family members about the changed behavior. Of course, it is also important not to take the behavior personally. Rather than coaxing or threatening in an attempt to engage the child, you'll need detached, patient observation. With younger children, you could initiate solitary play yourself (for example, with dolls in a doll house), which the child might join later.

Should I use structured interviews with children and adolescents?

Structured interviews for children and adolescents were developed to improve the quality of information obtained from mental health interviews. They also allow lay interviewers with instrument-specific training to obtain diagnostic information that has adequate validity and reliability for research purposes. Several such interviews are available for child mental health clinicians; all provide guidelines for their administration and cover a variety of symptoms, behaviors, and situations. These interviews offer differing degrees of flexibility in administration.

The most highly structured interviews specify the exact wording, order, and coding allowed, and minimize the role of clinical inference by the interviewer. Semistructured interviews are designed to be administered by clinically sophisticated interviewers who have received extensive training in their use; these interviews are less prescriptive and allow greater latitude for clinical decision making. Although we have listed some of these interviewing tools in Appendix 1, we believe that relevant clinical information can and should be obtained by an empathic clinician with experience in the science and art of interviewing young people. The flexibility inherent in an unstructured interview by a qualified clinician may also offer the best chance for building a sustained treatment relationship. That said, some self-report or parent and teacher questionnaires can help provide good quantitative data that can be tracked to measure improvement over the course of treatment.

CHAPTER 3

An Introduction
to Development

We do not intend to present full details of child and adolescent development. However, because both interview technique and diagnostic ability in child and adolescent psychiatry require a firm grounding in the stages of development and the achievement of developmental milestones, a brief review is appropriate.

We do intend this chapter as an introduction to the important subject of developmental concepts and the precepts needed to evaluate young patients at each stage along the way. We touch on some of the changes that characterize the march from earliest infancy to young adulthood. Table 3.1 summarizes many of the significant milestones.

Of course, there are no sharp demarcations; development flows seamlessly from one stage to the next. Moreover, changes involve not only the unfolding of biological maturation, but the effects of environmental influences. Height and weight, for example, result from the interactions of genetic programming with nutritional intake and general health status. Many of the environmental advances affecting today's children and their parents were unknown 100 years ago. In practice, the following material, so tidily contained in sections and paragraphs, is tightly interwoven.

We also caution that normal children vary tremendously in rate of development. As one example, twin A of a pair of boys began reading at age 3½, just after twin B learned to swim. Twin A did not learn to swim or twin B to read until nearly 2 years later; as teenagers, both boys swam and read well. The ages we report here are either averages or the consensus of experts; yet, as with the twins, the expected range within a normal population will be broad.

INFANCY (BIRTH TO 1 YEAR)

The period from birth to the first birthday encompasses the greatest changes in any year of development. It spans the time from total dependence to the first signs of autonomy, from

TABLE 3.1. Developmental Milestones of Childhood and Early Adolescence

Age	Gross motor movements	Fine motor movements	Affect/mood	Language/ speech	Relationships	Intellectual/ symbolic capacity
1 mo.	Raises head slightly when lying face down			Small noises in throat	Can identify mother by sight	
2 mo.	Can control head when held seated	Will grip an object placed in hand	Smiles (reflex)	Spontaneous babbling	Responds more to mother than to others	
3 mo.				Responsive cooing		
4 mo.	Can clasp hands together, hold rattle	Bats at objects	Smiles at others (social smile)	Laughs and squeals		Will look for an object that has vanished from gaze
5 mo.	Rolls over; plays with own foot	Will reach for an object and grip it	Will laugh, show excitement; displeased if toy is removed	Makes "raspberry" sounds		Explores objects with mouth
6 mo.	Remains seated when placed in position; good head control	Will shift an object from one hand to the other		Imitates sounds	Attached to adults who provide care	
7 mo.	Can hold two toys at the same time		Beginning to show stranger anxiety	Definite syllables, such as *ma* and *da*		
8 mo.	Pulls to seated position; feeds self a cookie			Comprehends *no*; says *dada* and *mama*, but not as specific names		
9 mo.	Crawls on hands and knees; holds own bottle	Will hit two objects together		Uses *Dada* and *Mama* as names; will look at an object when its name is said	Plays "where's baby?" and other games	

Note. This table generally lists those behaviors and accomplishments that a parent or a teacher might perceive in the course of ordinary interactions with a child, or that simple testing procedures would reveal. Many other accomplishments and attributes, including those in the areas of ethics, memory, sexual development, and development of attachment to parents, may be determined by in-depth interview or special testing.

Also note that authorities don't always agree on the ages at which specific tasks are first accomplished. The possible reasons for this lack of agreement include data from different populations or different eras, or perhaps dependence on impressions rather than data. The variability should warn us not to take any set of norms too literally, but to regard them as guidelines rather than standards.

Age	Gross motor movements	Fine motor movements	Affect/mood	Language/ speech	Relationships	Intellectual/ symbolic capacity
10 mo.	"Walks" if both hands are held	Will pinch an object between forefinger and thumb to hold it	Will express several emotions, such as affection, anger, anxiety, sadness	Can say at least one word other than *dada* and *mama*	Will wave "bye-bye"	Prefers certain toys
11 mo.	Walks by holding on to furniture	Will remove the cover from a box	Begins to have tempter tantrums	Understands about 10 words	Will offer toy to image in mirror	
12 mo.	First steps alone; will help with dressing (e.g., push foot into shoe)		May show separation anxiety	Understands simple commands with gestures		
13 mo.	Crawls up stairs			Can say five or six words other than *dada* and *mama*		Can find an object screened from view
14 mo.	Walks alone	Will scribble			Gives teddy bear a kiss	Imitates behaviors of parents
15 mo.		Will use spoon to feed self		Points to wanted objects	Returns a hug; likes to please parents	Likes to play with adult possessions
18 mo.	Can throw a ball; climbs up onto chair; walks up and down stairs unaided	Will imitate a single stroke with a crayon	Onset of negativism	Can say 10–50 words; points to own body parts; follows easy directions; points to pictures of common objects	Seeks loving attention; hugs doll or teddy bear with affection	Likes to explore closets and cabinets
21 mo.	Can squat and return to standing position	Can manipulate a spoon to eat		Can use two- or three-word sentences (usually verb + noun); uses words to ask for things	Possessive of toys	Recognizes self in a mirror

(continued)

TABLE 3.1 (*continued*)

Age	Gross motor movements	Fine motor movements	Affect/mood	Language/ speech	Relationships	Intellectual/ symbolic capacity
24 mo.	Runs well; can walk backward	Can draw circles, put on items of clothing		Can say up to 250 words; uses three-word sentences; uses *I, me, you*; uses own name; 25% of speech is intelligible	Play is mostly solitary (parallel play), though will show interest in others' play	Onset of fantasy play (e.g., with dolls); can remember one or two pieces of information (e.g., numbers or words)
30 mo.	Can jump a few inches to the floor; achieving control of bowels and bladder	Can hold a crayon between fingers and imitate vertical, horizontal lines	Expresses pride in own accomplishments	Uses full (four- to six-word) sentences with pronouns; names six or more body parts	Plays at helping with housework; relates to members of own family	Can imagine what another child might think or feel
3 yr.	Pedals tricycle; can hop on one foot; can feed self without spilling; grooms self; can throw overhand; begins to show hand preference	Can manipulate small objects skillfully; imitates plus (+) sign; can build tower (up to 10 blocks); draws a person with two facial features	Decline of negativism; enjoys showing off	Has a working vocabulary of ~1,000 words; can state use for objects (ball, pen); 75% of speech is intelligible	Plays with other children; interested in sex differences	Comprehends meaning of two or three of an item; can compare sizes (big vs. small); can state own gender; uses objects to represent people in play; can state own full name
4 yr.	Can jump forward; can dress self with supervision; can walk upstairs, left–right–left	Can draw a person with a face and arms or legs; can copy a square from a picture	May attempt to control emotions (e.g., crying)	Can name at least three colors; enjoys rhymes, follows three commands; can tell a story	Will take a role in play with others	Can make and honor an agreement
5 yr.	Can skip on alternate feet, catch a ball with two hands	Can copy a triangle from a model; draws a person with head, body, extremities		Can define simple nouns; asks the meaning of words	Can follow rules of simple games	Beginning sense of values (right vs. wrong, what's fair); can evaluate own capabilities with some accuracy; counts to 10

Age	Gross motor movements	Fine motor movements	Affect/mood	Language/ speech	Relationships	Intellectual/ symbolic capacity
6 yr.	Can bounce a ball on floor several times; can ride a bicycle	Can tie a bow or shoelaces; can print letters		Can tell left from right; corrects own grammar		Begins to develop ability to regulate own behavior (ability to wait, check aggression); understands that dreams are not real
7–8 yr.	Can hop, jump, run, skip, throw	Can copy a diamond; capability for cursive writing develops	Moods more stable; beginning capacity for empathy, worry	Verbally expresses fantasies, needs, wishes	Develops peer and best-friend relationships	Increasing curiosity, morality emerging; is concerned about opinions of others; recognizes that the whole comprises its parts
9–10 yr.	Increasing strength; individual and team sports			Expresses ideas with complex relationships between elements		
11–12 yr.			May develop animal phobias			Can reason about hypothetical events
15 yr.						Can hold in short-term memory seven or eight independent units (e.g., numbers or words)

dyadic regulation to the beginnings of self-regulation. This period also witnesses the development of the social bond that ties the infant to adult human beings.

A special note on birth order seems in order here. More than 80% of U.S. children have one or more siblings, who can influence a child's overall development. Parents tend to be more involved with and attentive to their firstborn children. Firstborns receive more parental stimulation, but the expectations and demands placed upon them are also greater. For these reasons, firstborns tend to identify with their parents (and with authority in general) more closely than do younger siblings. They will also conform more closely to parental values and expectations and be more strongly motivated toward school achievement, more conscientious, more prone to guilt feelings, and less aggressive than those born later. Perhaps in part because of these traits, many eminent scientists and scholars have been firstborns. But firstborns also tend to be less receptive to ideas that challenge a popular ideological or theoretical position.

In recent years, much has been learned about the remarkable capacities of a newborn infant. As lately as the 1940s, most developmental psychologists believed that infants were, in the words of William James, "buzzing, blooming beds of confusion." Because infants were perceived as sleeping most of the day and, when awake, only feeding, their exquisite sensory capacities were relatively unknown. However, sophisticated new methods of infant assessment, combined with the observational skills honed by animal behavior ethologists, have revealed that infant brains are prewired to recognize human signals almost from birth. There is rapid development of visual acuity, from 20/200 at 2 weeks of age to 20/70 at 5 months to 20/20 vision at 5 years. One-week-old infants can differentiate novelty from familiarity—they have learned to discriminate their mothers' odor from that of an unfamiliar lactating female, and they prefer their mothers' faces and voices to those of strangers. These sensory preferences launch the process of attachment that bonds them to their parents.

Of course, without adequate caregiving in early life, human infants will die. The attachment system ensures survival by providing them with a balance between security/safety and curiosity/exploration. Infants who do not have a sensitive, consistent adult devoted to their care often do not become securely attached to any one adult and are less socially sensitive. Some are less likely to smile, vocalize, laugh, or approach adults; others are indiscriminate in their constant search for attention, moving from adult to adult without showing any special preference. Such behavior has been observed both in children raised in relatively impersonal institutional surroundings and in monkeys reared in isolation.

The characteristics of the attachment relationship can be measured in a laboratory paradigm, the Ainsworth *strange situation*, when an infant is 1 year old. The strange situation involves a series of separations and reunions with a parent (usually the mother), both in the presence of a stranger and with the 1-year-old left alone in an unfamiliar room. A child who shows only moderate distress when the mother leaves, seeks her upon her return, and is easily comforted by her is assessed as *securely attached*. By contrast, a child may be *insecurely attached* in one of two ways. A child who does not notice the mother's departure, plays uninterruptedly while she is gone, and seems to ignore her when she returns is termed *avoidant*, whereas a child who becomes extremely upset when the mother leaves, resists her soothing when she returns, and is difficult to calm down is termed *ambivalent* (or *resistant*).

About 65% of U.S. children tested are classed as securely attached, 20% as avoidant, and 15% as resistant. All else being equal, it is believed that those children who demonstrate a secure attachment during the first 2 years of life are likely to remain more emotionally secure and to be more socially outgoing later in childhood than those who are insecurely attached. Although the data are not incontrovertible, insecurely attached children are probably at heightened risk for social or emotional problems later in childhood.

Each of the attachment styles described above is considered an *organized* attachment style. When the parent appears to provide both the source of and relief from stress, *disorganized attachment behavior* may develop on reuniting with the parent. Such behavior may be identified by contradiction (for example, showing indifference to the mother after her return), misdirection (seeking out the stranger instead of the parent), stereotypy (such as repeated hair pulling), or freezing (inability to move either toward or away from the parent, as if dissociated). Children whose attachment styles are disorganized may be at increased risk for later psychopathology.

Aspects of Development

The overall complexity of function is greater than the sum of increase in size, maturation of the nervous system, and the vicissitudes of the environment. The intersection of the child's innate potentials with parental influences has been referred to as *dyadic regulation*—an emotional process that is most obvious during the first year of life.

Physiology

A major task of the first year is to move from parental regulation of eating and sleeping to self-regulation. New parents are often astonished at the degree to which the household becomes organized around the needs of their infant. The young baby sleeps a majority of the day and night—as much as three-fourths of the time—and does not distinguish between daylight and night hours. During the first few months after birth, the struggle between the baby's innate sleeping schedule and that of the caregiving adults is ultimately resolved in favor of the demands of socialization. The eventual pattern of sleep—throughout the night, rather than in 4-hour increments—is established by the end of the first year.

Even a young baby has keen senses. As determined by the direction of head turning, a week-old infant can distinguish the odor of the mother's breast pad from that of another lactating woman, can discriminate the mother's face, and can distinguish her voice. (Researchers have even suggested that some familiar sounds are heard before birth.) Of course, throughout the early years of childhood, these early memory associations are reinforced many times over.

Temperament

How rapidly and how well the baby settles into the rhythms of life will depend in part on the fit between the child's and the parents' temperaments. *Temperament* can be defined as those innate characteristics that color an individual's character. It is inherent and to some extent biologically determined, as was demonstrated by Stella Chess and Alexander Thomas in the 1960s. They described nine basic dimensions of temperament: activity level; rhythmicity of biological functions; approach to (versus withdrawal from) novel stimuli; adaptability; sensory threshold of responsiveness to stimuli; intensity of reaction; mood quality; distractibility; and attention span/persistence.

Chess and Thomas characterized an "easy" child as one who easily adapts, readily approaches new stimuli, and has regular (rhythmic) biological functions and a positive mood of moderate intensity. It is obvious to what degree an easy baby can facilitate the task of parenting. A "difficult" child (10% of their sample) has irregular biological functions, has a mood that is intense and often negative, and withdraws from stimuli and adapts slowly or incompletely. They also describe the "slow-to-warm-up child" as one whose responses to new situations are mildly negative and whose adaptability is low, even with repeated contact. However, individual temperamental characteristics observed in babies don't necessarily predict later behavior accurately.

Motor Behavior

The first organized motor behavior, present even before birth and necessary for survival, is sucking. Next, early in life outside the womb, babies control their head movements so as to select stimuli that interest them. Of course, this suggests the importance of parental stimulation as a determinant of the speed and extent of motor development. Motor control proceeds from head to foot and from proximal to distal (example: shoulder to arm to hand to finger). There is a gradual progression from instinctive behavior (grasping an object placed in the hand) to reaching for an object to manipulating objects for a purpose (for instance, the child learns to assist with feeding by holding first a bottle and, a little later, a cup and spoon). Note again the parents' opportunity for influencing development by verbal and nonverbal encouragement (smiles and applause). The supply of materials for exploration can also promote development of fine motor coordination as the baby progressively practices grasping, transfers, and pointing.

Affective Behavior

As early as 8 weeks, the baby's smile fosters interaction and bonding with the parents. By 10 months, children have selectively attached themselves to several other people—parents, siblings, sitters. Fear of strangers appears at about 8–12 months, characterized by wariness when an unfamiliar person attempts to interact with the child. Separation anxiety begins a few months later and can be observed when a parent leaves. The child may fuss at the departure even when left with another familiar person. Also at about this age, the child begins to share emotional experiences with parents and to be influenced by the feelings of others nearby. This is known as *social referencing.*

Once mobility has been enhanced by crawling, the child can begin to explore the environment. Crawling to the parent upon request helps foster the bond between parent and child. The developmental sequence is from a recumbent, dependent position to an upright, "moving away" position. The attachment relationship (a basic survival mechanism, as noted above) fosters a balance between comfort and proximity during stress on the one hand, and exploration and curiosity during times of well-being on the other.

The development of attachment also relates to the process of differentiation of self from other nearby objects and people. Babies first explore the world by visually following the movements of others, and by reaching for objects and exploring them with their mouths. Self-stimulation begins by the fourth month and becomes a genuine part of play by the eighth month.

Communication

Infants smile, babble, and coo, capturing the attention of their parents. These early social stimuli elicit positive interactions centering around caregiving and play. There is little relationship, however, between the sounds produced during infancy and the child's amount or quality of speech at age 2. Development of speech depends on the maturing brain, as well as on a child's exposure to speech and cognitive stimulation through interaction with adults. Vocalization progresses from crying through cooing and random sounds to the beginnings of meaningful speech. When only 3 months old, the baby begins to vocalize in response to human speech; this leads to approval from parents, which reinforces the child's efforts to communicate through more speech.

Obtaining Information

Of course, in the usual sense of the term, no one ever truly interviews a tiny baby. Much of the information is obtained directly from the parent who has brought the infant to the session. This information is balanced with observations of the infant in interaction with the adult (infant evaluations should always be performed with the parent present).

Here are some questions of special interest in the evaluation of an infant: Was this a planned pregnancy? Were the pregnancy and delivery uneventful? How irritable has this baby been? How easy to soothe? How regular are feeding and sleeping schedules? Are the parents' expectations age-appropriate and realistic, or is this child at risk for eventual feelings of inferiority and guilt as a result of repeated failure? How have the parents dealt with abnormalities such as premature birth or a physical anomaly, either suspected or real? In such an event, do they accept the child's condition, or do they feel guilty and regard the problem as evidence of their own failure?

Most of the information you can derive directly from an infant will come both from observing the baby's interactions with others and from performing developmentally appropriate motor, sensory, and cognitive examinations (see Appendix 1). Often the infant responds most positively when sitting in the parent's lap. You should check for mutuality of gaze behavior; capacity for visual fixation and following; auditory responsiveness; and social (smiling, crying, avoidant) responsiveness. Note aspects of general development: Does the baby appear robust and healthy, or is there evidence of arrested development or failure to thrive? Are there any obvious physical characteristics, such as the classic appearance of Down syndrome? Does the older baby (or toddler) enthusiastically enter into simple games, such as peek-a-boo? Separation of the infant/child from the parent constitutes part of the standard evaluation of any young child. How does the child respond—with a brief whimper and a ready response to distraction, with inconsolable wails, or with indifference?

Finally, remember that because very young children tire quickly, more than one session may be necessary for the initial evaluation.

Symptoms

A number of characteristics, some of which may turn out to be symptoms, can appear even during the first year of life. Of course, most of them can also be manifested at later stages of development.

- Failure to gain weight and length (failure to thrive)
- Poor social responsiveness (paucity of smiles, failure to extend arms to be picked up)
- Problems with eating (fussiness about new foods, multiple food allergies, irritability when feeding, frequent regurgitation/rechewing of food, eating substances that are not food)
- Problems with sleep regulation (failure to establish a diurnal rhythm, excessive sleep during the day, excessive wakefulness at night)
- Relative lack of vocalization
- Response to strangers that is excessively fearful, intense, or prolonged, or failure to appreciate differences between strangers and familiar caregivers

DSM-5 Diagnoses That May Appear at This Age or Later

The diagnoses listed below typically first appear at about this age. See Appendix 2 for a more complete listing of diagnoses and ages at which they typically are encountered throughout childhood and adolescence.

- Intellectual disability (nonspecific but severe or profound, or specific syndromes such as Down syndrome); global developmental delay
- Rumination disorder
- Avoidant/restrictive food intake disorder (failure to thrive)

TODDLERHOOD (1–3 YEARS)

No sooner do children begin to form social bonds with caregiving adults than they start their decades-long struggle for independence. Even through young adulthood, as they establish their own families and careers, young people strive for significant autonomy—a sense of self. The toddler period is the stage of the "terrible twos," the first "no," even the first lie ("Who spilled that milk?"—"Not me!"). These are important and positive first developmental indicators of being separate, individual, unique.

Aspects of Development

This is also a period of tremendous curiosity, of joy in discovering what is possible. Expressing feelings is important, but so is accepting limits; thus parents need to foster the balance between exploration and consistent discipline. Toddlers need to be protected from violence and harm and to learn about safety—avoiding electrical outlets, busy streets, and anything that is hot. During these years, children develop the beginnings of self-discipline (for example, learning to leave items undisturbed on the store shelf, to look at but not touch ornaments on a Christmas tree).

Because babies and young toddlers are almost entirely egocentric, a major challenge for parents during this period is to help their toddler learn about sharing, taking turns, and waiting patiently. Toddlers begin to discriminate self from nonself. As they near their second birthday, they come to recognize themselves in a mirror, and can point to their own images and to those of other persons. They also become fascinated by other children. During this time, a toddler may acquire a new sibling; this offers the prospect of a built-in playmate and the opportunity to become a big brother or sister, but it also sets the stage for withdrawal of parental attention. Toddlers also acquire a fuller complement of affects. Nuances of mood and moodiness develop (lightning-quick changes, sadness, tantrums, whining); the response to limit setting may be negativity.

During these 2 years, language acquisition progresses at the rate of several new words per day, as vocabulary mushrooms from 1 or 2 words to about 1,000. At the same time, the use of language develops from single words to full sentences that employ the rudiments of grammar. By the end of this period, most children have learned to substitute verbal requests for pointing and crying.

Parallel to language acquisition, toddlers' motor activity progresses from uncertain, unsteady steps through climbing stairs to running, hopping, and pedaling a tricycle. Advancing motor skills enable the beginning of self-care. Young toddlers will help to undress and dress themselves (such as pushing a foot into a sock), learn to choose foods, and begin to feed themselves with a spoon and cup. The perception of mature behavior and the desire for proficiency drive much of this progress, which ushers in fantasy play as a rehearsal for grown-up behavior. By the end of toddlerhood, a toy begins to represent some object perceived as important in the adult world, instead of just an object to be manipulated.

Obtaining Information

Toddlerhood is (another) difficult age at which to obtain reliable information from a child; again, multiple, brief diagnostic sessions may be necessary. As with infants, all historical information comes from the parents, whose descriptions and concerns must be taken seriously. In the clinician's office, many children will not exhibit the symptomatic behaviors that are of concern to their parents (a generic warning that applies to patients well into their teens—and sometimes beyond). Repeated office visits to foster comfort and familiarity, or visits to the home or to the day care center (depending on where the symptoms are said to occur), may be necessary to the evaluation. Sometimes bringing a child to the office with the opposite-sex parent or even the entire family is illuminating.

As with an infant, it is important to observe a toddler's interactions with a parent and then to note the child's reaction when the parent briefly leaves the room. During this absence, you can attempt to engage the child in play. Observe relatedness, exploration of new toys, and apprehension with a stranger. How would you characterize the reunion once the parent returns? Assessing separation anxiety, which is normal at this age, should be part of every evaluation. A child who has previously experienced illness, hospitalization, or other separation may vigorously resist being interviewed alone. Early in the relationship, it may not be possible to interview the child at all unless the parent is present.

It is hard to sustain a conversation with toddlers, who need more verbal probes and structure in play than do older children. In posing questions or in proposing play, offer multiple choices, which increase the options for response. Even relatively nonverbal children may be able to respond to queries that relate directly to the play sequence they have just completed: "Is that the way it is [in this sort of situation] at your house?" However, it is extremely important not to play into the suggestibility of young children; they are eager for the approval of adults and may respond with "yes" to just about anything. Observe a toddler's ability to use language (vocabulary, complexity of sentence structure) and affect (range, predominant type, and appropriateness). Evaluate fine motor skills by having the toddler draw figures, squares, and diamonds. Assess handedness and footedness by having the child catch, throw, and kick a ball.

Excessive shyness or lack of inhibition may be apparent. How much control does the child require in the playroom setting—a simple "no," or repeated physical interventions?

Symptoms

Most of the same symptoms first identified in infancy can still be issues a year or two later. In addition, new symptoms may worry parents:

- Aphasia (loss of ability to understand or express written or spoken language)
- Disturbed consciousness (abrupt onset of inability to focus or sustain attention)
- Excessive crying, night waking, or refusal to go to bed at night
- Extreme misbehavior: temper tantrums, lying, refusal to cooperate, destruction of toys, cruelty, violence, rapidly fluctuating mood dysregulation
- Extreme shyness, presenting as withdrawal and apathy
- Inadequate social interaction (poor eye contact, restricted body language, inadequate fantasy play, limited ability to sustain a conversation or to share interests or enjoyment)
- Inflexible adherence to routine
- Language delay (for example, no language use by 18 months or no use of phrases by 30–36 months)
- Motor hyperactivity, which can occur in many problems or disorders
- Refusal to separate from parents or stay with sitters, a desperate need for attention, "being spoiled"
- Stereotyped movements
- Struggles over toilet training or new foods
- Testing limits, "being a devil," getting into everything, being "just like Dad or Uncle Ernie"

DSM-5 Diagnoses That May Appear at This Age or Later

- Intellectual disability (mild or moderate), global developmental delay
- Autism spectrum disorder

- Reactive attachment disorder, disinhibited social engagement disorder
- Delirium
- Posttraumatic and acute stress disorders
- Parent–child relational problem (Z-code)

PRESCHOOL AGE (3–6 YEARS)

During the next 3 years of life, children begin to develop the ability to observe, to think, and to mentally manipulate formed constructs in ways they will use later as they equip themselves for life as adults. These abilities form the basis for the existence of a private self within a child—one that is not readily discernible to the parents.

Aspects of Development

As development proceeds, children realize that there are adults other than parents and other immediate family members. Whereas relationships with parents were initially the main focus for interaction and for need fulfillment, children at this age gradually grow more interested in friends their own age—playmates at the playground, in day care, and in the neighborhood. They begin to attend birthday parties and other multiple-family events. Play, which becomes increasingly complex and symbolic, serves as a vehicle for wider socialization. Play relieves tension, works out problems, and helps children build a sense of identity and mastery over conflict. Differences between the sexes become especially pronounced in social situations. As same-sex friendships begin, activities tend to become gender-specific—dolls for girls, adventure toys for boys—though recent decades have witnessed a trend toward a greater degree of blended play.

By the end of the preschool years, all the elements of basic communication skills are in place. The child can converse in complete sentences that are logical and grammatically correct; eye–hand coordination allows printing, writing, and drawing; and the basics of numbers and colors have been grasped.

Locomotion becomes smooth, and all gross motor movements are better coordinated. Children at this age have boundless energy and curiosity, but their judgment is limited, so parents still need to guard against various types of accidents. Toward the end of this stage, there is a gradual reduction of impulsiveness.

As they near school age, children begin to adopt moral values. At first, these are rigid and lack subtlety—a sense of right and wrong, good and bad, fair play. Children also begin to demonstrate empathy for the distress of friends and parents. At this age, they want to please; as a result, loving discipline increasingly suffices to keep order. At the same time, they develop a capacity for jealousy and rivalry; secrets fascinate them.

Obtaining Information

A preschool child can provide some verbal information that is diagnostically useful, but most of what you learn will come from nonverbal facial and body language and from the quality of the child's interactions with you. Interviews most often focus on the present, and children's responses will consist of single-word or short-phrase replies to questions. Because of their age and inexperience, these children cannot supply much of the material vital to their own histories (especially family history and parental strife), but they may show surprising insight into the functioning of their nuclear families.

Start the interview not by discussing problems, but by asking confidence-building questions a child can answer easily—the child's own age, where the child lives, and with whom the child resides. Preschool children need encouragements to keep them going. Wait until rapport is established to ask what a child's feelings are about a parent or sibling. To address the child's wishes, body image, living situation, self-assessment, and other features, ask, "What would you like to change about yourself?" (An answer of "Everything" may indicate severe depression.)

The child's sense of the future and aspirations can be addressed by asking direct questions or by beginning a story that the child completes: "Once upon a time, there was a little child named [child's name]. What [name] always wanted to do was . . . " To assess mood, present the child with a simple scale: "How do you feel most of the time? Really sad, sad, sort of in the middle, happy, or really happy?" But unless you have formed a trusting relationship with the child, the response may be a clumsy attempt to please or to keep back information: "Really happy," the child may state in a subdued voice, while failing to make eye contact.

Young children also enjoy play interviews, which are used to obtain information that the children may not otherwise divulge (because direct questions may be seen as threatening). You can directly interact in play with a child; you can also observe the child's spontaneous play (with peers, on the playground, and so on). Carefully observe the child in interaction with others for the assumption of social roles (leader vs. follower, gregarious vs. isolated individual). In play, evaluate the child's choice of toys, affect regulation, activity level (normal exploratory curiosity vs. destructive, driven, reckless hyperactivity), concentration, frustration tolerance, mastery motivation, and persistence at a task.

Symptoms

- Anxiety upon separation from parents
- Elimination problems or genital complaints: enuresis, encopresis, pain, repeated

genital touching/masturbation, self-exposure (the latter complaints in particular may indicate sexual abuse)

▓ Extreme jealousy of a new sibling

▓ Few or no friends

▓ Impulsiveness of a self-harming nature (running into the street, grabbing knives, attempting suicide, ingesting medications or other substances)

▓ Inattentiveness

▓ Mood dysregulation

▓ Multiple fears (which may be manifested as excessively shy, withdrawn behavior)

▓ Nightmares, fear of the dark

▓ Refusal to follow directions

▓ Risk taking (recklessness, inappropriate fearlessness)

▓ Somatization of grief or stress (loss) reactions in stomachaches, headaches, "not feeling well"

▓ Symptoms that suggest anxiety: avoidance of play with same-age peers, frequent stomachaches, crying when taken to preschool, changes in appetite (anxiety may also be shown in play or dreams)

▓ Speech that is difficult to understand, stuttering

▓ Temper tantrums or aggressive outbursts

DSM-5 Diagnoses That May Appear at This Age or Later

▓ Communication disorders such as social (pragmatic) communication disorder, speech sound disorder, childhood-onset fluency disorder (stuttering), or a more general language disorder

▓ Stereotypic movement disorder

▓ Oppositional defiant disorder

▓ Pica

▓ Specific phobia and other anxiety disorders

▓ Breathing-related sleep disorders

▓ Non-rapid eye movement sleep arousal disorders, sleep terror and sleepwalking types

▓ Physical abuse of child, sexual abuse of child, neglect of child (T-codes)

SCHOOL AGE (6–12 YEARS)

Social relationships with peers become dominant as the child moves outside the family for interpersonal contact and reinforcement.

Aspects of Development

By the early grades of elementary school, preference for playmates of the same sex becomes dominant, with differentiation of styles of play and behavior by gender. At the risk of painting pictures in strokes that are too broad, it is common to see boys favor rough-and-tumble play in larger groups, oriented around shared experiences; they often play away from the immediate confines of home, exploring the environment. Girls, however, often play indoors or near home in smaller groups, oriented around shared confidences. For many children, socialization proceeds through peer group identification (such as Scouts and soccer). Games and play become much more rule-oriented. Activities at first occur close to home (Cub Scouts, Brownies), but take older children farther afield for hikes, overnight camping trips, and out-of-town sporting matches. Social relationships become important; the earliest signs of bullying behaviors and victim roles occur.

Although for over a century this age has been called the *latency period*, these children have significant developmental tasks to master. Indeed, *mastery* (competence) and *competition* are two of the watchwords of the years that precede adolescence. A child's focus moves outside the family to include schoolwork, which provides practice that lays the foundations for later, life-sustaining work. Of course, mastering basic educational skills (reading, writing, math) occupies much of the child's attention. At least as important are developing good study skills and feeling positive about learning—experiences that are balanced by the competing demands of games and other play, entertainment, and hobbies. Self-esteem, competence, and self-confidence become important attributes.

For the first time, a child may shift allegiances to a new authority figure—a teacher or coach—often forcing a reevaluation of the parents' values (especially about education). School-age children become progressively able to keep reality and fantasy distinct, and in general to view the world from the perspective of increasing experience and developing judgment. Before the age of 8, children describe others in terms of physical appearance; later they will use more abstract terms. They develop the verbal ability to express complex ideas and relationships between elements (cause and effect), and to show off their improving use of language with plays on words.

Children at this age have an increasing ability to retain and operate on information (for example, to keep a string of digits in mind). At first rigid and moralistic, children may express feelings of guilt or remorse when they fail to attain a given standard. (It may not be until the late teenage years, if ever, that they accept a lesser standard of performance in themselves.) During this period, they also become able to modulate their own affects and to show emotions different from what they feel inwardly. Moreover, they experience completion of the development of gross motor skills: running, jumping, and throwing with accuracy and increasing strength.

Obtaining Information

Although you still need to speak first with parents and teachers, school-age children can relate considerable historical information. Although many older children can talk about themselves nearly as well as adults can, play is still a useful facilitator of communication, especially in the grade school years. Studies have demonstrated that behavior in play reflects a child's everyday activities and concerns. Games and drawing can also facilitate communication.

Each evaluation should begin with some preliminaries. First, perhaps, offer an introduction along the lines of "I'm Ms. Smith, and I'd like to get to know you by talking and playing with you," or "I'm a doctor who works with children." You might ask whether the child knows the reason for the interview. A little explanation of the process can help allay the anxiety that many younger children will feel when confronted by a new environment and a strange adult who asks a lot of questions. Straightforward, simple explanations of expectations and confidentiality usually work best. Above all, a child should experience any clinical interview as both nonjudgmental and nonthreatening. Use smiles, eye contact, and other physical signs of welcome and ease to communicate comfort and the feeling that it is safe to reveal information.

Allowing the child to lead the interview (especially in play) fosters a sense of control, which tends to facilitate communication. Cautious use of humor can help build rapport. At the same time, avoid being excessively friendly; you want to learn how the child typically forms a new relationship. "Tell me about your family" isn't likely to net you much; instead, ask the child to describe a typical activity, such as washing dishes—who washes, who dries. Try using a just-reported issue to learn how the child might respond in other circumstances: "Instead of your mom making up the rules about chores, what if you got to make them up?" Asking to hear "three wishes" can help reveal aspects of the child's fantasy life and view of the future. And here are some other ways you can encourage the child to reveal private viewpoints: "What would you do if you were in charge of your family?" "What would happen if nobody had to go to bed on time?" "If you were oldest, what would you do?" "Suppose someone fell down? What would you do to help?"

Children tend to be more accurate in reporting facts (what actually happened) than in making judgments (whether an event or behavior was good or bad, whether it occurred frequently or infrequently). Therefore, you aren't likely to learn much from asking "why" questions, which may only make a child feel puzzled, threatened, or incompetent. The "why" of things is deduced gradually from the accretion of evidence obtained from other informants, patient interviews, and testing. In play or in verbal interaction, it is important to gauge both the spontaneity and the logical, goal-oriented nature of the communication. Young children will recall more accurately if open-ended questions are used, but their information won't be as complete as that provided by older children. If they are only asked yes–no questions, children under the age of 10 accurately report their fears—but not much else. If a child does not answer a question, you will need to shift topics or get the answer in play.

Speech, language, and learning problems, such as articulation defects or problems with comprehension, can be evaluated by direct observation during the initial interview. Samples of writing and reading should be obtained as a further assessment of language proficiency. You can test spelling and writing by asking the child to label a just-completed drawing of family members. What do you observe about the child's thought progression and logic? Of course, much of *any* interview is nonverbal, so observe the child's temperament, frustration tolerance, and ability to relate to you.

Depressed affect, with tearfulness, feelings of worthlessness, and (sometimes) aggression, can be expressed verbally or in play. A child's moods will be reported better by the child than by parents, but as with adults, contemporary diagnosis of depression and other negative affects requires more than cross-sectional observation. Historical and behavioral data are also needed from parents and other informants.

Various writers have suggested methods for dealing with the threat that negative feelings pose for children:

- Suggest that many other children feel the same.
- Present two or more acceptable constructs: "Do you like school pretty well, or would you rather not go?"
- Express the assumption that all children sometimes engage in negative behavior (such as fights with siblings).
- Suggest an acceptable reason for bad behavior: "Maybe you ran away because you needed to show someone how you felt."

Throughout an interview, though you may not agree with a child, it is important to respect the child's defense mechanisms. This is especially true for younger children, whose need for approval can be both intense and immediate.

In the mental health interview, play serves three functions. It can be a therapeutic tool that engages a child's imagination with fantasies that present conflicts and their resolution. It can also serve as a topic for conversation. Finally, toys or games can ease tension while the interviewer and patient engage in conversation. Experienced clinicians most often use combinations of play and talk—straight play, straight talk, and talk facilitated by play—to keep the momentum of a session going. It is usually not difficult to decide which technique(s) should be used. At first, you might try all three to see how the child responds, then proceed with whichever seems easiest for the child. If one method works for a while but then progress stalls, try another.

Try to establish the fewest rules possible, but use them consistently. If behavior becomes unruly, you may need to protect the child as well as the environment. You can say, "I won't let you hurt me or destroy things in the office." When behaviors get out of control and the child's attention cannot be diverted, the session can be stopped or the child can be physically held (but see sidebar below). It is important to set the limits clearly in advance and to define the parameters of intervention. (Be sure to inform the parents of these limits and the methods available to enforce them.) If you suspect that a session may end prematurely, ensure that a parent is available to take charge of the child.

The important themes to watch for in play are similar to those an older patient might talk about as trauma or conflict. Loss and grief, anger, fears, feeling unloved, low self-esteem, isolation, and alienation all commonly appear in play. These can be manifested in specific play scenarios with animal or human figures; in drawings, they may be indicated by the choice of colors, shapes, and sizes, by order versus chaos, and by the presence or absence of key figures. Children may tell as much by what they leave out or avoid in play as they do through inclusion. Normal children have a variety of themes, affects, and play preferences, and share their interactions and experiences easily in play interviews. Psychopathology in play is most evident in rigid, fixed themes, affects, and preferences, whereby the child excludes you or other participants entirely, or is inappropriately compliant, seductive, or combative. Watch for the affect. Bland themes may be as telling as violence or chaos.

> Two issues confer a degree of potential risk, for clinician as well as patient.
>
> Sometimes moving the interview away from the office by walking or sitting outdoors makes a child feel more at ease. However, no one wants to be the clinician responsible for allowing an impulsive child to dart off into traffic. Where and when you will take a patient out of the office needs to be clearly outlined and parental consent obtained in advance. And even with permission, no child who is acutely upset should be allowed where you will have increased difficulty controlling the child's behavior.
>
> The second situation—when you are tempted to hold a child to manage aggression or prevent the child from bolting out of the office—has been much debated. Some point out that it could potentially elicit traumatic memories and possibly violent reactions. Once again, this is the sort of issue that should be worked out in advance with parents. Find out how they manage this sort of situation. Explain what circumstances could necessitate a holding intervention, and obtain their consent.

Symptoms

In addition to the symptoms mentioned previously, inquire about and watch for the following:

- Absence of speech in specific social situations
- Angry mood
- Anxiety in children (especially girls) who physically develop early
- Bullying or being a target of bullying
- Deliberately blaming others
- Depression
- Enuresis
- Hyperactivity, fidgeting, talking excessively
- Impulsiveness (inability to take turns, intrusiveness)
- Inability to focus attention during class
- Learning problems
- Loss of temper, arguing, defiance, spite
- Nightmares
- Panic attacks
- Repetitive motor behavior that is nonfunctional
- Rituals or magical beliefs associated with unreasonable fears
- School refusal
- Shyness/fearfulness that is excessive
- Somatization
- Substance use
- Stuttering and other verbal fluency problems
- Temper outbursts
- Tics
- Trouble with reading, math, writing
- Withdrawal or isolation

DSM-5 Diagnoses That May Appear at This Age or Later

- Anxiety disorders (including phobias)
- Attention-deficit/hyperactivity disorder
- Autism spectrum disorder
- Conduct disorder

- Disruptive mood dysregulation disorder

- Learning disorders

- Encopresis

- Enuresis

- Obsessive–compulsive disorder

- Separation anxiety disorder

- Selective mutism

- Tourette's disorder and other tic disorders

- Sleepwalking

EARLY ADOLESCENCE (12–15 YEARS)

Although the drive to achieve independence from parents continues and even accelerates during early adolescence, the family remains a preeminent influence for adolescents. This may appear contrary to popular belief, but several studies have reported that most adolescents have relatively few serious disagreements with their parents. Whereas adolescents and parents often disagree (sometimes sharply) on issues of contemporary social concern such as politics, use of social media, substance use, and sexuality, these are mostly differences in the intensity of an attitude rather than its direction; gulfs between generations usually reflect different levels of support for the same position.

In the end, there isn't much evidence supporting the myth of adolescence as a period of inevitable storm and stress. Most teenagers continue their close and supportive relationships with their parents; in their relationships with peers, they tend to embrace parental values rather than to reject them. However, there can be no doubt that adolescents do test limits; think omnipotently; succumb to peer pressure; and often support culture heroes, philosophies, or lifestyles that are upsetting to the parents.

The onset of adolescence is so variable that no exact age can be given. *Early adolescence* is marked by the onset of puberty, which in some girls can begin as young as 10. *Middle adolescence* usually refers to a period that begins 2–3 years later, with *late adolescence* beginning

The age of consent for treatment of a non-emancipated minor varies from state to state. In most jurisdictions, an adolescent (ages ranging from 12 to 17 are listed) can consent to treatment for sexually transmitted diseases, contraception, pregnancy, substance abuse, and emotional distress. The legal age of consent for treatment can also vary, depending on which condition is the focus of treatment. Know the local laws pertaining to where you practice and the conditions for which an adolescent is seeking evaluation or treatment.

another few years after that. Typically, early adolescents will be 6th–8th graders; middle adolescents will be 8th–10th graders; and late adolescents may be in the 11th grade through the first 2 or 3 years of college. Somewhat arbitrarily, we have chosen age 15 as the crossover point between early and late adolescence. We simply cannot find behavioral and emotional distinctions that clearly mark the limits of the middle phase. And, in reality, the ages in each of these stages can vary by several months or years.

Aspects of Development

Adolescence marks the emerging comprehension of one's sexual orientation and, for most, the beginning of the shift from same-sex to opposite-sex preoccupations and activities. If these changes do not take place early during this period of development, they will occur within the next few years. An adolescent feels a powerful adherence to the peer group; cliques and clubs are critical to the sense of belonging, which also fosters a need to stay in touch with peers by phone, texting, social media, through after-school sports and social events. Getting ready to drive a car heightens the sense of moving away and belonging to a new group.

Sibling rivalry can sometimes become intense, especially if siblings are the same sex, are close in age, or have similar interests. Stepsiblings in blended families are especially at risk for rivalry and territoriality. Outside the family, competition intensifies in a variety of areas, including athletics, attractiveness, and academic/intellectual pursuits. Preeminence in sports supersedes the mere development of skill.

Early adolescents experience a growth spurt. In boys, it begins at about age 12. In girls, growth accelerates a year earlier, with menarche occurring at about 12½ years (3 years earlier than was the case in 1900). Whereas for boys, early maturation can promote self-confidence in interactions with peers and adults; for girls, peer pressure and concerns about body image can disrupt self-concept.

By the midteens, intellectual development is nearly on a par with that of adults. Children of this age can define complex scientific terms and reason about theoretical events or constructs. Despite increasing prominence of moral distinctions and a sense of what is right or good in others (particularly their parents), adolescents' judgment about their own behavior is often their downfall. The typical adolescent illusion of invulnerability promotes risk taking, which leads to experimentation with drugs, sexuality, or illegal behavior so often as to constitute almost a rite of passage for young people.

Obtaining Information

The first years of adolescence mark the age when information from the patient becomes predominant in the mental health workup. Adolescent patients know more of their own histories and can communicate in an interview on a more nearly equal footing than is true for younger children. Usually the patient should be interviewed first; the subsequent parent interview is often better accomplished when the teenager is present.

Developing trust and rapport with a teen is critical. At the outset, it is especially important to explain about confidentiality and its limits. Try to establish a trusting relationship that will increase the likelihood of obtaining reliable data and set the stage for future therapy. It is often useful to balance the need for trust against the need for truth with a statement such as this: "There are some topics uncomfortable to share. If one of them comes up, let me know and we can put it aside for the time being. I don't want you to feel you have to lie because something makes you uncomfortable." Sometimes adolescents will talk about experiences that their friends have had, while denying (falsely) that they themselves have been involved.

In an interview with a teen, you should be friendly and interested, but respectful of your age difference. Whereas it's nice to know something about culture heroes, athletes, and rock stars, our experience has been that showing a genuine interest in learning about these topics can be just as useful in developing a strong working relationship with a young person. Beware, however, of being overly friendly or of trying to act too "hip" (itself a dated term by now!); teenagers can often see through artifice like a pane of glass.

You will especially need to assess these issues:

- The family situation, from the dual perspectives of adolescent and parents; presence or lack of support in the primary family system

- Sexual knowledge, including sexual experiences, both heterosexual and gay/lesbian/ bisexual/transgender; pregnancy; use of safe-sex practices

- Use of tobacco, alcohol, and both prescription and illicit drugs

- Delinquency, truancy, and participation in gangs

- Self-harmful behavior

- Being a bully or a target of bullying

- Being the victim of physical or sexual abuse

- Friendship patterns and activities with peers

- Issues of dependence–independence; developmental readiness to meet the demands of society

- Identity formation ("Who am I? What will be my place in the world?")

- Self-esteem—a big concern for the preadolescent and adolescent

- Empathy (how sorry does the adolescent feel when a sibling or friend has a problem?)

- Conscience ("What would you do if . . . ?")

As with an adult, try to end your interview with a teen by providing some sort of summing up. As positively as possible, state your initial impressions. What do you propose for treatment? For future meetings? What will you tell the parents?

Symptoms

- Adherence to fads of food, clothes, and style, including hair dyeing and tattooing/body piercing (the latter are increasingly normative, but may worry parents and other significant adults)
- Anxiety symptoms in boys or girls who experience late onset of puberty
- Impulsiveness
- Loneliness, depression, suicidal ideation
- Overt aggression, destruction of property, theft, rule violation
- Poor school attendance (either truant or avoidant)
- Rebellion against authority (at its highest during these years)
- Somatic complaints

DSM-5 Diagnoses That May Appear at This Age or Later

- Major depressive disorder
- Persistent depressive disorder (dysthymia)
- Bipolar disorders
- Generalized anxiety disorder
- Body dysmorphic disorder
- Gender dysphoria
- Circadian rhythm sleep–wake disorder, delayed sleep phase type
- Substance use disorders
- Eating disorders

LATE ADOLESCENCE (15–21 YEARS)

Although we have stated the limit for late adolescence as age 21, in reality it can last much longer; the final leg of the march to independent life often extends through college and a graduate degree or two. But by age 21 (more or less), the adolescent's personality has been established, and the inclination toward marriage (or long-term partnership) and the bearing and rearing of children has been determined.

Aspects of Development

As adolescents move toward the completion of their education, they increasingly take on adult responsibilities and viewpoints. Of course, the exact timing and sequence can vary widely; many young people are late bloomers. Depending on social milieu and parental mores, dating usually begins early in this time period; sexual activity is the norm by the end of the teen years. The young adult develops the capacity for mature love. Judgment improves, and as the end of the teens looms, the typical adolescent becomes serious about work or further education.

Obtaining Information

Older adolescents may present themselves for evaluation, without the immediate prospect of information from outside resources. As for any other patient, collateral information should be sought and evaluated whenever possible. The material covered, including the mental status examination, will be essentially the same as for an adult.

Symptoms

- Concerns about masturbation, other sexual behaviors
- Appetite symptoms
- Mood symptoms
- Symptoms suggesting trauma
- Anxiety symptoms
- Substance use problems
- Emergence of psychotic symptoms
- Onset of realization of same-sex orientation (earlier for males than for females)

DSM-5 Diagnoses That May Appear at This Age or Later

- All major adult diagnoses except some neurocognitive disorders (such as neurocognitive disorder due to Alzheimer's disease)
- Most personality disorders (antisocial personality disorder is first diagnosable at age 18)

A Variety of Interviews
with Children and Adolescents

CHAPTER 4

The Infant/Toddler Interview

PURPOSES AND GOALS OF THE INFANT/TODDLER INTERVIEW

Most infants and toddlers referred for mental health evaluation *won't* meet criteria for a DSM-5 diagnosis. Exceptions include autism spectrum disorder; disorders of eating, sleeping, and elimination; reactive attachment and disinhibited engagement disorders; and movement disorders. Yet for several reasons, clinicians need to feel comfortable and competent in evaluating these very young children: (1) to institute treatment early enough to avert permanent developmental consequences; (2) to assess the potential risk of similar conditions in siblings and other children in a household; and (3) to identify problems in parents. Of course, infants and toddlers can only receive an adequate evaluation in the presence of their primary caregivers.

Most often, the persons interviewed will be one or both parents, grandparents, or foster parents. (As in other chapters, however, we use the term *parents* here to stand for all primary caregivers.) Usually they are concerned about lack of developmental progress or a disturbance of regulation—significant problems with sleeping (the most common of all), crying, feeding, or limit setting. Many clinicians feel that such abnormalities may foreshadow anxiety disorders, disorders of attachment, neurocognitive disorders, and autism spectrum disorder. Clinicians need to help parents differentiate normal variations in development from important problems that need intervention.

A mental health clinician evaluates an infant and parent with three goals in mind. One is to develop rapport with the parent; another is to obtain a clear picture of the nature of the symptoms and concerns. The third is to observe a variety of clues to the nature of interactions between the infant and parent:

- Does the infant clearly signal either pleasure or distress, making it easy for the parent to understand the communication?

- How sensitively and consistently does the parent respond to the infant's signals and bids for attention, as well as to expressions of pleasure and satisfaction?

- Does the parent appear depressed? Frustrated? Angry? Or even cognitively impaired?

- How does the parent handle the infant's expressions of frustration or lack of interest that may result from the interactions?

- When the infant cries, is the reason clear?

- Does the infant smile readily? Is the infant easily consolable?

- Will the infant engage with the examiner?

- Does the infant show clear preferences for certain individuals and toys?

- Does the infant seem hypersensitive to loud noises, bright lights, or rapid transitions?

- Does the infant seem to have the temperamental characteristics of an "easy," "difficult," or "slow-to-warm-up" baby (see the discussion of infant temperament in Chapter 3)?

The following interview with a toddler demonstrates many of these points. The material in **boldface** indicates some of the areas the interviewer tries to evaluate in this brief interview.

Joan is a 14-month-old child who is just beginning to toddle. Her pediatrician has referred her because her mother is worried that she is excessively shy, especially with strangers. The referral note indicates no history of important problems during the pregnancy (poor nutrition, illnesses, smoking in the home, use of drugs or alcohol) or perinatal period (postpartum depression, single-parent status, low family income).

Once they enter the examination room, the examiner sits on the floor and points to a set of toys placed within easy reach. Following this lead, the mother also sits on the floor. At the beginning of the interview, Joan sits quietly on her mother's lap, looking about cautiously; after a few moments, she allows herself to be placed on the floor. At first, the interviewer does not attempt to engage Joan directly, but stacks some blocks and observes her from a slight distance. Joan will be permitted to join in at her own pace.

INTERVIEWER: Hello, I'm Dr. V. You must be Ms. T. And this must be Joan. She is all dressed up for her outing. Let's begin by seeing how Joan is doing these days in terms of her development. It looks like she's walking.

In an initial attempt to establish rapport and to indicate that observations are an important part of the interview, the interviewer acknowledges that Ms. T. has made a special *effort in preparing her infant. The interviewer notes that Joan's **general development** is that of a normal, healthy-appearing child who shows no evidence of arrested development or failure to thrive. Neither does she have the **physical characteristics** of some intellectual disability syndromes (such as Down syndrome), or hand flapping or other unusual behaviors that could suggest autism spectrum disorder. Although shy at the outset, Joan is definitely engaged in the process. During this earliest part of the interview, the interviewer observes how secure Joan seems to feel while seated on her mother's lap and how much stimulation her mother provides.*

MOTHER: She's started to walk, but she's afraid to let go. She's been cruising [walking while holding on to furniture] for a long time, but she won't just get up and walk. If you distract her, she'll sometimes take a few steps on her own, but even then she tries to hang on.

The mother immediately expresses a concern about Joan's developmental progress. Her anxiety is evident, both in the care she has taken with Joan's dress and in this initial expression of concern.

INTERVIEWER: She seems to be able to pull herself to a stand. So physically, she's right on schedule?

MOTHER: Yes.

*The interviewer observes and underscores Joan's developmentally appropriate behavior and strengths, commenting on the normal **motor development** (walking at a developmentally expected age, absence of hyperactivity). This strategy is an attempt to reassure the mother and to foster the therapeutic alliance, thereby shifting her focus from developmental failure and pathology to normality and progression.*

INTERVIEWER: And how about her schedule—does she sleep and awaken at regular times?

MOTHER: She eats regularly. She sleeps through the night, but sometimes she'll nap and sometimes she won't. The most she'll do is two naps about an hour and a half each, and most nights she screams when you put her to bed. She'll fall asleep, but she always screams.

*In response to questions about her infant's routines, the mother, as before, emphasizes potential problems, not strengths. For the time being, the interviewer again steers away from possible pathology to focus on what the child is doing well. Note how the interviewer uses the mother's own words as a bridge to another topic. Questions about **eating** and **elimination** form a part of every infant/toddler interview.*

INTERVIEWER: Tell me about her eating regularly.

MOTHER: She has cereal in the morning and a bottle and juice. She eats almost anything.

INTERVIEWER: Anything?

MOTHER: Pretty much anything that is finely chopped.

INTERVIEWER: Cookies?

MOTHER: I try not to give her any, but if I do, she likes them.

INTERVIEWER: Candy? [Meanwhile, Joan has pulled herself to a standing position, but still clings to her mother's shoulder and avoids eye contact with the interviewer. She has not begun to explore the age-appropriate toys on the floor.]

The interviewer is trying to see what limits the mother may be setting for the child. In the evaluation of any infant, there is the possibility that at least a part of the problem relates to the nature of the **dyadic relationship** *between the child and parent. What is the quality of their shared attention and intimacy? How well can the adult tolerate tension while skillfully returning the infant to a state of comfort?*

MOTHER: She doesn't get very much of it, but for Halloween she started chewing on the bowl of Halloween candy.

INTERVIEWER: How would you describe her temperamentally? Is she an easy child, or is she difficult?

MOTHER: I think she's a little bit of a mixture, because she's very intense and she's very stubborn. Her emotions are very intense.

INTERVIEWER: So when she cries, she really cries?

MOTHER: And if something happens that she doesn't like—like the other day she was trying to push the buttons on the TV, and she couldn't get them to do what she wanted—she just started screaming. She's not easily soothed. She's really happy except when she gets mad.

The interviewer notes the two adjectives stubborn *and* intense. *They may prove important to the assessment of Joan's* **temperament**. *But her mother quickly points out that Joan's* **basic mood** *is neither depressed nor anxious, but happy. It is important to determine whether infants can communicate their needs and feeling states clearly. Through her intense emotions, Joan seems to communicate readily; however, her mother views these same intense emotions as a problem. Infants who are difficult to comfort often challenge the competence of their parents and trigger feelings of inadequacy.*

INTERVIEWER: Today she's cautious in a strange situation, but when she's at home, she's out there exploring?

MOTHER: At home, she's constantly exploring and moving around. She loves music; she'll start dancing.

INTERVIEWER: Really! Does she watch TV?

In a child so young, a formal assessment of intelligence will be pretty unreliable. Instead, the interviewer asks about such qualities as curiosity, persistence, attention, and task mastery, which may give clues to Joan's **cognitive development**.

MOTHER: Yes, there's a morning show for children. She'll stop whatever she's doing and watch.

INTERVIEWER: How is she at home? Does she play with toys?

MOTHER: Her favorite thing is to mess up the house. She'll take all the clothes out of the drawers and all the pots out of the cabinets and rummage through the trash, if she can.

INTERVIEWER: [To Joan] You're so curious at home, all the time playing and exploring things. What do you think I'm playing with here? Do you want to play with me? [At last, Joan timidly takes a block and puts it into a cup. She seems about to engage. Almost immediately, her mother moves back, first a few inches. Then, over the next few minutes, she retreats further; she eventually gets up from the floor and sits in a nearby chair.]

Such interactions can provide an opportunity to evaluate how very young children play with toys, as well as how they respond to strangers, to direct gaze, and perhaps to being picked up. Engagement, mood, "leading versus following," creativity, spontaneity, motor skills, and attention span can all be assessed in the course of simple games. In play, the interviewer follows Joan's lead, placing blocks in a cup. This type of parallel play is less threatening for an inhibited, anxious child, as Joan is reported to be. However, the mother's early, somewhat rapid withdrawal poses a potential threat. So the interviewer tries to maintain the tie to the mother by continuing to question her, which also serves to take the pressure of direct engagement off the child.

INTERVIEWER: Does she like books?

MOTHER: She loves books. She'll let me read a book to her at almost any time.

JOAN: [Babbles.]

INTERVIEWER: [To Joan] Everything is interesting to look at. [To the mother] Does she speak words yet?

The interviewer has observed Joan beginning to explore and, for the first time, comments directly to her from a slight distance, rather than interacting and possibly driving her away. Her babbling prompts questions about speech development. Even in a prever-

bal child, an interviewer should look for early evidence of **language difficulties,** *such as slow onset of speech sounds or, later, problems with pronunciation.*

MOTHER: Just a few—*Mama* and *dog.* She loves the dog. She fights with the dog for the same toys.

INTERVIEWER: [To Joan] Can I have that?

Now the interviewer attempts to interact with Joan by asking her for an object. The play engagement proceeds slowly, however, suggesting shyness and inhibition. If these are temperamental traits, these qualities could be strengths, even though the mother may view them as problems. However, if the infant's inhibitions reflect overcontrolling interactions on the part of the mother that are anxiety-driven, they probably indicate a relationship problem. A third possibility is that a strange, unfamiliar setting such as the clinician's office produces caution that is appropriate. If that's the case, the infant should slowly begin to warm up. The interviewer's task is to attempt to differentiate the several possible sources of Joan's caution.

INTERVIEWER: Do you think she'd play here all day?

This suggestion that Joan is beginning to enjoy herself is designed to reassure the mother; it may also reassure the infant through their mutual nonverbal social referencing.

MOTHER: She might.

INTERVIEWER: Is she in day care?

MOTHER: No, she's at home with her nanny.

INTERVIEWER: [To Joan] Well, let's see if you can put these blocks in the cup. [Beginning to interact with Joan more directly, the interviewer intentionally shifts positions to block Joan's view of her mother. Joan experiences the anxiety of separation and at once begins to cry vigorously, even though her mother remains seated nearby.]

Perhaps the interviewer has moved too quickly. However, evaluation sessions are usually time-limited, and some observation of "separation," even in a parent's presence, is important.

INTERVIEWER: She's been holding it in.

The interviewer comments that Joan has been a reluctant participant, holding in her anxiety about the evaluation. She has not fully engaged with the interviewer, bravely trying, but in fact beginning to cry almost immediately after the interviewer starts to interact with her directly. On the positive side, Joan's ability to **discriminate significant figures** *can be in no doubt.*

JOAN: [Cries loudly and inconsolably.]

MOTHER: Joan! It's OK, honey, you can play.

INTERVIEWER: As long as she is playing by herself, she's fine.

JOAN: [Ignores the sound of her name and continues to cry. Her mother holds her, tries to reassure her, and finally picks her up and rocks her, all to no avail.]

So far, the most striking features of this interview are the intensity of Joan's crying and, as her mother has described previously, her inconsolability. An older child of 2 or 3 might be testing limits by indicating behaviorally, "No, I won't listen." At Joan's 14 months, her selective attention and reluctance to engage suggest not defiance, but a need to control her separation anxiety by shutting out all novel stimuli and other sources of comfort, focusing exclusively on her mother.

MOTHER: It's OK, honey, it's OK. [Continues rapidly rocking Joan, who cries harder and begins to kick and arch away, clearly resisting being comforted.]

At this point, the mother might excuse herself from the interview for a moment and comfort Joan in private. She might also comment on how difficult the interview is for Joan, or for both of them. Rather, eager to please the interviewer, she continues to rock mechanically and answer questions, seemingly unaware of how to respond to the child's needs. As a result, Joan's crying escalates.

Caregiver response *to a very young child's needs is a core characteristic for any clinician evaluating an infant or toddler to observe. In this case, the mother seems almost agitated in her need to soothe Joan. At this developmental stage, stress with new settings, experiences, and strangers can be expected. But Joan's distress seems to be, at least in part, a response to her mother's affective signals.*

INTERVIEWER: If you have strangers in your home, how is she?

MOTHER: It depends on who's there. She loves women about my age and other little kids. If she's with relatives she hasn't seen in a while, she's very slow to warm up, but if I'm there it's OK, and once she gets used to them she's OK.

Some infant symptoms are transient and may appear only with a specific caregiver. When the other parent or a grandparent is present, an evaluator may see a different picture. In evaluations of infants and toddlers, the critical issue is to determine which behaviors are age-appropriate and normal (thereby representing transient parental concerns) and which are likely to cause significant future problems. For this reason, the interviewer wants to learn whether Joan's behavior occurs in multiple contexts and social situations. Despite the child's almost constant clinging and refusal to explore and engage, it is not clear how far these behaviors generalize to other settings. Later the interviewer will need to ask about Joan's interactions with her father and her nanny.

INTERVIEWER: What about going into a grocery store—do you think she does OK then?

[Begins playing with the blocks, clinking them together, but Joan continues to whimper. Although she has finally stopped crying, Joan obviously does not care to return to the play.]

It is important to ask about the child's behaviors—and **parents' expectations**—*in different settings. Even shopping in a grocery store can become an overstimulating outing. If parents expect behaviors that are not age-appropriate, they will judge a child's actions as inadequate.*

MOTHER: People come up to us and it doesn't bother her. I think she doesn't like women in their 70s with lots of makeup on. I think they scare her. She'll start crying. She's used to going out to stores, though.

INTERVIEWER: Ah, good. Well, perhaps we've done enough for today.

A brief session is often dictated by the limited attention span of a very young child who has become tired. Several sessions over a period of weeks or longer may be needed for infants and toddlers, whereas a single session is often sufficient to evaluate older children and adolescents.

MOTHER: What do you think is wrong with her?

INTERVIEWER: I understand your concern about the intensity of her emotional responses. We saw that here today. We also saw how difficult she can be to soothe and how stubborn she can be, but I'm not sure yet that there is anything fundamentally wrong with Joan. Of course, we'll need to evaluate her some more to see how she acts in other settings and with other people. But there will be a few things we can talk about that could help you with her. [Mother and child get ready to leave. Joan brightens at the prospect. Despite her mother's encouragement, she refuses to wave goodbye.]

Although such a preliminary conclusion might bring relief to some parents, others might disagree with the clinician as to the seriousness of the behavior they observe in their infant or toddler. A parent should help determine whether a more extensive evaluation is indicated. Such an evaluation might include a home visit, a visit with the infant and other parent, and a talk with both parents without the infant. Often two parents have differing views of a child's problems and the best approach to resolving them. Of course, the clinician should always listen attentively to parental concerns. For parents who do not wish a complete evaluation, reassurance should be framed in the context that they can come back in a few months if they are still concerned. In any event, time may yet prove Joan's mother correct: Extremely shy young children often grow into older children who have anxiety disorders.

CHAPTER 5

Play Interview
with a 6-Year-Old Girl

As we have described in Chapter 2, examiners interviewing young children frequently use play material to enhance interaction; to observe the children's physical, emotional, and cognitive capacities; and to elicit areas of conflict or trauma. Play provides distance from anxiety-provoking situations and allows a child to communicate indirectly. Feelings can be expressed without verbal acknowledgment, although the interviewer needs to confirm suspected play communications with direct questions. However, when a child has been playing comfortably, it is likely that pretend feelings or experiences will match those the child experiences in real-life situations. Play sessions like the one presented here are most helpful in evaluating school-age children. However, toddlers, some early adolescents, and children of any age with developmental delays also respond positively to play techniques.

Some children move right in and begin to explore; others require time (or a nearby parent) to warm up to the interview situation. In either case, an amount of time suited to a child's own interactive style should be allowed for engagement.

At age 6, Susan has been brought for evaluation because her teacher is concerned that she is bossy at school with her friends. The teacher is also concerned that Susan does not sustain attention appropriately for her age, at times seeming lost in her own fantasy world. Susan's mother also worries about excessive sibling rivalry.

INTERVIEWER: Hi, you must be Susan. My name is Dr. Q. Did your mother tell you why you are here today? [Susan nods affirmatively.] What did she tell you?

SUSAN: That you could help me with my problem.

INTERVIEWER: What kind of problem do you have?

SUSAN: My mom says I don't get along with my sister, but I don't think so.

INTERVIEWER: Well, I hope I can help in understanding whether or not there is a problem. I like to play with children. It helps me to understand the problem. Do you like to draw?

Throughout, the interviewer uses smiles, eye contact, and other nonverbal signs (difficult to depict on the page) to communicate concern for Susan's comfort and well-being. Above all, a child should experience any clinical interview as both nonjudgmental and nonthreatening.

SUSAN: Yeah.

INTERVIEWER: Well, I've got some Magic Markers here. I'd like you to draw a picture of your family. Do you understand?

SUSAN: OK.

[Using bright colors, she begins to draw figures, neatly and appropriately proportioned for her age. The interviewer observes and says little, except to ask who the figures represent and the names of the siblings and dog. Susan proudly shows off her spelling and writing abilities by printing the names boldly next to the figures.]

Younger children often don't really understand the meaning of the word understand. *To ascertain a child's comprehension, an interviewer can ask for a repetition of the task. Susan, however, seems to have no such problem. (If Susan were an older child, asking her to draw the floor plan of her home might serve as an icebreaker.)*

INTERVIEWER: That's really excellent. Who taught you how to spell like that?

SUSAN: My mommy.

INTERVIEWER: Really? And who's this?

SUSAN: My dad.

INTERVIEWER: And who's that?

SUSAN: My sister, Denny, and my baby brother, Isaac.

INTERVIEWER: How do you spell Denny?

SUSAN: D-E-N-N-Y.

INTERVIEWER: How old are the three of you? Can you write your ages? [Susan writes the ages above the child figures in the drawing: 6 above her own name, 4 above Denny, and 6 months above baby Isaac.]

Here and for the next few moments, the interviewer tests several aspects of Susan's development by asking her to spell, to write, and to talk about her family.

INTERVIEWER: You have very good writing. And this is your dog? What kind of dog is Roscoe?

SUSAN: A yellow Lab.

INTERVIEWER: How old is Roscoe?

SUSAN: She's 4 or 5.

INTERVIEWER: Where does she sleep?

SUSAN: She's an outside dog—she stays in the back yard.

> *Names of siblings, friends, and animals provide anchor points to help focus later discussions; they also serve to make those discussions more real for the child. Information about relationships with animals often provides an indication of the child's capacity for empathy.*

[All this while, Susan has been finishing her drawing, filling in colors and details of clothing. The interviewer has been observing, praising her skills, and asking questions about her picture. Susan has readily answered.]

INTERVIEWER: I see you've put sunglasses on Denny.

SUSAN: 'Cause she likes them.

INTERVIEWER: She likes them? [Instead of offering more information about these sunglasses, Susan takes a new piece of paper and begins to draw more people.]

INTERVIEWER: And these are your friends?

SUSAN: Uh-huh.

INTERVIEWER: What are their names?

SUSAN: Melody, Vanessa, Johnny, Mara—these are twins.

INTERVIEWER: So there's one boy, Johnny?

SUSAN: Johnny and Mara are twins.

INTERVIEWER: Do any of them live near you? [Susan nods while continuing to draw.] They all live by you? [She nods again.] And do you go over to their house to play with them?

SUSAN: They come and play with me. And sometimes I go to their house.

INTERVIEWER: Can you draw a picture of your house?

SUSAN: Yeah.

INTERVIEWER: Has it been raining a lot at your house?

> *The interview is taking place during a time of local flooding; the interviewer is assessing Susan's awareness of current events.*

SUSAN: Yeah.

INTERVIEWER: Have you had any flooding?

SUSAN: No.

INTERVIEWER: It looks like you like to draw. Do you draw in school, too?

SUSAN: Yeah.

INTERVIEWER: You're a good artist. Who else in your family draws?

SUSAN: Denny.

> Using this medium, in just a few minutes the interviewer has obtained a lot of information about Susan's experience of her family, friends, and home environment.

INTERVIEWER: Do you get your own room, or are you sharing it?

SUSAN: I have to share my room with Denny and hear her snoring at night.

INTERVIEWER: And hear her snoring at night?

SUSAN: Yeah.

INTERVIEWER: Oh, my. What time does Denny go to bed?

SUSAN: The same time I do, 7:30.

INTERVIEWER: Then she falls asleep and starts snoring, and you can't get to sleep?

SUSAN: She starts snoring in the middle of the night and wakes me up.

INTERVIEWER: Do you guys have bunk beds, or are the beds next to each other?

SUSAN: Bunk beds.

INTERVIEWER: Who's on top?

SUSAN: Me.

> The actual facts about who sleeps where and when are less important than ascertaining the overall thematic structure of the household and flavor of personal relationships. Note that the interviewer has used a number of closed-ended questions in this interview. Of course, by allowing a child to respond from the universe of personal experience, open-ended questions will yield more information that is valid; however, young children will give less information in free recall than will be the case with older children and adolescents.

INTERVIEWER: Where does Isaac sleep?

SUSAN: In the room next to ours. He has his own room.

INTERVIEWER: You said Roscoe sleeps outside. You never let her in the house?

SUSAN: No, never.

INTERVIEWER: And your mom and dad have a big bedroom. Is it next to yours?

SUSAN: It's next to Isaac's.

INTERVIEWER: [Pointing] What's that—a fence?

SUSAN: That's to keep Roscoe in the yard.

INTERVIEWER: If she gets out of the yard, does she run away?

SUSAN: Yeah. Then we have to try and catch her. We have to call her a thousand times.

INTERVIEWER: You said you have bunk beds—tell me more about your room.

> *The interviewer begins to explore the sibling relationship with Denny, who "lives" in the bed below and who snores. Asking Susan to describe her room helps the interviewer obtain a feeling for her surroundings.*

SUSAN: Yeah.

INTERVIEWER: Do you have your own dresser and your own clothes? [Susan nods "yes."] And what about your toys? Where do you keep them?

SUSAN: In our cupboard. We share them.

INTERVIEWER: You share?

SUSAN: Our room is always a mess.

INTERVIEWER: Messy? And does your mom say, "Clean up your room, girls"?

SUSAN: Yeah.

INTERVIEWER: And who cleans it up.

SUSAN: Me! Denny starts playing a game and I say "No, Denny, we have to clean up, not play." And she says, "But I want to play, not clean up."

INTERVIEWER: She doesn't obey you very well, does she?

> *The interviewer repeatedly comments on what Susan says. Such comments show children that they can talk to adult professionals about what bothers them and that they will be listened to.*

SUSAN: No, she doesn't.

INTERVIEWER: Do you ever beat her up a little bit?

> *In eliciting information about aggression, it may work well to use terms commonly understood by most children, such as "hit," "kick," and "yell." However, if a phrase such as "beat her up a little bit" is used by a child or informant, it would pay to explore its meaning.*

SUSAN: No.

INTERVIEWER: No. Does she ever hit you?

SUSAN: Yeah, a lot.

INTERVIEWER: She hits you and takes things away from you?

SUSAN: Uh-huh.

INTERVIEWER: How does that make you feel?

> *The interviewer already knows much of this material, but studies have shown that children themselves are the most accurate reporters of their own feelings, moods, and inner experiences. On the other hand, parents and teachers more accurately report children's behavior.*

SUSAN: I don't know, kinda mad. But maybe, not very . . .

INTERVIEWER: Since you're the oldest, I guess you have to set a good example. You have to behave yourself and not get into any trouble?

> *By framing the question as "I guess," the interviewer provides an opportunity for Susan to answer negatively.*

SUSAN: I do get in trouble.

INTERVIEWER: What happens?

SUSAN: I keep yelling at her if she doesn't mind me. She never stops playing.

INTERVIEWER: And then do you get in trouble, or does she get into trouble?

SUSAN: We both get into trouble.

INTERVIEWER: Well, here's an idea. Pretend like this is your sister and I'm going to be you, OK? I'm going to be playing with these toys here and behaving myself and just having a little tea party here, and what does your sister do? [While continuing to talk, the interviewer sets two teacups on saucers and pours pretend tea into the cups. Susan immediately takes her assigned role as little sister.]

> *Giving Susan the opportunity to play-act Denny may indicate how "pesky" and unmanageable her sister really is. Role playing, often with dolls or hand puppets, is often useful to help children divulge material that they cannot or will not express in other ways. In this case, the interviewer uses information obtained earlier to set up themes of play.*

SUSAN: Oh, I want to play with you, too.

INTERVIEWER: No, go away. I want to play with my . . . Hey, you can't hit me. What are you doing? I might just hit you right back. Now you behave yourself. Do you hear me?

> *In the role of the younger sister, Denny, Susan immediately becomes combative. The interviewer, in the role of the older sister, threatens justifiable retaliation (Susan has previously said that she never hits Denny). The interaction, however, suggests two pos-*

sibilities: (1) Denny is quite provocative and immediately invokes physical altercation; (2) Susan carries a significant amount of pent-up anger toward her sister. Of course, these possibilities may coexist.

SUSAN: Who cares?

INTERVIEWER: Who cares? I care. I'm having a tea party here. You want a cup of tea?

Susan continues in the role of the bratty younger sister. The interviewer switches gears from threats to an invitation to join in. The switch allows "Denny" to start playing cooperatively. Does Susan's version of Denny have this capacity?

SUSAN: Yeah.

INTERVIEWER: OK. Here. But clean up after yourself. Don't make a mess.

SUSAN: Uh-oh, I spilled my tea. Can you go get me a washcloth?

"Denny" does indeed switch, but the interviewer immediately throws out a challenge, which "Denny" creatively meets with another immediate provocation.

INTERVIEWER: Why don't you go get your own washcloth?

SUSAN: 'Cause I don't know where Mom hides them.

INTERVIEWER: OK, here's a washcloth. Clean up your mess. Thank you very much, now go away and stop bothering me.

SUSAN: OK. [Giggles.]

Susan is obviously involved and enjoying the game, which may well reflect real-life interactions with her younger sister.

INTERVIEWER: You want another cup of tea?

SUSAN: Yeah. I'm going to play Barbies, though.

INTERVIEWER: But they're my Barbies. I don't want you to play with my Barbies.

SUSAN: I have my own under my bed.

INTERVIEWER: Well, don't play with mine, all right?

SUSAN: OK.

Notice how Susan has now taken control of the theme. The interviewer has suggested the tea party, but Susan wants to play with dolls. The interviewer has tried to generate a conflict between the sisters, but Susan has deflected an argument by stating that she has her own dolls. As the game progresses, the interviewer will notice whether Susan insists on maintaining control or is willing to share.

INTERVIEWER: [In an adult voice] Do you want to play with a girl Barbie or a boy Barbie?

In the written transcript, it is hard to keep track of who is playing whom, but the participants themselves have no trouble. As Susan and the interviewer get into their respective roles, their play is likely to reflect the everyday interactions of these two sisters. The interviewer changes to an adult voice to provide distance momentarily from the pretend situation. This is an attempt to realign the play roles according to Susan's preference.

SUSAN: Will you play with my Barbies with me, please, please?

INTERVIEWER: Oh, you are such a pest, Denny, but I will play with you a little while, all right? Oh, this is a lovely Barbie. Let's play house.

SUSAN: I'm the mommy.

Now Susan changes from the role of Denny to that of Mommy. In three words, the interviewer makes the transition.

INTERVIEWER: I'm the sister.

SUSAN: [As Mommy] You go clean up your room!

INTERVIEWER: [As Denny] Do I have to, Mommy?

"Mommy" becomes a little bossy, both in tone and in direction. The interviewer's "Denny" pouts and acts resistant.

SUSAN: Yeah. Now.

INTERVIEWER: How come? Can't I just play a little while longer? I'll do it later, all right?

SUSAN: An hour longer. In an hour you've got to take a bath.

INTERVIEWER: I hate baths.

SUSAN: You got dirty in the mud yesterday.

INTERVIEWER: Yeah, but I'll take a bath tomorrow.

SUSAN: You still need to make your bed—now!

INTERVIEWER: Well, if I make my bed all muddy, Susan will clean it up for me.

SUSAN: She won't have to clean it up. She's going to school.

INTERVIEWER: No! I don't want her to go to school. I want her to play with me.

The theme is control, with the interviewer playing the role of the resistant, entitled younger sister, attempting to evaluate the kinds of reprisal that "Mommy" might invoke. We note that "Mommy" and "Susan" appear understanding, patient, and benevolent. From this play interaction, compromise and resolution, rather than physical punishment and yelling, seem the preferred modes of interaction in this household.

SUSAN: I'm sorry, she must go to school. Goodbye.

INTERVIEWER: Goodbye, Susan, have a nice day at school.

SUSAN: Now you go play and take a bath.

INTERVIEWER: Oh, boy! I love this bathtub. I'm going to make a big mess in here. I'm going to splash around and make a mess.

SUSAN: Did I hear you say *mess*?

INTERVIEWER: Nope.

SUSAN: You're going to clean that up.

INTERVIEWER: I'm not going to clean it up, 'cause I'm having too much fun playing in here.

SUSAN: Your brother's coming in to take a bath with you.

> *Again, "Mommy" is not provoked into an argument by "Denny's" challenges, but shifts focus by introducing the baby brother. In this way, she avoids a confrontation over "Denny's" mess.*

INTERVIEWER: OK, but I don't like him. He's such a baby. He put soap in my mouth.

SUSAN: You can behave, or I'm going to put soap in your mouth.

> *Here, for the first time, "Mommy" threatens retaliation if any harm comes to the baby.*

INTERVIEWER: No, I'm behaving, but he's bothering me.

SUSAN: He's doing nothing except playing there in the tub.

INTERVIEWER: He's crying, he's screaming, he's bothering me.

SUSAN: You get out now. Get out now!

INTERVIEWER: OK, Mommy.

> *The theme of Susan's younger siblings' being irritating and provocative is constant, fueled by the interviewer's role playing that supports sibling rivalry. However, Susan as Mommy (previously as Denny) could have changed themes or tone. At the end, "Mommy" finally becomes firm and insistent.*

INTERVIEWER: Mom?

> *"Denny" starts again. The interviewer and Susan are really involved in a life drama. The interviewer is trying to push the limits, in order to observe Susan's responses as she play-acts them through the behavior of her younger sister.*

SUSAN: What?

INTERVIEWER: I'm hungry.

SUSAN: You already had dinner. No more snacks.

INTERVIEWER: Oh, please?

SUSAN: No.

INTERVIEWER: Couldn't I have a little snack?

SUSAN: No.

INTERVIEWER: Please? I'm hungry. How about a cookie?

SUSAN: You can have carrots.

Another demonstration of patience and compromise.

INTERVIEWER: No, I don't want carrots. I hate carrots. I want cookies.

SUSAN: No sweets after dinner!

INTERVIEWER: Oh, please? I promise to brush my teeth.

SUSAN: You'll have to brush 'em 14 times.

INTERVIEWER: Fourteen? OK, just give me one cookie and a little milk.

SUSAN: Here you go.

INTERVIEWER: You threw my cookie in the bath. It's all wet. Help! Let me out of here. I'm clean. Help! Help!

SUSAN: OK, you can get out. Go to bed—you're being mean.

INTERVIEWER: But I'm not tired. You told me I could stay up late tonight.

SUSAN: Well, it's 9:00.

INTERVIEWER: No, I want to watch TV. One more program.

SUSAN: OK, but that's it.

The foregoing drama reflects conflict and resolution, provocation and compromise—interactions typical of everyday family life. Struggles centering around eating, bedtimes, and cleanliness are universal and often serve as a focus for play interactions. In more disturbed children, violence becomes a fixed theme early in the play. Profanity, sexualized interaction, catastrophic accidents, and risk-taking behaviors are more ominous signs of serious psychopathology.

INTERVIEWER: I don't want to go to bed. You know why?

SUSAN: Why?

INTERVIEWER: Because my sister snores.

SUSAN: Susan?

INTERVIEWER: Yeah, Susan. She snores, and I don't want to go in there.

In reality, Denny snores, but Susan accepts the switch and continues to respond as Mommy.

SUSAN: I'll set you up in the baby's room.

INTERVIEWER: Thank you very much, but I won't go in there, either.

SUSAN: All right.

INTERVIEWER: I'd like to come in your room, Mommy.

SUSAN: OK. Bedtime.

INTERVIEWER: Guess we'll sleep next to each other.

SUSAN: [Makes a snoring sound.]

INTERVIEWER: Oh, gosh! I can't sleep here. There's so much noise. Stop snoring!

SUSAN: Sorry, that's the only thing I can do to sleep.

INTERVIEWER: I'm scared. It's like a thunderstorm.

SUSAN: I'm not a thunderstorm.

INTERVIEWER: You *are* a thunderstorm! [Changes to an adult voice.] When you snore, do you know what that means?

SUSAN: What?

INTERVIEWER: Sometimes it means that you have a stuffy nose. And sometimes it means that when you sleep, you breathe through your mouth instead of your nose.

SUSAN: Children, put your stuff away.

Either the interviewer's educational intervention is premature or the play is too much fun. Susan switches to cleaning up, rather than going to sleep.

INTERVIEWER: Mom, you do it. We don't want to clean up. You clean up.

SUSAN: I'm gonna call Dad in on this.

INTERVIEWER: [As Dad] You kids clean that up and stop fighting.

The interviewer takes on the role of Dad, who speaks in a commanding tone. By bringing Dad into the play, Susan has expanded the cast of characters, and the interviewer jumps on board to see whether any new information can be obtained. Such expansions and switches are common with children who have active imaginations and can maintain their orientation and focus. Such flexibility would not be characteristic of a child with a psychotic or depressive disorder, a severe anxiety disorder, or intellectual disability.

INTERVIEWER: Here, have a cookie. Do you want some juice?

SUSAN: Yeah.

INTERVIEWER: Well, here's your juice. Now you kids turn the light off and go to sleep. I'm not coming in here again. You hear me?

SUSAN: OK.

INTERVIEWER: Good night. And no snoring!

SUSAN: [Makes snoring sounds.]

INTERVIEWER: What did I say? No snoring!

SUSAN: Sorry, Dad, I just couldn't help it.

INTERVIEWER: Denny, I'm telling you. You stop snoring, or you're gonna have to sleep outside with Roscoe.

SUSAN: Susan did it.

> By accepting blame, is Susan here being protective of her sister, who is being threatened by "Dad," or is she showing how Denny shifts blame upon her? Notice the fluidity of the role playing as Susan and the interviewer move in and out of all four family member roles.

INTERVIEWER: Are you snoring, Susan?

SUSAN: Yes, but I'll try not to. Can I stay up a little later?

INTERVIEWER: No, it's a school night. You've got to go to school tomorrow, and you need your sleep.

SUSAN: Who says I can't?

INTERVIEWER: Dad says you can't. You want to fight with Dad?

SUSAN: I'm going to go get Mom.

INTERVIEWER: [As Mom] Who's calling me? What's the matter, Susan?

SUSAN: Go get Dad and tell him I want to stay up a little later.

INTERVIEWER: [As Mom] She wants to stay up a little later. [As Dad] Well, I said she has to go to bed. Now, who's the boss? [As Mom] I told her earlier that she could stay up a little later. [As Dad] All right.

SUSAN: Thanks, Mom.

INTERVIEWER: You can stay up a little later, but just a few minutes.

SUSAN: A few minutes. OK, Mom. I want a cookie. Where are they?

INTERVIEWER: It's too late for cookies now, honey. No more snacks now. It's time to get ready for bed.

SUSAN: Now?

INTERVIEWER: Is that all right?

SUSAN: OK.

INTERVIEWER: Good night, girls. No snoring. I'll see you in the morning, and sleep well. I'll give you each a kiss good night.

As with the other play sequences, bedtime has ended with everyone consoled and asleep. Negotiation and compromise have largely resolved the control and limit-setting issues. Susan recognizes the end of the sequence, but wants to continue to play.

SUSAN: Let's play something else.

INTERVIEWER: OK. Now let's play school. What's your teacher's name?

The interviewer has chosen the next topic to explore how this child experiences her school life. It would have been useful to let the child pick the next topic to see what she identifies as an important aspect of her world.

SUSAN: Mrs. G.

INTERVIEWER: Mrs. G.? This is Mrs. G. [Takes another doll and plays the role of the teacher with yet another voice.] Well, good morning, Susan. It's nice to see you.

SUSAN: [Yawns.]

INTERVIEWER: Ooooh. You're very tired. I bet you stayed up late last night, huh? You're supposed to go to bed early.

The interviewer maintains an authoritarian demeanor. Susan attempts to stand up for herself, but the interviewer persists. Ultimately, as before, she retreats from confrontation.

SUSAN: I'm not tired.

INTERVIEWER: You were taking a nap. I'll have to tell your mom to get you to bed earlier. Did you do your homework?

SUSAN: Unh-unh. I was sleeping.

INTERVIEWER: Well, we're having a spelling test today. Are you ready for a spelling test?

SUSAN: I think so.

INTERVIEWER: I'm going to pick a hard word. How do you spell *father*?

The interviewer is attempting to assess some of Susan's cognitive skills; with young children, this is often best done in a play context. The chosen word may be too hard for most 6-year-olds, though some children memorize it early.

SUSAN: F-A-T-H-E-R.

INTERVIEWER: You get an A. Very good.

SUSAN: [Pleased] Ooooh!

INTERVIEWER: Now we're going to have math.

SUSAN: M-A-T-H. [Giggles.]

INTERVIEWER: Do you know what 7 plus 6 is?

SUSAN: No.

INTERVIEWER: Do you know what 3 plus 1 is?

> *The interviewer starts with a task that is difficult, then follows with a more age- and grade-appropriate problem. Other clinicians might start with easier problems to build confidence.*

SUSAN: Four.

INTERVIEWER: Do you know what 6 plus 2 is?

SUSAN: Eight.

INTERVIEWER: Very good. Do you want to learn how to play Squiggles? If I make a squiggle like that, can you make a picture with my squiggle?

> *The Squiggle game, first described by Donald Winnicott, is an attempt at projective test-ing with young children who like to draw. The child or the examiner draws a squiggly line or shape; the other adds to it, making it a meaningful drawing. After a few turns each, the child is asked to "tell a story" linking the squiggles. If possible, the examiner's completed squiggles should try to reflect some of the child's presenting conflict areas.*

INTERVIEWER: Great. A flower. Now you make a squiggle and I'll draw a picture. [Susan complies.] You made a hard one. [Turns the paper on which Susan's squiggle is drawn around and around, trying to visualize a completed drawing, then com-pletes the squiggle.]

> *Like most children, Susan has grasped the concept easily and appears to enjoy the game.*

SUSAN: What's that?

INTERVIEWER: I drew a horse. So what do we have? A flower, then a horse. Now it's my turn. [In all, Susan and the interviewer draw a flower, a horse, a tree, a lady with curly hair, diamonds, and a house with smoke coming out of the chimney. Susan's mother enters the room before they get to the storytelling part of the game.]

INTERVIEWER: Well, Susan, I see we've run out of time. We have to stop playing. Thank you for coming. Goodbye.

CHAPTER 6

Play Interview
with a 7-Year-Old Boy

It is especially challenging to obtain meaningful information from a child who has a disturbance of emotion or behavior. It requires simultaneously following the child's lead; trying to establish and maintain meaningful engagement; and obtaining information that relates to distractibility versus attentiveness, focus versus impulsiveness, cooperation versus control, curiosity versus inhibition, rigidity versus flexibility, and engagement versus isolation. The use of age-appropriate play materials often facilitates the process.

The play interview that follows illustrates the great difficulty even an experienced interviewer can have in maintaining a relationship with a challenging patient. In the comments, we note in **boldface** 10 important qualities that should be observed in any child interview: activity level, attention span and distractibility, communication facility, coordination, frustration tolerance, impulsiveness, mannerisms and other peculiarities of physical motion, mood state, response to limit setting, and response to praise.

Seven-year-old Norman has been a patient in a day treatment program for over 2 years. Initially, following his parents' divorce, he experienced irrational fears that he would be abandoned. The current referral has stemmed from tics, hyperactivity, distractibility, and aggression not adequately managed by medication. His working diagnosis is attention-deficit/hyperactivity disorder comorbid with Tourette's disorder.

Curious and extremely active, Norman enters the examination room unaccompanied. (Neither parent is present, because he has come from his day treatment classroom.) On the floor is a bucket of toys, which immediately attracts his attention. At first, he darts from toy to toy and explores the room.

INTERVIEWER: Hi, Norman. I'm Dr. S. Come and look at some of the things I've got here.

The interviewer, at once noting Norman's high **activity level,** *begins with a smile and an invitation to explore and play with the play materials. These are efforts to put the child at ease.*

NORMAN: What's this—costumes?

INTERVIEWER: I'll show you. This one is a puppet.

NORMAN: What?

INTERVIEWER: Put your hand in it.

NORMAN: [Sniffs the puppet.] Smells funny. What's this? [Removes a doll from the toy pail.]

INTERVIEWER: It does?

NORMAN: Yes.

> *Norman does not take to the puppet in the usual way. Rather, he sniffs it (a mannerism?) and immediately goes to another toy. The interviewer is unable to sustain his interest and thus shifts with Norman to the next object.*

INTERVIEWER: What does he look like?

NORMAN: Looks like a Barbie doll.

INTERVIEWER: Except he's lost a shoe.

> [Norman drops the doll and keeps moving on to new toys. He asks a barrage of questions about each of the items he has handled: "What's this?" "What does this do?" "How do you use this?" However, he doesn't really listen to the interviewer's responses. Finally, Norman impulsively picks up a camera, then darts to the video-recording microphone and pulls at the wires. Now the interviewer sets limits and asks Norman not to touch the microphone. Norman responds by expressing his desire to leave the session. After the interviewer urges him "to play for a little while longer because I want to play with you," Norman returns to the toy box but remains focused on the microphone.]

> *Norman's **impulsiveness** and short **attention span** are plainly evident in this sequence of events, along with his need for (and resistance to) **limit setting**.*

NORMAN: What's the microphone for?

INTERVIEWER: So that people can hear what we're saying when they watch the movie. Didn't your teacher take a movie of you? Don't touch it, please. No, you have to leave it.

NORMAN: Yeah.

INTERVIEWER: Was it a video?

NORMAN: [Turns his attention back to the toy camera.] I wish there was film in here. How do you open this?

INTERVIEWER: Do you like cameras?

NORMAN: Yeah. How do you open it?

INTERVIEWER: Here. [Opens back of camera.]

NORMAN: I like cameras. Ready? [Snaps the shutter and then runs to the microphone mounted on the wall, bends down, and shouts into it.] Are you ready?

INTERVIEWER: [Attempts to distract Norman from the microphone.] There's no film in the camera. Do you like to draw? Do you like to draw pictures?

NORMAN: No film? Well, let's get some film.

INTERVIEWER: Well, we can't right now. We could get some film some other time. Please leave the microphone. Let's see what we've got here.

NORMAN: We can talk in this. Are you ready? [Shouts into the microphone.] I'm going to go back to my class now.

INTERVIEWER: Well, I just wanted to play with you for a little while. Look at all these things. [Dumps the container of toys onto the floor.]

*Norman's **distractibility** is shown in his attraction to the recording equipment. He resists interacting directly with the interviewer and repeatedly threatens to end the session and return to the classroom. The interviewer keeps trying to engage him with toys.*

INTERVIEWER: Let's see, a doctor and a nurse. What else do we have here?

NORMAN: Why are they so mad?

INTERVIEWER: Are they mad?

NORMAN: Uh-huh. [Whispers something.]

INTERVIEWER: Well, we'll go back in a few minutes, all right? I want to play with you for a little while.

Several times now, Norman has made it clear that he wants to go back to his class. It is not unusual for a child to show resistance early in an interview; some children become frozen with anxiety, whereas others will cry and refuse to let go of a parent's hand. Persistence and considerable ingenuity may be needed to keep a child in the room long enough to become engaged.

*Norman's question about the neutral doll's being mad may be an indication of **affect**. Is he annoyed that there is no film in the camera? That he can't touch the microphone wires? That he can't leave the playroom to return to his classroom? Before the interviewer can respond further, Norman veers off in yet another direction.*

NORMAN: What's this?

INTERVIEWER: Oh, it's one of those things that doctors use. What do you call it?

NORMAN: A needle. Why do people have to have a shot?

INTERVIEWER: Because they're sick. Norman, did you ever get a shot?

NORMAN: Ready? [Turns off the light.]

INTERVIEWER: No, leave the light on. Can you put it back on? Can you put it back on, please?

NORMAN: We don't need a light.

INTERVIEWER: Yes, we need the light. [Firmly] Please turn the lights back on for me! Thank you.

Questions about medical interventions fail to engage Norman, who now runs off and begins to turn the light switch on and off. Despite the goal of allowing a child relatively wide behavioral latitude as a diagnostic measure, it happens with some frequency that **limits** *must be firmly set—even to the point of physically restraining a child who hits or damages furniture or equipment.*

INTERVIEWER: [Turns back to the dolls.] They're sick. You're going to have to give them a shot. All right? Do you want to do it? You want to be the doctor? I hope he doesn't cry. Don't cry, little boy, because you're sick. Where should I give it to him, in his arm?

NORMAN: I'll take his picture.

INTERVIEWER: Oh, you're going to take a picture?

NORMAN: Yep. See?

INTERVIEWER: Take another one! I'd better take his clothes off.

NORMAN: He's sick?

INTERVIEWER: I have to find his arm. Where . . .

NORMAN: How do you know he's sick?

INTERVIEWER: I don't know. Let's make up a story. What's wrong with him? [By this time, the interviewer is lying almost full length on the floor, trying to engage the child in play.]

The interviewer again suggests "illness" in an attempt to solicit identification from Norman and possibly to judge his capacity for empathy. Note, however, that when interviewing an impulsive child, it's important to avoid physical positioning that could limit your ability to prevent the child from bolting out of the room.

NORMAN: I don't know. [Takes up a transformer (see Chapter 2, p. 39), which he manipulates into its several identities.]

INTERVIEWER: Norman, what's that?

NORMAN: What is it? I don't know. What is it? How does it work?

INTERVIEWER: Can you make it change shape?

NORMAN: Yeah.

INTERVIEWER: Oh, you're good, Norman. You know how that works?

NORMAN: I know how it works.

INTERVIEWER: Great! Can you show me?

[Norman does so, and continues to play with the transformer.]

Part of an experienced interviewer's stock in trade is allowing a child to demonstrate expertise at operating a piece of equipment; this should promote a sense of mastery and boost the child's ego. The technique also works well when the child brings in a show-and-tell item that embodies a scientific principle or historical event that can be "taught" to the interviewer. **Responding to praise,** *for the first time Norman begins to answer questions, all the time forming and reforming the transformer.*

INTERVIEWER: Norman, how do you feel today?

NORMAN: Um, fine.

INTERVIEWER: Are you happy?

NORMAN: Yeah.

INTERVIEWER: Good. Do you feel sad?

NORMAN: Yeah.

INTERVIEWER: Do you feel sad today?

NORMAN: I don't feel sad today. I feel happy because . . .

INTERVIEWER: Because what? Because you're here?

The interviewer suspects that Norman may not be pleased to be involved in the interview, so attempts to elicit a negative reaction, but is surprised to get a positive one.

NORMAN: Yeah.

INTERVIEWER: Did you want to come here yesterday?

NORMAN: Yeah.

INTERVIEWER: Yeah! Hey, you're doing great with that transformer. [After considerable discussion about the transformer, yielding much praise, the interviewer attempts to draw Norman's attention to some more meaningful human figures—doll figures in the doll house—but is once again rebuffed. Ultimately, a pair of scissors and a folded piece of paper turn the trick.]

INTERVIEWER: Do you know how to cut with these scissors? I was going to make a pattern.

NORMAN: Yeah.

INTERVIEWER: You know about the Mario Brothers?

NORMAN: Is that what you're making? Is that Mario?

INTERVIEWER: Yeah.

NORMAN: Where's his legs?

INTERVIEWER: What's the other guy's name? Uh, do you remember what his name is? The other guy? I'll make him, too. [Creates patterns in the folded piece of paper with the scissors, and shows the patterns to Norman. Over the next several minutes, their play centers around the theme of various Nintendo characters—Mario, Luigi, and the Princess.]

Child mental health professionals must remain current in children's popular games, music, and cult heroes.

INTERVIEWER: What do you think?

NORMAN: I don't know. Is he happy?

INTERVIEWER: He's a little angry.

The interviewer is attempting to match Norman's feelings.

NORMAN: Why?

INTERVIEWER: I don't know. Somebody isn't doing what he wants to do.

NORMAN: Why?

INTERVIEWER: And they don't want to play with him.

NORMAN: They don't want to play with him?

INTERVIEWER: Yeah. But the Princess, now, she wants to play with him. [Cuts the Princess out of the paper, while Norman continues to play with the transformer. But Norman is engaged in the play theme.] This is a very fancy Princess.

NORMAN: Is she happy?

INTERVIEWER: Yes. But not Mario and not his brother, Cuomo. I think his brother's name is Cuomo.

NORMAN: I think it's Luigi.

INTERVIEWER: Luigi! That's his name, not Cuomo!

NORMAN: Yeah, Luigi.

INTERVIEWER: What a good memory you have, Norman. Mario and Luigi are not going to play with the Princess. What level is she locked up on?

NORMAN: The Dragon level.

INTERVIEWER: Yeah, the Dragon level. And . . .

NORMAN: Why is she locked up on the Dragon level?

INTERVIEWER: Ah, because somebody evil has kidnapped her.

The interviewer is pushing the themes of good and evil, of anger, and of separation and reunion. Norman finally seems actively engaged in this plot. The Nintendo figures are well known to him.

NORMAN: Yeah?

INTERVIEWER: And locked her up.

NORMAN: Yeah.

INTERVIEWER: And Mario and Cuomo—what's his name?

NORMAN: Luigi.

INTERVIEWER: Mario and Luigi have to rescue her. But there's a lot of enemies in the way. Right?

NORMAN: Right.

INTERVIEWER: I think there's all those things that try to come down and shoot them and bomb them. Can you help to get the Princess out?

NORMAN: Yeah

INTERVIEWER: And save her? You cut it out. I can't do it.

NORMAN: You can do it.

INTERVIEWER: I can't do it. I did it crooked. You do it. Just do this side.

NORMAN: I'll try.

INTERVIEWER: Try to save her. [Norman finally takes the scissors and begins to cut the paper.] Yeah, you're a good cutter. The Princess is great! [Puts the cutout Princess into the doll house. Norman crawls over to the table on which the doll house is standing and stands up. Each takes a toy figure.]

The interviewer finally has Norman playing in an unstructured, fantasy mode. Now Norman introduces a theme.

NORMAN: Yeah! I'll be the kid.

INTERVIEWER: You be the kid. And I'll be what?

NORMAN: The teacher. Time to get up for school!

INTERVIEWER: What's the kid's name?

NORMAN: Johnny. But there's something flying up in the sky!

INTERVIEWER: What is it? What is it, Johnny? What's flying?

NORMAN: A space ship. [Reintroduces the transformer into the play, zooming it around.]

INTERVIEWER: Ah! Is it a friendly one?

NORMAN: Yeah.

INTERVIEWER: Oh, good. Then he can come into our house. [Begins to talk in a play-act voice, taking the part of the mother. Norman is actively engaged in playing with the doll house.]

NORMAN: What's the spaceman called?

INTERVIEWER: Zorro.

NORMAN: I am a nice robot. [Talks in a mechanical, spaceman voice.]

INTERVIEWER: Thank you for coming into our house. Did you bring anything with you from outer space, Zorro?

NORMAN: Yeah. A race car.

INTERVIEWER: A race car?

NORMAN: That's right.

INTERVIEWER: What's the matter, Zorro?

NORMAN: Something happened to me.

INTERVIEWER: Are you broken?

NORMAN: Broken? I'm turning myself into a spaceship.

INTERVIEWER: Oh.

NORMAN: I'm getting him into a spaceship. You can help me.

INTERVIEWER: I'll try. Do you want to make a rocket ship like that?

NORMAN: Could you fix him?

INTERVIEWER: Oh, I'll try. You know, this is so hard for me to do. You're very good at it—I don't know how to exactly do it. It goes right in here, doesn't it?

Although Norman is now involved, it is the mechanical manipulation of the trans-former, in a manner inappropriate for his age, that dominates his interest. His verbal *responses are generally limited to brief, single sentences; clearly, his **ability to communicate** is restricted. It is noteworthy that for the first time, he has asked for help. However, with time running out, the interviewer tries to switch to information gathering. This is met with some (albeit limited) cooperation from Norman.*

INTERVIEWER: Do you remember my name?

NORMAN: Yeah, you're Dr. S. [Turns the transformer back into his rocket ship.]

Two activities are going on simultaneously as the interviewer attempts to persuade Norman to cooperate in further tests of cognitive and motor skills.

INTERVIEWER: Do you remember Dr. C.?

NORMAN: Yeah, I do. Do you? I have to leave now. I'm going to space. Bye.

INTERVIEWER: Oh, please don't go. Come back again.

NORMAN: I will, I promise. After supper.

INTERVIEWER: [To doll] Johnny, Zorro went away. Now it's time to get into the school bus and go to school.

NORMAN: I have to go back now.

INTERVIEWER: Oh, I'm going to miss you. Are you going back to outer space?

NORMAN: We're there now.

INTERVIEWER: Oh, Johnny, we're going to miss Zorro so much. [Norman is flying the spaceship around the room, but is actively playing with the interviewer.]

The theme of leaving and reunion remains prominent. Norman has picked up on the interviewer's cue that the time of the session is nearing an end.

INTERVIEWER: You're back. Are you back from outer space?

NORMAN: Yep.

INTERVIEWER: Hooray! Zorro's back!

NORMAN: Can I go back?

INTERVIEWER: Go back where?

NORMAN: My class.

INTERVIEWER: OK. Can you do one thing for me? Do you know how to jump? Can you jump off this?

NORMAN: No.

INTERVIEWER: Try it.

NORMAN: No. I'd just like to go back. [Begins to fly the transformer back into space.]

INTERVIEWER: Just give it a try for me. I'll show you. [Puts away the materials, then gets up onto the first step of the stair climber and jumps down.]

In this and subsequent tests, Norman's **physical development and coordination** *appear to be at a level a year or two younger than his chronological age of 7.*

NORMAN: OK.

INTERVIEWER: Oh, you're going to do it from the top step. Oh, boy, you're a good jumper. OK, wait a minute. Do this. Can you hop on one foot like that?

NORMAN: I'll do it from up here.

INTERVIEWER: No, just do it down here. Good. Now do the other foot.

NORMAN: Ah, I can't do that one.

INTERVIEWER: Oh, you can't?

NORMAN: If I jump on that foot [pointing to his left], can I hold on to something?

INTERVIEWER: Here, hold on to me. OK, can you catch? Here comes the ball. Put the transformer down for a minute. Now throw it to me.

NORMAN: [Misses the ball and picks it up.]

INTERVIEWER: Good. Try it again. You've got it. Do it again. Whoa, here comes one. Oh good, you catch great. And you throw great. Once more.

NORMAN: [Drops it.] We're all done.

INTERVIEWER: All right. We're all done. Do you know what I'm going to do, Norman?

NORMAN: What?

INTERVIEWER: I'm going to get some film, and I'll bring my camera back and let you take some pictures. But we have to stop now.

NORMAN: Yeah.

INTERVIEWER: OK? Let's go see what your class is doing.

NORMAN: No, I want to stay here.

INTERVIEWER: Not now. We have to stop.

NORMAN: We can't stop right now, 'cause we're playing.

INTERVIEWER: I know, but I need to stop now because we don't have any more time. But you did a good job.

NORMAN: No, no, no, no.

INTERVIEWER: Come on.

NORMAN: Let go of my hand.

INTERVIEWER: Thank you for coming. [Exits, with Norman in tow.]

*In the space of an hour, the interviewer has managed to engage reluctant Norman's interest to the point that he now wants to stay and play. All of Norman's presenting problems are evident in this play interview: anxiety and distractibility, difficulty becoming involved with a toy or with the interviewer, continual disruption of the session, and preoccupation with mechanical toys in preference to animal or human figures. There has been no real opportunity to observe Norman's **frustration tolerance,** though the interviewer's is excellent.*

CHAPTER 7

Interview with
a 9-Year-Old Girl

Julia comes for an evaluation because her mother feels that she has too few friends and spends too much time alone daydreaming. She is a bright child, mature for her age, who easily answers all of the questions put to her. Two interviewers are involved—a graduate student, who uses drawings to facilitate a question-and-answer interview, and a faculty member, who continues the interview by using play techniques. Nine-year-old children are on the borderline between using play techniques and responding to direct questions. The interview demonstrates that a child of this age still enjoys play and can share her fantasies through this medium.

TRAINEE: Hello, my name is Dale. I would like to get to know you a little. Do you mind chatting with me?

JULIA: No.

Most interviewers usually state more about themselves and give some idea of the interview's purpose. There is some controversy about use of first names versus surnames. Teachers at school are rarely addressed by their first names; the same is true of pediatricians and family doctors. There probably is no right or wrong approach, but this trainee might say, "My name is [Dr., Mr., Ms.] Smith, but it might be easier for you to call me by my first name, Dale. Have you been told why you are here today?"

[The trainee and Julia both sit on the floor amidst some soft pillows and toys. The interview proceeds for some minutes, the trainee asking a great number of questions that are mostly closed-ended. In brief answers that she does not amplify, Julia reveals that she is a 9-year-old third grader who likes recess the best at school, though she won't say why. She has friends (though not in her class), and two brothers, one older, one younger than she. Finally, the trainee asks whether Julia likes to draw. A nodded "yes" leads to proffered paper and Magic Markers.]

TRAINEE: Why don't you draw a picture of your family?

[While Julia is drawing, the trainee continues the questioning, asking whether she has her own room, what colors it is painted, and whether she has privacy there. Julia's mostly one-word answers reveal that her older brother does not play with her, but teases her a lot. She feels closer to her younger brother; however, she spends a lot of time in her room listening to her iPod. Her family has only lived in this area for the past year.]

TRAINEE: Did you move because of somebody's job?

JULIA: Dad's.

TRAINEE: Did you have trouble making friends here?

JULIA: No, I have better friends here.

TRAINEE: How did that happen?

JULIA: I don't know. It just did.

TRAINEE: How do you get to school?

[Julia states that she walks to school. It appears from her replies to subsequent questions that she prefers this school because it is less structured. She previously attended a private school where teachers were strict and children behaved well. There is some confusion: She doesn't exactly acknowledge that children in her current school misbehave, but she expresses some concern about disruption and lack of teacher control in the new school. She also reveals that her mother is at home after school, and that she has fewer friends to play with than at her former home.]

Julia's intense focus on her drawing may help her avoid fuller responses to questions. It is often better to let a child finish drawing before continuing with an interview—a principle that applies to play of all sorts. When a clinician and child are engaged in a play activity—either structured, such as a game of checkers, or unstructured, such as doll play—it should be the focus of the therapist's attention, as it is of the child's. The clinician should be fully involved. If more specific information is needed, a clinician might say, "Let's stop playing now so that I can ask you some questions." Like a bridge between topics in an adult interview, such an intervention focuses mutual attention on the questions to follow.

Although playing and questioning at the same time should generally be avoided, this principle has its exceptions. Occasionally a child may answer questions more reli-

ably and feel more relaxed and comfortable with a minor distraction, such as fiddling with a transformer.

INSTRUCTOR: Hi. Can I join you? Are you working on a picture of your family? [Julia nods.] Let's see, who is that? And that? [Julia writes names over the brightly colored figures of her mother, father, and two brothers.]

The interviewing instructor, who has been observing from a slight distance, joins the two on the floor and refocuses on the drawing. As an interviewer should do with all drawings done by children, the instructor carefully notes the colors, sizes, and shapes of objects, and their positions on the page. Drawings may be used to assess age-appropriate skill levels, but, more importantly, may be used as a projective technique to elicit thematic material.

INSTRUCTOR: Is your older brother really that tall? He looks almost as big as your father.

JULIA: No, he's not really that big.

INSTRUCTOR: You said that you moved here from another school. [Julia nods.] How do you like this school?

JULIA: Some things are good, and some things are bad. [Stops drawing.]

INSTRUCTOR: Tell me more about that.

This is an exploratory, open-ended question. Once the instructor begins to ask questions, the drawing stops. Julia tries to please the interviewer by answering with more detail, but the conversation remains unrevealing.

JULIA: Well, there are better climbing structures here, and there are no bugs or ants here.

INSTRUCTOR: Do bugs make you nervous? [Julia shakes her head.] What's the matter with ants?

JULIA: They make me itch.

INSTRUCTOR: What about the kids?

JULIA: There are some really mean kids in the school. Also, when it rains, the water comes inside the classroom.

INSTRUCTOR: Do you have to wear a raincoat and boots in the room? [At this smiling attempt at humor, Julia returns the smile and shakes her head "no."] What happened in your old school if some kids were mean?

JULIA: Well, the teacher would call the parents and tell them that they had to stop, and the kids would not be mean any more.

INSTRUCTOR: And what happens here?

JULIA: There aren't any mean kids here.

Julia is reluctant to engage in emotionally charged, potentially upsetting dialogue. Pursuing more specific questions only makes her more defensive. The instructor takes the cue and, in the next exchange, changes topics, learning that the family's move a year ago may be a source of Julia's current problem. Getting the name of a best friend in the old school, and then learning that she has had no contact with her past friends, strengthen this hypothesis.

INSTRUCTOR: You mentioned that you had a best friend in your old school. What's her name?

JULIA: Erin.

INSTRUCTOR: Have you visited her since you moved here? [Julia shakes her head.] Have you written or called her? [Another denial.] You haven't called her? How come?

JULIA: Well, I tried calling her once, but she didn't call me back. And I wrote her five letters, but she never wrote back.

INSTRUCTOR: What do you think happened?

JULIA: [Dejectedly] She doesn't know my address.

INSTRUCTOR: What a shame. Maybe something can be done to help get you guys together.

The instructor attempts to be helpful, not really believing that her best friend couldn't contact Julia if she really wanted to remain in contact. This statement needs further exploration. By conveying warmth and the possibility of help in the future, the instructor attempts to establish a positive therapeutic alliance.

INSTRUCTOR: [Takes up a spider hand puppet.] Do you want to play with some of my toys? I've got some puppets here. Hi, I'm a friendly spider. Do you want to be my friend?

[Selecting a turtle, Julia eagerly takes to the hand puppets. Adopting a different voice from normal in playing the spider, the instructor approaches the turtle, waving one of the spider's many arms.]

INSTRUCTOR: Ms. Turtle, I'm going to be moving away and I wanted to come by and say goodbye. I will miss you a lot. Will you write me a letter? I don't want to move away. Do you promise to stay my friend?

The instructor sets the tone of the interaction as a follow-up to the previous discussion. It is important in fantasy play to seek as much distance from the source of trauma as possible without losing sight of the core issue. Toys, especially puppets, dolls, and animal family figures, are ideal stimuli for evoking imaginary material. Pretend voices help in the distancing; playful, childlike antics also often break the ice. When play content turns serious, however, the clinician should also become serious. Children deserve respect for their painful material, just as adults do.

JULIA: [Also using a pretend voice] What's your name?

INSTRUCTOR: My name is Ms. Spider.

JULIA: OK, I won't forget your name. Goodbye, I'll miss you too.

INSTRUCTOR: Could I give you a little kiss goodbye?

JULIA: No, not a kiss. You can shake my hand. Bye-bye.

Ms. Spider has moved in to give Ms. Turtle a farewell kiss, but even in play Julia clearly defines her boundaries: no kissing, just friendly handshakes.

INSTRUCTOR: Hey, Ms. Turtle, how come you didn't write me? You moved away a month ago and I haven't gotten a single letter from you, and that makes me sad. [Ms. Turtle immediately hands Ms. Spider the picture she has been drawing.] Oh, you have sent me a letter. What a pretty picture. This is your family. I like getting it. Can you write again? [Ms. Turtle immediately draws a picture of a sunrise and hands it to Ms. Spider.]

This immediate compliance suggests that Julia wants to close down the painful feelings of separation. Even in play, Julia's need to deny painful experiences is obvious. The instructor respects Julia's defenses and avoids premature interpretations.

INSTRUCTOR: Ms. Turtle, I don't like my new house. Can I come back and visit you in our old neighborhood?

JULIA: OK.

INSTRUCTOR: It's so nice to be back here. I don't ever want to go to my new house again. Will you write my parents a letter for me and tell them that I don't want to go back?

Using clinical intuition, the instructor pursues the theme of separation. Though the instructor is now directing most of the scene and setting up the themes, once Julia begins to take the initiative, the instructor can begin to follow her lead.

JULIA: [Starts to write, but then takes an alligator puppet from the toy bag and speaks with a gruff voice.] You have to come home.

INSTRUCTOR: Who are you, Alligator?

JULIA: I'm the dad.

INSTRUCTOR: Hi, Dad. Can I stay with my friend Ms. Turtle for a couple of months?

JULIA: No, you have to come home immediately.

INSTRUCTOR: No, I won't go. I hate my new home.

JULIA: Well, you have to go home right now.

INSTRUCTOR: No. [To Ms. Turtle] Please hide me. Where can I hide?

JULIA: [As Ms. Turtle] Hide under the bed.

> *Although Julia has taken the lead by introducing Dad into the play and giving him the role he took in real life (forcing the family to move), the instructor attempts to explore the depth of Julia's feelings about the move by showing marked resistance to it (to the point of hiding from Dad).*

[Now a chase sequence begins in which the alligator chases Ms. Spider all over the house. Finally the alligator grabs Ms. Spider in his mouth and carts her off.]

INSTRUCTOR: I'm hungry. Do you have anything to eat?

JULIA: [Takes a bunny puppet.] Would you like to go on a picnic?

INSTRUCTOR: Who are you, Bunny?

> *Children can easily play-act (and keep straight) multiple roles. Sometimes the interviewer must also play more than one role. It is appropriate for the interviewer to interrupt the play from time to time, if confusion arises, by using a natural adult voice and to ask for clarification: "Wait a minute. I thought I was the little girl. Who are you right now?" The principal task for the interviewer is to get in touch with the "inner child" and let that child play with the patient, while also observing the interaction from an adult perspective. These are the two roles that all child therapists must entertain simultaneously.*

JULIA: I'm the mommy. Do you want to go on a picnic?

INSTRUCTOR: Oh, yes. Thank you, Mommy.

JULIA: We have to make some sandwiches.

INSTRUCTOR: I love peanut butter sandwiches. And can we bring marshmallows?

JULIA: Sure!

INSTRUCTOR: Oooooh, I love picnics, but I hope we don't run into any ants on this picnic. I don't like ants.

JULIA: Sometimes you can't help it when ants come.

> *The instructor reacts positively to the idea of a picnic, but sets the tone for a little trouble. Earlier in the interview, Julia has stated that she doesn't like her new school*

because of "bugs and ants." By introducing the abstract construct of ants at the picnic, the interviewer provides a bridge to learn what may be wrong with the new school. In other words, the picnic may become a metaphor for her new school. It appears that Julia may understand the ant analogy.

INSTRUCTOR: [Begins to fly by with a toy helicopter and carries on with the game.] The ant 'copter's coming with ants.

JULIA: [Begins to populate the picnic area with toy figures as she sets up the play theme.]

INSTRUCTOR: Who are these guys? Do they get to come to the picnic?

JULIA: These are my mom, my dad, and my brother. They can come on the picnic.

INSTRUCTOR: I'm comin' with more ants. [Flies the helicopter by, spraying ants all over the place. Julia, seeming to enjoy herself, vigorously brushes them away.] You can't stamp 'em out fast enough. You're gonna itch and itch, and it's gonna get into the picnic. [Julia grabs a dinosaur figure and begins to approach.] Uh-oh, here come the dinosaurs. I'm out of here. 'Bye. [The helicopter flies away.] Go away, Dinosaur. OK, you got me. No more ants. Hurray, the dinosaurs save the day! Now we can all play and have a wonderful picnic. Is the dinosaur gonna eat a marshmallow?

Earlier, Julia has described her response to ants as "They make me itch." Is this Julia's metaphor for stress and pain? Julia has resolved the problem of "itch" by calling into play a powerful force that drives the problem away. She also now reveals some of her heightened neediness.

JULIA: Since I got rid of the ants, I get to eat all the food.

INSTRUCTOR: Oh, a little greedy, aren't you, Mr. Dinosaur? I'm gonna have to take you on and bring some more ants around. Pssssssssssssssssssss. [Returns with the helicopter and sprays ants all over the dinosaur.] That's what you get for eating all the food and not letting anybody else have any.

Here the instructor may be committing an error by confronting Julia's defense directly and attempting to label her hunger and neediness as greed. To counter this misinterpretation, Julia sets the source of her difficulty back on her father.

JULIA: I'm the dad. [Puts the dinosaur figure down and takes up the father figure.]

INSTRUCTOR: [Quickly shifts roles from helicopter pilot and ant spreader to hungry child.] I'm hungry. Can I have a marshmallow?

JULIA: No, you can't.

INSTRUCTOR: But I want some marshmallows, too. Please, Dad, can't I have a marshmallow?

JULIA: No, sweetheart, it's too much sugar for you.

INSTRUCTOR: Oh, come on, Dad. Don't be such a fussbudget!

JULIA: You can have a hot dog.

INSTRUCTOR: I don't want a hot dog. I want some marshmallows, Dad. Please!

JULIA: Well, you can't.

> *By this time, there is some indication that one of the stresses at home may be struggles over limits. Dad is again portrayed as being strict and unbending.*

INSTRUCTOR: Well, here comes the big bird. You think you're gonna take the marshmallow, mister? No way!

JULIA: Oh, yeah? [Enlists the help of another animal-monster figure.]

INSTRUCTOR: No way, it's mine! [They begin to struggle over the marshmallow.] Oops! Who's that? Are you the monster? Who are you?

JULIA: I'm the mother, and I say no fighting, you two.

INSTRUCTOR: OK, Mom, you're the boss. [Then in a regular adult voice] I think our time is up and we will need to stop for today. Thanks for coming in.

> *At the end of this sequence, the mother has restored peace. Perhaps this is her usual role in this household. When the hour is up, a clinician often must end a session abruptly. It may be good to suggest that the play can continue next time (if so, the same toys and play setups should be available). If a child is in the midst of a drawing, it is important that the clinician keep the artwork for the next visit. In a therapeutic relationship that is going well, play themes may continue over many sessions.*
>
> *To avoid sudden transitions, a clinician should manage time to allow preparation for ending the session. It can provide insight into a child's reactions to limit setting, and to the experience of having to say, "Goodbye until next time."*

CHAPTER 8

The Adolescent Interview

It's a truism that an adolescent is neither a small adult nor a large child. By the teenage years, toys and games have usually outlived their usefulness in an interview situation; however, an initial game of checkers or chess may help get some younger adolescents started. A snack or drink may also help facilitate dialogue (remember to ask parental permission first).

Depending on the patient's level of maturity, most of the interview techniques that are used with adults can be applied to the adolescent interview. Regardless of age, an informant can help set the stage for the evaluation of a hospitalized patient. However, as with an adult outpatient, an adolescent office patient should usually be interviewed before information is obtained from the parents. At some point, you may want to follow up the individual interviews of adolescent and parents with a family session to learn how the parents and their child interact.

As you will note in the interview presented in this chapter, the clinician spends much time trying to develop rapport. This is not unusual with adolescent patients, who often develop trust in the clinician more slowly than is true of either adults or younger children. In what follows, we have summarized some passages of dialogue.

This interview takes place on an adolescent inpatient unit. (It is safe to assume that in this case it is not the patient who has initiated the evaluation—an issue that should be clarified at the beginning of any adolescent interview.) The interviewer has never met the patient before and does not have the benefit of his prior history. Casey is dressed somewhat sloppily in baggy jeans, sweatshirt, and baseball cap turned backward. He lounges in his chair and pays as little attention as possible to the interviewer.

> INTERVIEWER: Hello, my name is Mr. W. I want to thank you for agreeing to be interviewed today. Did your doctor tell you why I wanted to meet with you?
>
> *This rather formal introduction may seem foreign to some clinicians who work with adolescents. We feel it is important to find a middle ground between excessive formality*

and inappropriate familiarity. Adolescents need to feel that the adults in their world have the maturity and experience to handle their problems and to ensure their safety. Seductiveness, excessive informality, or attempts (usually unsuccessful) to dress or talk like teenagers can repel an adolescent patient as surely as condescension or lack of engagement can.

CASEY: Yeah . . .

INTERVIEWER: And why was that?

CASEY: I don't remember.

INTERVIEWER: Well, that's OK. Let me try and explain. I work with Dr. Z., and I would like to get to know you a little better so I can help Dr. Z. understand your problems better. Is that all right with you?

CASEY: [Long pause] Yeahhh . . .

INTERVIEWER: Could you tell me why you came here?

CASEY: I dunno. [Silence]

INTERVIEWER: What sort of problems were you having?

CASEY: Nuthin' . . .

INTERVIEWER: It sounds like you're not too keen to talk.

CASEY: [Prolonged silence]

The interviewer's good attempt at an open-ended beginning has been consistently rebuffed by a patient who is, at best, uninterested in conversation. If possible, the interview must now be salvaged by closed-ended questions, with careful attention to opportunities to form some sort of relationship with Casey. First, the interviewer presents some ground rules.

INTERVIEWER: Let's talk a little bit about what we're trying to do here. You're here in the hospital when you don't want to be, and we're trying to learn what it will take to get you out. Dr. Z. has already heard something from your folks about why you're here; now we want to hear your side of it. Anything you say that will help us may get you out of here more quickly. Do you understand?

CASEY: [Nods his head and steals a glance at the interviewer.] Uh-huh.

INTERVIEWER: We also need to agree on this: I'm going to try to be sensitive to your feelings, but I will have to ask a lot of questions. If I ask a question that you don't feel you can answer truthfully, just ask me to talk about something else. But don't just make something up. Any time you don't tell the truth, it will confuse us. And you could be here longer. OK?

CASEY: [Nods.]

INTERVIEWER: Still another thing: What you tell me I will treat as confidential. That means I won't tell anyone, without your permission. The only possible exception, I think you'll understand, is if you're planning to harm yourself or someone else. Then I'd have to make sure you and others are protected. OK?

CASEY: Sure.

With these statements, the interviewer has emphasized three important points: (1) a philosophy that the patient is not the entire problem, (2) the need for truth, and (3) the need for safety. These are fundamental to every interview, whether the patient is an adolescent or an adult; they may have to be stated more than once. In addition, the interviewer has addressed the adolescent's need for assurance that his possibly embarrassing thoughts and feelings will not be divulged without his express consent.

INTERVIEWER: How old are you?

CASEY: Fourteen.

INTERVIEWER: How long have you been in the hospital?

CASEY: This is my second week, I think.

INTERVIEWER: And you were an inpatient before at another hospital?

CASEY: Yeah.

INTERVIEWER: How long were you an inpatient?

CASEY: Nine days.

So far, the interviewer has been asking simple questions that this recalcitrant patient can answer in a word or two. The patient's slouched posture, brief answers, and initial refusal to cooperate all signal the absence of rapport.

INTERVIEWER: Was it helpful to you?

CASEY: No. I didn't like it. I thought it was just torture.

INTERVIEWER: Torture?

By repeating a word offered by the patient, the interviewer encourages an open-ended response. This technique is one of the most useful for guiding the direction of an interview while encouraging verbal output.

CASEY: Yeah. They treated me like a criminal. Almost exactly the same as in juvenile hall.

INTERVIEWER: Have you been to juvenile hall?

A lapse: Instead of saying, "Tell me more," which would keep the dialogue open-ended, the interviewer asks a yes–no question.

CASEY: I've seen it. Yes.

INTERVIEWER: From inside or outside?

CASEY: From inside.

INTERVIEWER: Boy, you've seen a lot of things! But you look kind of sad today.

The interviewer focuses on affect by making a statement ("You look sad") rather than by asking a question ("Do you feel sad?"). The statement avoids argument and reinforces the use of words to communicate (especially appropriate for younger children).

CASEY: Well . . . yeah. Just today. I'm getting into trouble with Cherub [another patient]. She is just provoking me until I say something to her, and she doesn't get into any trouble. They even notice it. I mean, she's calling me all these names.

INTERVIEWER: Do you feel they're picking on you?

CASEY: No, it's just really Cherub, and Johnny has done some stuff, too. He's thrown my dominoes out the window. I've seen him do that, and then he lies to me. And that makes me mad.

INTERVIEWER: I can understand that. Let me ask you this: Have you ever been in this place before?

The interviewer wants to move ahead, but an abrupt subject change may not be the best way to proceed, especially with a yes–no question.

CASEY: No.

INTERVIEWER: How many times were you in juvenile hall?

CASEY: I wasn't in there.

INTERVIEWER: I thought you said you were?

CASEY: I saw it.

INTERVIEWER: From the outside?

CASEY: No, I was inside for a probation hearing.

Interviewer and patient are sparring, testing each other's veracity and trustworthiness. The patient continues to be guarded, but the interviewer responds with another attempt at open-ended questioning.

INTERVIEWER: What were you doing on probation?

CASEY: I robbed this lady's house a couple of times. I went with someone the first time—an older guy. We took some cigarettes and some liquor and money.

INTERVIEWER: Uh-huh.

A barely uttered encouragement keeps the ball rolling without getting in the way of the patient's stream of thought. Adolescents often handle negative mood states (anger, anxiety, depression, guilt) through counterphobic acting out. Clinicians, like this interviewer, must be careful to respond with acceptance without appearing to condone the behavior in question. At the same time, they must dig beneath the behavior to search for its psychological underpinnings.

CASEY: Well, it wasn't much. She lives a few blocks away from me, and we just walked in. The back door was open.

INTERVIEWER: [Waits in silence for many seconds until the patient, feeling the need to fill the void, begins to speak again.]

CASEY: He . . . he was my homeboy, and I just went along. It was a couple of months ago, beginning of the school year. He stole a car. I didn't steal the car, but I was in it. Now he's on probation. He—

INTERVIEWER: And when do you get *off* probation?

To keep the focus on the patient, the interviewer interrupts, but uses the patient's own word to make the transition.

CASEY: I think it's going to be 3 years.

INTERVIEWER: And since then, have you been going to school regularly?

CASEY: Yes. Sometimes I ditch, but I've been going. Even if it's a lot of bullshit.

INTERVIEWER: Look, let's change our focus a bit. Tell me if there was ever a time in your life when you weren't getting into trouble. Were there happy times in your life, or has your life been kind of shitty all along?

This interviewer has obtained some information concerning Casey's relationship with his peers—an important topic for any evaluation of a teenager. The interviewer next tries to look for any history of untroubled, positive family experiences. Although this transition is abrupt, it is announced ("let's change our focus") to let the patient know that they will be pursuing a different course and that the interviewer is assuming more control of the process. The mild vulgarity may be an attempt to use language the patient will relate to. Of course, it is important to speak so that the teen will understand, but an adult who tries to imitate teenagers' language too closely risks rejection. Clinicians sometimes feel that they must choose between relating to an adolescent patient as a peer and sounding like a censorious parent. In reality, a middle ground is almost always possible.

When the going is a little rough, as it has been intermittently in this interview, clinicians sometimes consider switching to a structured interview. Although in some cases that tactic is reasonable (perhaps essential), here the clinician avoids the temptation and is subsequently rewarded with a relatively smooth interview that produces both information and a degree of rapport.

CASEY: Depressing, because of what happened at school. It was really one teacher, one bad teacher who started the whole thing.

INTERVIEWER: Uh-huh.

CASEY: This teacher—it was first grade—picked on me, and I had her all the way through sixth grade. She was a jerk. She'd pick three people out of each class, all these people she didn't like. Every time she came in, she'd make them sit outside just because she didn't like them. I was one of them.

INTERVIEWER: So it started in first grade, and it followed you because of that one teacher?

CASEY: Yeah.

INTERVIEWER: And you couldn't break the habit or change their minds?

Several summary statements verify that the interviewer understands.

CASEY: It wasn't that. It was the teacher. She was real mean. I accidentally broke a pencil once, and she got real mad at me and sent me down to the office. She says, "The school pays good money for these pencils, and you go around breaking them. You've got to go to the office." They did this stuff all the way through sixth grade.

INTERVIEWER: And then what happened?

Now the interview is moving along well, but the clinician is still concerned at the relative lack of affective material. It is fairly usual for an adolescent to portray all the problems as emanating from without. Denial of responsibility suggests character pathology in an adult, but may be normal for an adolescent.

[Casey relates more material about his progress through school.]

INTERVIEWER: When you started thinking about grade school, it seemed to me that you started to cry a little bit. Was it a hard time for you?

CASEY: I started to cry? What do you mean? I'm crying because of what's going on in that other room. [Gestures next door, where loud voices can be heard.]

Some facts have emerged about Casey's long-standing difficulties in school, but only a little rapport has developed. When the interviewer attempts to focus on affect, the patient shies away and returns to the present.

INTERVIEWER: You keep thinking about Cherub?

CASEY: And how I'm getting in trouble for things that she did.

INTERVIEWER: That's a pattern. People sort of pick on you, and you get into trouble. How come that happens to you?

Here the interviewer attempts an interpretation in the form of a question. In general, we agree with the conventional wisdom that it is best to avoid early interpretations. They are often wrong, and even when correct, they may prevent the revelation of more intimate material. In this case, however, the patient responds positively.

CASEY: It's because they know I'll get angry at them if they set me off, so they do.

INTERVIEWER: They try to set you off?

CASEY: They get me in trouble by doing that.

INTERVIEWER: So when you get angry, what happens? Do you hit them?

CASEY: No. Well, sometimes, but usually I start cussing at them and stuff. I did with Cherub and I got in trouble for it, even though Cherub was saying really disrespectful things, like "Oh, you have no friends." Stuff like that. She wasn't getting into trouble with that, and I'm really angry because I got in trouble.

INTERVIEWER: You got into trouble; she didn't. She got off free?

The interviewer is still trying to establish rapport with statements and questions that empathize with the patient's feelings of being scapegoated. This is a strategy that can backfire in the long run, because the patient surely understands on some level that he contributes to his own troublesome interactions. However, in this initial interview, the interviewer still wants to develop reliable, diagnostically useful information. The information needs to include not only the symptoms of the illness and the facts of the past history, but also data about the patient's capacity for insight and for forming therapeutic relationships.

CASEY: Yeah. And she gets to leave the program today, and she barely goes to any of the groups. I go to the groups. I don't stay in my room and refuse to go to them.

INTERVIEWER: And she doesn't have to?

CASEY: No.

Some meaningful facts have been obtained, and some degree of understanding of this adolescent boy's minimal insight into his problems has been observed. The interview is proceeding smoothly, and a reluctant patient has revealed much more information than might have been expected. By this time, the transition to a different subject has been reduced to a single syllable, "Now."

INTERVIEWER: Now, how did you get yourself into the hospital here?

CASEY: I got really angry at school and spit at one of the teachers, and they suspended me, and my mom said, "That's it. You're going to a hospital."

INTERVIEWER: Do you think it's been helpful?

CASEY: I don't know, really. I'm *saying* it's been helpful because I want to get out of here, but I think it's just been torture.

INTERVIEWER: Do you have to take any medicine?

CASEY: I take lithium and Zoloft.

INTERVIEWER: How do they make you feel?

CASEY: Lithium makes me shake a lot, and Zoloft, I don't know.

INTERVIEWER: Do they help you control your temper?

CASEY: Sometimes, yeah, but when Cherub does that kind of stuff to me, I still get angry.

INTERVIEWER: When you're mad and get into fights, have you ever hurt anybody?

CASEY: Yeah. I don't fist-fight or anything too often, though.

INTERVIEWER: Give me an example of someone you hurt.

CASEY: This one kid at school, I whacked him across the face and hurt him really bad. I think I gave him a bloody nose, but that was all.

INTERVIEWER: Do you have friends in school?

CASEY: At B— High I was really popular, and I was hanging out with the popular students there. Then I got put in C— High, and I don't even know anyone there.

INTERVIEWER: What's C— High? Is that where the problem kids are?

CASEY: No. It's a really preppy school.

INTERVIEWER: Is it a private school?

CASEY: No. It seems really preppy, and I don't really like it.

INTERVIEWER: Why did you get put there?

CASEY: Because my mom felt that I was getting in too much trouble at B— High.

INTERVIEWER: Tell me about your family—your mom and dad.

Using a bridge supplied by the patient, the interviewer moves to another area.

CASEY: They're OK, I guess.

INTERVIEWER: Do they work?

CASEY: My dad does. He's an engineer.

INTERVIEWER: And your mom stays home?

CASEY: Yeah.

INTERVIEWER: Have you ever heard them fight?

CASEY: Yeah, I have, but they don't do it too often.

INTERVIEWER: So they get along pretty well?

CASEY: Yeah.

INTERVIEWER: Any brothers and sisters?

CASEY: I got a sister.

INTERVIEWER: Tell me about her.

CASEY: She's 12.

INTERVIEWER: Does she look up to you—try to do what you do?

CASEY: Not all the time. She doesn't smoke or anything, and if I smoke, she doesn't. I hope she doesn't copy me.

When talking about his sister and his family, Casey seems to soften, and even expresses the hope that the sister will not take after him. This may be evidence of a capacity for empathy—a subject that is very important to evaluate in any adolescent patient.

INTERVIEWER: When did you start smoking?

CASEY: This past summer.

INTERVIEWER: Did you start drinking then, too?

CASEY: I drank a little bit. I drank a lot of wine and stuff before that, but that's when I started drinking hard alcohol.

INTERVIEWER: Did you ever have any problems from drinking?

CASEY: What kind?

[After further questioning about possible academic, medical, and personal problems from smoking and drinking, followed by some questions about street drugs, the interviewer learns where Casey was born and why the family moved to the current location. Casey also discloses some facts about his grandparents.]

INTERVIEWER: Did you ever think about going back to D— to live?

CASEY: Yeah, I really want to go back to D—, but my mom says no.

INTERVIEWER: [Softly] It could be like a new start.

CASEY: Yeah. Everybody in my family wants to go back to D— except for my dad.

This has been Casey's first really enthusiastic response in the interview, and the interviewer builds on it. It is especially vital with an adolescent patient to project the clinician's genuine fondness for the patient. Because of Casey's initial hostility and resentment at hospitalization, it has taken much of the interview to get to this point.

INTERVIEWER: When your mom said no, did she mean she didn't want to, or she didn't want to because of your dad's job?

CASEY: She told me she did. She told me she'd like to move back to D—, but Dad's got a good job.

INTERVIEWER: So when you were 5, your family moved to this area, or did you move around a little bit?

CASEY: We moved here.

INTERVIEWER: You've had the same house that you've always had since you were 5?

CASEY: Yeah.

INTERVIEWER: Do you have any pets?

CASEY: Yeah, I have two cats.

INTERVIEWER: No dogs?

CASEY: I want a dog.

This is the second positive statement of the interview. The interviewer uses it as a springboard to the discussion of other positive feelings.

INTERVIEWER: You do? A dog would be good for you. What kind of dog would you have?

CASEY: A golden retriever.

INTERVIEWER: Yeah, they're great. Say, do you think things are better between you and your mom and dad since you've been in the hospital?

CASEY: Yeah, and I haven't gotten yelled at by my dad.

INTERVIEWER: Are you mad at your dad?

CASEY: I get mad at him sometimes.

INTERVIEWER: Does he get mad at you? Does he hit you?

CASEY: Yes. Well, not hard.

INTERVIEWER: When you were smaller, did he hit you?

CASEY: No. Well, he spanked me.

INTERVIEWER: Did he—or anyone—really abuse you? Beat you up?

This could be a place to ask explicitly whether the patient has ever been a victim of sexual abuse.

CASEY: No, nothing like that.

INTERVIEWER: Tell me a little bit about how a day is for you when you're not in here. You said you're at C— High. What time do you have to be there?

CASEY: At 8:00.

INTERVIEWER: How do you get there?

CASEY: My mom drives me.

INTERVIEWER: Are you in school all day or half a day?

CASEY: All day.

INTERVIEWER: And how do you get home?

CASEY: My mom picks me up.

The interviewer now has a pretty good idea of Casey's relationship with his family; it is much more positive than might be expected of a troubled teenager. Learning how other family members interact with teens, and how independent the teens have managed (or want) to become, can be a difficult task for clinicians. Casey's evidence will still have to be evaluated against that of his parents.

INTERVIEWER: What do you do after school?

CASEY: I usually hang out with friends.

With more time, the interviewer would want to ask Casey to elaborate on his activities with his friends. What do they do? Where do they do it? Who is involved? Why does he like/admire certain friends? Some interviewers ask, "What would your best friend say if I asked about you?" You can ask children and younger adolescents, "What would you like to change about yourself?" (This is the equivalent of the classic request for "three wishes," asked of even younger children.) All such information provides a fuller picture of the more positive aspects of personality and interests, and the questions help cement the therapist–patient relationship by demonstrating an interest in the patient as a whole individual, much as do the questions about sports and hobbies that follow.

INTERVIEWER: Do you have a lot of homework?

CASEY: No.

INTERVIEWER: Are you on any kind of teams? Did you play soccer or anything like that?

CASEY: I did, but don't any more.

INTERVIEWER: Why not?

CASEY: Because I don't like soccer very much.

INTERVIEWER: Do you have any hobbies?

CASEY: Yeah, I bowl.

INTERVIEWER: You bowl? What's your score?

CASEY: My highest score is 147.

INTERVIEWER: That's pretty good. Better than me. What else? Does your family go camping or do anything like that?

CASEY: No, we don't go camping.

INTERVIEWER: You're from the East; you must like snow?

CASEY: Yeah, I like snow.

INTERVIEWER: Snowboarding? Do you have a skateboard?

CASEY: [Shakes his head "no" to each question.] I did, but someone stole it.

INTERVIEWER: Do you spend time on a bike?

CASEY: Sometimes.

INTERVIEWER: Mostly you just hang out with your buddies smoking and drinking?

CASEY: Yeah.

INTERVIEWER: Got a girlfriend?

CASEY: No.

INTERVIEWER: Have you had any girlfriends?

> This question could also be phrased, "Have you had any romantic relationships, with girls or with guys?"

CASEY: I don't think so. Well, kind of. When I was in E— Hospital.

INTERVIEWER: Have you ever been really close to any girl?

CASEY: [Long pause] I don't think I want to talk about that.

INTERVIEWER: OK. I'm glad you told me. So E— Hospital was where you were an inpatient before?

> Casey has complied with an earlier request of the interviewer, who will mark the area of sexual knowledge and experience as important to revisit later.

CASEY: Yeah.

INTERVIEWER: And what was that for?

CASEY: It was a couple of months ago. That was because I got into a fight with my dad.

INTERVIEWER: Do you remember what you were mad about?

CASEY: No, I don't.

INTERVIEWER: Besides that time in the hospital and this one, have you been in other times, too?

CASEY: No.

INTERVIEWER: Have you ever tried to hurt yourself or kill yourself?

CASEY: No. And I know what you're going to ask—I've never thought about it. Not seriously, anyway.

INTERVIEWER: Have you ever tried to hurt your parents or your sister with a knife or gun?

CASEY: I frightened my mom with a knife, but I wasn't going to hurt her. [Wipes his eyes.]

By now, the interviewer has addressed three areas that are vital to every patient assessment: sex, substance use, and suicidal ideas and violence. They have not been adequately evaluated yet (details of whatever thoughts Casey may have had about self-injury should be explored in depth), but the interviewer feels that the patient is safe. And the ground has been prepared for further questioning later.

INTERVIEWER: You keep getting tearful. What are you sad about?

CASEY: I don't know just what's going on in there. [Points to the next room.]

INTERVIEWER: You can't let that go?

CASEY: It's hard to. I just get into trouble a lot when people do things to me.

INTERVIEWER: You're a nice kid, and you still get into trouble.

CASEY: I get into trouble.

INTERVIEWER: You try hard, and they don't appreciate you.

CASEY: Yeah.

INTERVIEWER: I don't understand that. I don't understand why they don't appreciate you. It's just that your temper gets out of control? They trigger something, and boom, you're gone? Is that the problem?

The interviewer now attempts again to form an alliance with the patient, and finally seems to be succeeding. The patient answers the next series of questions with more affect and conviction.

CASEY: Sort of.

INTERVIEWER: Sort of. Have you ever broken things, put your fist through the wall?

CASEY: I kicked a hole in the wall.

INTERVIEWER: What else? Broken windows?

CASEY: I broke my screen and jumped out the window.

INTERVIEWER: You mean to get out of the house? [Casey nods "yes."] Have you been involved in other stealing, besides breaking into that house those two times?

CASEY: I shoplifted a couple of times.

INTERVIEWER: And the car? Stealing the car.

CASEY: Yeah.

INTERVIEWER: Do you know how to drive?

CASEY: Yeah.

INTERVIEWER: Have you driven by yourself?

CASEY: Only with my friends.

INTERVIEWER: Do you like it? Are you a good driver?

CASEY: Yeah, I'm OK.

INTERVIEWER: Probably too fast.

CASEY: I'm too scared to go fast.

INTERVIEWER: I was going to ask you about that. Do you get scared?

A good transition to questions about his feelings.

CASEY: Yeah.

INTERVIEWER: What sorts of things scare you?

CASEY: Sometimes I get scared when I have to go to school. Some people, they came over and tried to beat me up and stuff, and they had a gun and stuff, and they were going to shoot me, and I got scared about that.

INTERVIEWER: Are these people in gangs?

CASEY: Yeah.

INTERVIEWER: Are you in one?

CASEY: No, I'm not.

INTERVIEWER: Now I need to ask you about some other feelings and experiences lots of people sometimes have. Do you ever get really scared, like when you go to high places, in elevators, or in crowds?

The interviewer signals another change of topic, and lets Casey know that these routine questions do not mean that he is suspected of having had such experiences.

CASEY: No. Well, when I get into big crowds and tight places, that scares me.

INTERVIEWER: Does your heart pound and you sweat?

CASEY: Yeah.

INTERVIEWER: You've had that? Tell me more.

CASEY: Sometimes I just begin to shake when I get scared. Then I can't breathe. I sweat a lot and my heart pounds.

INTERVIEWER: Does that happen very often?

CASEY: No, only once in a while when I'm in a panic. A bunch of guys are going to get me.

INTERVIEWER: Is it only when someone's trying to hurt you, or does it also happen when you're in tight places or crowds?

CASEY: Um, I guess just when I'm afraid of someone.

INTERVIEWER: Would you describe yourself as either especially neat or especially messy?

CASEY: I'm in the middle.

INTERVIEWER: But do you like everything in a certain order?

CASEY: No.

INTERVIEWER: What about voices? Do you ever hear voices that don't seem real?

CASEY: No.

INTERVIEWER: Do you ever see things other people don't see?

CASEY: No.

INTERVIEWER: What about high moods? Like you feel really terrific, *too* good, and there's no reason for it?

CASEY: No, unh-unh.

INTERVIEWER: Or been terribly overactive—maybe you didn't need to sleep much for days on end?

CASEY: No.

INTERVIEWER: Or have you ever felt so bad you had thoughts about harming yourself, killing yourself, maybe?

CASEY: Not really.

INTERVIEWER: What does that mean?

CASEY: You know, I guess lots of guys think about it. But I never *wanted* to or anything.

As we would hope, the interviewer has circled back and obtained more information about the topic of self-harm.

INTERVIEWER: OK. How's your appetite?

CASEY: It's good now. But sometimes it's bad.

INTERVIEWER: How long is it usually bad?

CASEY: I dunno. Just when I'm feeling lousy. Depressed, you know.

INTERVIEWER: Have you lost weight?

CASEY: I'm not sure. I don't think so.

INTERVIEWER: Are you about the right size, or are you small for your age?

CASEY: I'm small for my age.

INTERVIEWER: How do you feel about that?

CASEY: Bad and lonely, sometimes. But I do have some good friends.

INTERVIEWER: Do you talk to them about feeling lonely?

CASEY: I talk to them.

INTERVIEWER: When you're feeling depressed, how long does that last?

CASEY: I dunno—not long. Maybe a day or two.

Adolescents' moods tend to be short-lived and labile. When clinicians don't appreciate this fact, they sometimes prescribe unnecessary medications and other treatments. As we carefully evaluate possible mood disorders, we must keep in mind that young patients typically lack perspective as to changes in their own moods. Repeated interviews across time are essential.

INTERVIEWER: Our time is almost up, and I would like to ask you just a few more questions. They may seem boring, but I would appreciate it if you would try to answer as best you can. OK?

In the hands of an experienced clinician,* a complete, formal mental status exam (see Table 1.1) is not necessary for every adolescent patient, any more than it is for every adult. Completeness is indicated whenever there is a question of severe mental pathology (for example, cognitive, psychotic, mood, or substance use disorders), or when, for legal or other purposes, the record needs to reflect a complete baseline evaluation. Of course, the behavioral aspects of mental status should be noted for every patient— general appearance and behavior; affect (apparent mood); flow of thought—for these require no special set of questions. Questions necessary for much of the remainder—

---

*Of course, clinicians in training should do a complete mental status exam on every patient they evaluate.

content of thought; insight and judgment; and aspects of the sensorium (memory, attention span, fund of information)—will come up as other matters are pursued. Note that in pursuing a formal assessment of Casey's mental status, this interviewer doesn't make the common beginner's mistake of describing the mental status tasks as "silly," which would convey the impression that they are not important.

CASEY: OK.

INTERVIEWER: What's the name of this hospital?

CASEY: F— Hospital.

INTERVIEWER: What day is it today?

CASEY: Thursday.

INTERVIEWER: Do you know the date?

CASEY: It's December.

INTERVIEWER: And the date?

CASEY: I don't remember.

INTERVIEWER: What year is it?

CASEY: [States it correctly.]

INTERVIEWER: That's good. Do you remember my name?

CASEY: No.

INTERVIEWER: OK. What sort of work do I do?

CASEY: You're the consultant. You're supposed to help me get out of here.

INTERVIEWER: Good. Here's three words that I want you to repeat back to me and then remember. *Apple, clock, mustang.* Can you repeat them for me right now?

CASEY: *Apple, clock, mustang.*

Before going ahead with the test of short-term memory, the interviewer ascertains that the patient has understood the items and that his immediate recall is intact. The interviewer does not invite rehearsal by alerting Casey that he will be asked to repeat these items a few minutes later.

INTERVIEWER: Good. Here's a question: What's the same about an apple and an orange?

CASEY: I don't know. Nothing.

INTERVIEWER: Try to think about it a little bit more.

CASEY: You eat them.

INTERVIEWER: Sure! That's good! Anything else?

CASEY: No.

INTERVIEWER: How about a chair and a bed? What's the same about them?

CASEY: I can sleep in them both.

INTERVIEWER: [Chuckles.] I guess so! Anything else?

CASEY: Well, they're both furniture.

INTERVIEWER: Excellent! Here's a saying: "People who live in glass houses shouldn't throw stones." What does that mean to you?

CASEY: Stones break glass.

INTERVIEWER: Good. Anything else?

CASEY: No.

INTERVIEWER: OK. Do you remember those three things I told you to remember?

CASEY: I remember *apple,* but that's all.

INTERVIEWER: Are you sure? Try to recall the others.

CASEY: I can't.

INTERVIEWER: That's OK. You've done just fine. Now I want to go back to something we talked about earlier—the car theft. How would you deal with this now, if you were with your friend and he wanted to do it?

CASEY: You mean would I go along with it again?

INTERVIEWER: [Nods.]

CASEY: I dunno . . . I hope I'd say "No," but I dunno . . .

INTERVIEWER: Why "hope"?

CASEY: Well, it's sure caused me a lot of trouble.

INTERVIEWER: OK. Well, I really appreciate the time you've spent with me. Thank you.

Questions of the form "What would you do if . . . ?" serve as a check on judgment that have more relevance for teenagers than asking them to state three wishes or to describe what they would do if they found a stamped letter. Such questions serve as a means of evaluating character and personality, and as a check on the congruence of an adolescent's values with those of mainstream adult society and culture. A similar sort of question, with many of the same advantages, takes the form "Tell me what you did in [a given situation]." This situation will usually describe an interpersonal problem the patient has already mentioned, though the interviewer may instead suggest a problem with a hypothetical relationship. Casey's responses to the last two questions asked of him address both insight and judgment.

CHAPTER 9

The Parent–Child
Initial Interview

A clinician often conducts an initial interview with one or both parents and the child together. Because children, especially young ones, are so responsive to their environment, it is rare for a child to be the only individual in distress. It is not unusual for a family, however, to present one child as the identified patient. A couple of generations ago, the family assessment was usually carried out by several different professionals. A psychiatrist might interview the child; a social worker might interview the parents; and a psychologist might use formal tests to assess the child's cognitive and emotional capacities.

More typically in recent years, a single professional completes the initial evaluation and makes referrals for specialized services only when indicated. Because children, parents, and teachers often tell different stories, it is especially important to obtain information from multiple sources. Interviewing a parent and child together—or the whole family, when possible—provides an opportunity to reconcile discrepancies. It may also be therapeutically beneficial for each family member to hear the others' concerns. (For obvious reasons, a traditional family interview is contraindicated in cases of suspected physical or sexual abuse.)

GOALS OF THE PARENT–CHILD INTERVIEW

The family interview is not inherently superior to other types of interviews, but it does have its advantages. It allows you to get different viewpoints about the problem and to meet all the players and observe them interacting. The people the child talks about become real in your mind. When successful, a parent–child interview answers several questions:

1. What family dynamics can direct observation reveal? Some possibilities include the following:

   - Enmeshed relationships, in which boundaries between family members are poorly defined, leading to a low degree of privacy and independence

- Disengaged relationships, in which there is little sharing of communication or live experiences
- Discord/hostility between the parents
- A possible alliance between a child and the weaker of two parents
- Overprotection of a "sick" child
- Scapegoating of a "bad" child

2. How does the family cope? Does it adapt by changing the alignments, boundaries, or distribution of power within the family to reflect altered circumstances (such as entry or exit of a member, development of children into adolescence)?

3. How do family members work together to solve problems?

4. How do they communicate with one another? Does each take a turn, respecting the rights of others to be heard? Does one member do most of the talking? Or do all talk at once, seldom listening to what others are saying?

5. How can the family's decision-making process be characterized? The answer to this question can run the gamut from authoritarian to democratic to permissive.

6. What cognitive distortions (inaccurate perceptions of any aspect of a child's conduct, character, or capabilities) bear on the relationships among family members?

7. Do any members openly denigrate a child who is present? How does the child react?

Although a family interview elicits some information relevant to the mental status of the identified patient, individual interviews generally produce more detailed, high-quality information of this nature. This is easy to understand: The presence of other family members may inhibit the disclosure of certain types of sensitive material, even by a patient who is very young. When a family interview is desired as a part of the evaluation of an individual patient, it is often better to interview the family first. You will obtain information from the group more easily before you have developed a relationship with one individual.

CONDUCTING THE PARENT–CHILD INTERVIEW

Some clinicians like to begin the interview by introducing themselves by profession ("physician," "social worker," "psychologist," "nurse") or by a more generic term ("counselor," "clinician," "therapist") who wants to get to know the child and the family in order to help with problems. Whatever introduction you use, make it clear that your job isn't to find someone to blame, but to "learn how your family works and help it work better."

You might start with an open-ended request, such as "Who would like to begin?" or "Who wants to tell us why we are all here today?" When the identified patient is a younger child, the person who begins will almost always be a parent, but you will have delivered the message that contributions are welcome from all. When talking with a parent, you should note the child's nonverbal as well as verbal communications. Ask whether the child agrees or disagrees with the parent's description of a behavior, feeling, or sequence of events. As the interview proceeds, attempt to involve the child, continually balancing and integrating the child's and parent's contributions.

INTERVIEW WITH ERNEST MONAHAN AND HIS MOTHER

In the interview that follows, a family physician has referred Ms. Monahan and her 10-year-old son, Ernest, to evaluate his chronic physical complaints. Though tall for his age, Ernest is thin and slightly built. His mother is also tall, but overweight and somewhat overbearing. (When invited to attend, Mr. Monahan explained that he could not be present this time but would participate in a subsequent interview.)

As in Chapters 4–8, the dialogue includes *italicized comments*. Here, these comments actually serve three functions. In some cases, they interpret the statements of Ernest and his mother. In others, they explain what the interviewer says or does. Finally, they sometimes give voice to the interviewer's internal working speculations about family dynamics.

INTERVIEWER: So what brought the two of you here?

The opening question is not "What is Ernest's problem?" or "What's wrong with Ernest?" Instead, the interviewer frames the problem as one affecting at least two people. Ms. Monahan provides the initial response.

Ms. MONAHAN: We first figured out that Ernest was going to be sick for a long time 2 years ago, right at about March or April. We already knew that you [addressing her son] had been sick since maybe February. What happened was, right at Thanksgiving weekend, Ernest came down with what appeared to be a viral cold—headaches, fever, not a severe fever, 102, 103, a really bad sore throat, achy all over, no GI or gastric symptoms, just a bad cold. We thought, "Oh, great, our local cold for this winter." As we went into the second week, some of the symptoms got better, but he was still sick—feeling really bad, body hurt all the time. So about the end of the second week I said, "OK, this has gone on long enough, now let's go see the doctor," and she said, "Yep, it looks like one of those bad colds going around, just keep him home until he gets well." But by the end of the fifth week, we went back and said, "This isn't getting any better." Ernest had changed to the point where he was running periodic fevers up to 100, was in bed exhausted, and his body and throat hurt all the time, yet nothing was positive.

The very long run of speech allows the informant maximum scope to tell her story in her own words. There is a hint of dissatisfaction with the family physician. Also note that Ms. Monahan dominates the opening: She "tells" Ernest how he felt and what happened. At this point, Ernest sits passively, not interrupting.

INTERVIEWER: Mono?

MS. MONAHAN: Mono screen was negative.

ERNEST: I already had mono—

Ernest has been listening quietly and tries to interject. But his mother interrupts and finishes for him.

MS. MONAHAN: Yeah, you'd had mono . . .

ERNEST: Second grade.

MS. MONAHAN: Second grade. And so, um . . .

INTERVIEWER: [To Ernest] Can you get mono more than once?

The interviewer wants to engage Ernest and ensure that his mother doesn't hold the floor too long, so responds to his interjection with a related question.

ERNEST: I don't think so.

INTERVIEWER: You're right. I was just testing.

ERNEST: Doesn't your body build up antibodies?

INTERVIEWER: Yep.

The interviewer maintains a relaxed, almost bantering style that might not be used if this interview were solely with the mother. It serves to engage the patient, even though his mother provides most of the information.

MS. MONAHAN: So at this point people are throwing up their hands and saying, "What's wrong?" So the doctor had a leap of clinical intuition and had him tested for CM [cytomegalovirus]. His blood titer came back as positive, and he was spitting out a very high titer of live CM virus in his urine. So now we knew that he had a significant CM virus.

ERNEST: Mom, they did blood tests after I was sick a few months.

Ernest is still trying to tell his version. Although Ms. Monahan has dominated the interview, the interviewer chooses not to intervene. Ms. Monahan has made it clear earlier that she becomes disappointed with physicians fairly readily, and the interviewer, content to watch the relationship unfold, is not threatened by being dominated.

Ms. Monahan: The first time she picked it up, he had been sick about 2 months. At that point, we knew that we couldn't treat him with anything. The only thing, since there weren't any antiviral drugs, was the old "Keep him comfortable, take him home, treat him well, feed him well, da da da da, and wait for it to go away; he will get better." It's now been 15 months.

Again, the mother's frustration with the medical profession is apparent.

Ernest: But I'm so much better than I used to be, *so* much better!

Ms. Monahan: Oh, yes, goodness. Anyway, we'd been home-schooling Ernest from Thanksgiving through March, but the stress was just too great, and he just wasn't getting well, and so we decided, "Screw it; we're just going to take him out of school, let him rest, really make this a therapeutic time." We brought in lots of funny movies; we brought in humor; we brought in—

Interviewer: Had you read Norman Cousins?

The interviewer is assessing Ms. Monahan's health care knowledge. Cousins's book Anatomy of an Illness as Perceived by the Patient *(New York: Norton) is an autobiography of personal recovery from an unknown viral illness, similar to that described for Ernest. It is narrated with a strong antimedical bias and was a top seller when it was first published in 1979.*

Ms. Monahan: I did. I'll tell you, I read everything I could get my hands on. We did humor; we did whole foods; we did fruits; I mean, we just—

Interviewer: This was starting in March?

By now Ms. Monahan's circumstantiality threatens to derail the interview, so the interviewer cuts her off with directive questioning.

Ms. Monahan: Yeah, then as soon as he was strong enough, we started walking; the first time, he was just dragging. But he learned how to ride a bicycle that May.

Ernest: No, I think it was, no—

Ms. Monahan: Maybe the beginning of May you started riding your bicycle?

Ernest: The beginning of June.

Ms. Monahan: Beginning . . . so right before Bright Star you learned to ride your bicycle?

Interviewer: What's Bright Star?

Ms. Monahan: That's a summer recreation day care program, and it starts the third week in June. School's out the 10th and it starts the week after, and we've been in it for years. So we just kept building towards this, and he kept getting better and better and better, but he'd have these days where he'd smack up against this wall [she emphasizes with a loud handclap], and you could just see him go whack and boom, and he would just sag and he'd be out for 2 or 3 days—what, about every 2 weeks?

ERNEST: Every once in a while.

MS. MONAHAN: In the fall, we put him in several new schools, first one, then another— Crest View.

INTERVIEWER: Wait a minute—from Thanksgiving he wasn't in school, then Bright Star summer recreation, and now Crest View?

The interviewer makes a summary statement to clarify, and also to try to stay on track.

MS. MONAHAN: Right, I'm sorry. Jimson Day. And let's see, this week you had an episode of weakness, Monday, Tuesday, and half of Wednesday, but I was trying to remember when your last episode was. It was about, what, 3 weeks ago, a month ago?

ERNEST: You mean when it lasted, like, 4 days?

MS. MONAHAN: Yeah.

ERNEST: But that was different, because I had a really bad cold.

MS. MONAHAN: OK, I was thinking of the last time you were absent just for fatigue.

ERNEST: Um, a couple days ago.

MS. MONAHAN: Well, I mean before then.

ERNEST: Oh, before that? Almost a month.

Mother and son again battle over clarity. Their inability to agree on events, and their inability to resolve discrepancy, reveal a significant power struggle. The mother is domineering and overwhelms Ernest (and the interviewer) with trivial detail. She controls Ernest and others around her with confrontation and interruptions.

MS. MONAHAN: Yeah, I think so. The episodes are getting farther and farther apart, so our attitude has been "OK, yes, we're getting better. Yes, this is slow, but at least we're getting better." So that's where we are today. He's back in school, but had one episode this week. What stimulated our visit was that, starting way back at the beginning of the process in March, April, May, I realized that we had a kid on our hands who is extraordinarily bright, has wonderful capabilities, and is now saddled with this chronic fatigue and pain.

ERNEST: It's sad.

MS. MONAHAN: And his throat hurts.

INTERVIEWER: [To Ernest] What did you say?

ERNEST: I just said "sad."

INTERVIEWER: Sad.

> *Picking up on one word used by Ernest, the interviewer tries to change the direction of the interview, but the mother interferes.*

MS. MONAHAN: Sad, and you get sad, too. You feel really depressed during those times.

ERNEST: No, I don't.

MS. MONAHAN: OK.

ERNEST: It just looks like it, since I'm in pain.

MS. MONAHAN: Yeah, I think you're a little sad too, but, you know, it's not bad.

> *Once again, the interviewer is excluded as mother and son try unsuccessfully to resolve their differences.*

INTERVIEWER: So did Ernest start in public school, then—

MS. MONAHAN: We started, we had him in kindergarten and first grade, and just—it was horrible. The public school system, despite its reputation, is atrocious. In particular, the elementary schools are absolutely horrible. They were—

INTERVIEWER: So second grade through—

MS. MONAHAN: Second grade through the current grade, he's been in private schools. Second and third he was in Jimson Day; then he skipped fourth—we had him tested to skip fourth into fifth—and it was in that fifth grade, that Thanksgiving that he first got ill. So he missed that fifth grade. So he's now with his age group, which is so funny, because we just jumped through so many hoops to get him skipped, and—

> *Ms. Monahan is not only discontented with the medical system; in her view, Ernest's education has also been fraught with confrontation and disappointment. She tends to externalize, blaming others for the family's problems of living. The interviewer has begun to wonder whether Ernest's physical symptoms may be an expression of his frustration with his mother's need to control his education.*

INTERVIEWER: So you're back to where you started?

MS. MONAHAN: Yeah.

INTERVIEWER: [To Ernest] You're a fifth grader?

ERNEST: Yes.

INTERVIEWER: And the reason to leave Jimson Day . . . ?

Ms. Monahan: Every time the teacher would walk out of the room, the kids were all over the place.

Ernest: You never did go in the room.

In contrast to his mother, Ernest tries to tell a balanced story.

Ms. Monahan: So then I learned about Crest View, which is for gifted children. You can't get in without testing. They have behavioral guidelines and expectations, and you have kids that are really interested in learning. You're not messing around with bums.

Ms. Monahan's message to Ernest is this: "Either you maintain a high standard of excellence or you are a bum." What alternative is there for him? To become sick and not compete? Although it is much too early to comment openly, the interviewer notes Ms. Monahan's apparent need for control as she lives vicariously through her son and denies her own inadequacies.

Interviewer: You like it?

Ernest: Yeah, I really enjoy the school.

Ms. Monahan: Tell him about Mrs. Johnson.

Ms. Monahan continues to assert control over the interview, even as the interviewer tries to develop an alliance with Ernest.

Ernest: My teacher, Mrs. Johnson, is 3 inches shorter than I am.

Interviewer: You're pretty big for your age, aren't you?

Ernest: Yeah, which makes me the tallest person in my class. And she's round and plump, and is always very stolid in front of parents and adults, but really loosens up when there are no other adults around.

The interviewer mentally files away Ernest's unusual (for his age) use of the word stolid *as fodder for the mental status evaluation.*

Interviewer: She's fun?

Ernest: Yeah, she's really fun.

Interviewer: What sort of courses are you taking this year?

Ernest: Well, we're doing math—but, unfortunately, for the fifth grade they didn't have any sciences except computer science, which is really cool. So we have math, spelling, reading.

Interviewer: What are you doing in math?

Ernest: We just finished up proportions.

INTERVIEWER: Fractions?

ERNEST: Yeah, we're doing all sorts of stuff with fractions, and she's teaching us all the different uses of canceling numbers.

INTERVIEWER: Do they have a lot of homework?

ERNEST: Medium, but when it comes to reports and book reports—all different kinds of reports—and oral presentations, which we also have, it becomes a huge amount.

INTERVIEWER: And weekends?

ERNEST: On weekends if there're reports; otherwise, they're pretty easy on you.

> *The subject of schoolwork does not create conflict or threaten Ms. Monahan, who has briefly fallen silent. But the topic of weekends is more threatening—information about the family might be revealed—and, true to form, she now takes over. Her use of we and us when talking about Ernest's homework suggests the exceptional degree to which she identifies with her son.*

MS. MONAHAN: One weekend we were accidentally trapped out of town because our car conked out. We fortunately had taken all his homework with us. We had 5 hours one day, just working on a state report.

ERNEST: And then 3 hours the next day.

INTERVIEWER: Let me go back to the pains and weakness. It seems like these episodes are spreading out a little bit. Do you feel like you're back to normal again?

ERNEST: Sometimes. But I'm almost always pretty tired, and once in a while I get sore, but other than that, between the episodes I'm feeling . . . [long pause].

INTERVIEWER: Pretty good.

> *The interviewer finishes up; this is not recommended as a rule, but here Ernest appears lost in thought. A better intervention might be to paraphrase his last few words: "Between the episodes you're feeling . . . " and give Ernest another opportunity to finish his thought.*

ERNEST: Yeah.

INTERVIEWER: Do you have trouble sleeping?

> *The interviewer attempts to return with Ernest to the earlier reference to sadness and possible depression, but Ms. Monahan chimes in with her son.*

BOTH: [Simultaneously] Yes.

INTERVIEWER: [Directly to Ernest] Can you tell me about that?

ERNEST: Well, it takes me a long time to get to sleep.

INTERVIEWER: Do you sleep in your own room?

ERNEST: Yeah.

INTERVIEWER: What time do you go to bed?

ERNEST: I have a deadline. I have to go to bed by 9:00. It's called "lights out." My parents just let me read to about 9:30, but then they just come in, and I close my book and turn off the light.

INTERVIEWER: But you're still not sleepy?

ERNEST: No, actually I'm sleepy, but I can't sleep.

INTERVIEWER: OK. And then what happens?

ERNEST: And then I . . . [long pause].

INTERVIEWER: Do you lie there awake in the dark?

ERNEST: I just kind of lay there until I go to sleep, and . . . [long pause].

> *The pauses suggest that there are topics Ernest may not wish to discuss in the presence of his mother. For now, the interviewer fills in to move the interview along, but will return to these subjects in a later private interview with Ernest.*

INTERVIEWER: Do you have a sense of how long that is?

ERNEST: Yeah, sometimes I can be awake until 11:00.

MS. MONAHAN: And what I need to interject here is that I do research. And my business for the last 25 years has been illness patterns. And what I've noticed in him is that when he starts to have several late nights in a row where he'll say, "Oh, gosh, Mom, I just couldn't sleep last night," it will be just before one of his relapses.

> *Ms. Monahan now asserts her academic credentials. Not feeling threatened by her expertise, the interviewer respectfully asks her professional opinion, in order to maintain the alliance.*

INTERVIEWER: Do you think that this is a biorhythm problem? Is his biological clock normal?

MS. MONAHAN: I don't know what's triggering it, but I know that one of the symptoms I watch for is several nights in a row where he is very late in getting to sleep. I don't know if the sleep drives it. Does the fatigue drive the sleeplessness?

INTERVIEWER: Is he hard to wake up in the mornings?

MS. MONAHAN: Not when he's doing well. Then he wakes up with a big smile.

ERNEST: And I just hop up.

INTERVIEWER: Do you need an alarm?

ERNEST: I'm groggy sometimes.

Ms. Monahan: You know we had a joke in the family, because Mom and son both wake up really slowly. Dad is opposite. He's gotten really good about sneaking out in the morning so he doesn't wake us up.

According to this description, the mother and son share characteristics, whereas the father is different; this suggests that the team of Ernest and Mom may exclude Dad. Such forms of enmeshment are not uncommon in families that somaticize.

Interviewer: Do you ever have bad dreams?

Ernest: I don't really remember my dreams.

Ms. Monahan: We've noticed that he can't sleep over at anybody else's house, because they go and have a great time, and the next day he can't get out of bed.

Interviewer: Well, are you too tired to be athletic?

Ernest: I love to ride my bicycle, but I hurt. I don't really like to go on recreational walks, but—

Interviewer: Do you play soccer or do anything else?

Ernest: I used to play soccer, but when I got sick, I stopped.

Ms. Monahan: One of the things—this is not a criticism, sweetheart—Ernest is not a smooth runner; he's always been a clumper. It's like he's got three left feet down there and they interfere with each other, so he's not really well coordinated.

Once again, the mother denigrates Ernest's abilities; is she trying to keep him from participating in the wider world?

Ernest: It's *two* left feet.

Ms. Monahan: And he didn't have the coordination to ride a bicycle until he was 8; it was last year, 9, I guess. But you're superb when it comes to video games and computer games and—

Interviewer: Fine motor skills.

Ms. Monahan: He's writing—he's going to be writing our home page for our business. We go to my office on the weekends if he wants to do that.

Interviewer: You're at the college?

Ms. Monahan: Yeah.

Interviewer: In what department?

Ms. Monahan: Biology. So the main reason that I wanted to get counseling for Ernest is—how should I put it? He's extremely talented; he's a highly intelligent child with a fabulous future. He has the capability to be anything, to do anything in this life he wants.

INTERVIEWER: There's a "but" coming here.

MS. MONAHAN: And my goal in life is to make sure that he's educated and prepared. That's why my goal is to keep him going in school, to make sure he's got fun and exciting things in school. I've had absolutely *no* backup on my diagnosis of chronic fatigue syndrome. In all the reading I've done, he fits every single profile. Not a single physician that I've talked to has said, "Yes, chronic fatigue syndrome."

INTERVIEWER: It's hard to diagnose in children. It's hard to diagnose in anybody.

Ms. Monahan finally begins to talk about why she has sought a mental health interview when her view so strongly supports a physical illness and no psychological problems have been described. She has never stated that Ernest has a possible somatic symptom disorder. The trap is that if she has failed in achieving her aspirations, and is expecting to achieve her goals vicariously through Ernest's efforts, she will again be disappointed. The interviewer remains supportive, but avoids concurring with the mother.

MS. MONAHAN: Well, the thing that made me most angry was, we went to see the pediatric infectious disease CM specialist. I blocked her name because she made me so mad. She spent 3½ hours with this child on a cold table, buck naked, with a sheet around him. And she looked at me at the end of all of this and said, "There's no biological reason for his condition. I think he's been abused."

INTERVIEWER: Abused?

MS. MONAHAN: Abused! Scared the living hell out of me. I was crying and Ernest was crying. We went home; we had a cup of hot chocolate; and I said, "OK, honey. Has anybody ever touched you, or beaten you, or done anything?" And we talked about this for 2 or 3 days, and I am absolutely confident in my heart of hearts and a mother's suspicious mind—never has he ever had any problems of this nature. It just fried me. This woman kissed off his entire physical condition by saying, "No biological cause." I want to find a physician who will work with us and take a look at the profile. I've been a patient little mom. I'm done being patient. I want somebody who's going to work with us.

The mother has now completed (and restated) her case: "Agree with me, or I will go elsewhere." The interviewer remains supportive, but does not necessarily accept the diagnosis of the mother, who also predicts lifetime morbidity.

[After some more discussion of Ernest's recent health, the interviewer moves to other parts of the evaluation.]

INTERVIEWER: How was your pregnancy?

MS. MONAHAN: Superb. I—

INTERVIEWER: It was an easy 9 months and a full-term delivery?

MS. MONAHAN: Yep, right to the day. I knew when I got pregnant because it was a planned pregnancy. I was a single mom—a single woman and I wanted a child, so a good friend of mine donated the sperm, and so I know exactly when I became pregnant. And I had a great pregnancy.

The mother casually mentions her artificial insemination and her planning to be a single mother—facts of which Ernest appears already aware. The interviewer leaves this for a later meeting.

INTERVIEWER: Are you married now?

MS. MONAHAN: Yeah. I got married when Ernest was 4, to a college sweetheart. He and I got back together again, the flames were still there, and we got married.

INTERVIEWER: And he's adopted Ernest?

MS. MONAHAN: Yep. April 11 is our family day.

INTERVIEWER: Do you have other children?

MS. MONAHAN: No.

INTERVIEWER: Not a smoker?

MS. MONAHAN: Nope, I didn't smoke or drink. I haven't smoked since I was 21. I don't drink, don't do drugs.

INTERVIEWER: How did you get to this town—did you grow up here?

MS. MONAHAN: No, I came here to go to the university.

INTERVIEWER: Do you have an advanced degree?

MS. MONAHAN: No, I have a BS degree in biological science. I would have loved to go to medical school or to graduate school, but I ran out of money.

INTERVIEWER: Where did you grow up?

MS. MONAHAN: South of here. My father was a scientist.

INTERVIEWER: Is he alive?

MS. MONAHAN: Yes, medically retired. I believe that I've had chronic fatigue syndrome since 1980. I've also always had PMS. I developed a very bad case of pneumonia in 1980. Immediately thereafter I had terrific trouble with fatigue and concentration. I just recently read an article about a genetic susceptibility in chronic fatigue syndrome. And I thought, "Oh, goody, great birthday present." But that leads me to think that this could very well be caused by me. [To Ernest] Sorry, guy!

INTERVIEWER: Do you get pains too?

MS. MONAHAN: It's interesting. For the last 4 years, I've had a terrible increase in symptoms, but I'm very, very private. I'm excellent at hiding my symptoms.

INTERVIEWER: So you don't miss work.

MS. MONAHAN: I miss 1 or 2 days a month, because I'm home shivering wrapped in a blanket because I can't move. I've just changed doctors again, because I was getting discouraged at the lack of progress. For 20 years, I've been patted on the head and sent to psychiatrists. I've been drugged and counseled, and, and—

INTERVIEWER: And now you're bringing Ernest to a psychiatrist.

MS. MONAHAN: Because I'm at my wits' end. I'm not getting any support.

INTERVIEWER: But he's doing well. I don't understand.

MS. MONAHAN: He's not doing well. Monday and Tuesday he was sick as a dog, in bed, weak from pain.

INTERVIEWER: But you know what it is. It happens to you too.

With somatic symptoms that interfere with her life, Ms. Monahan is even more like Ernest than she has previously acknowledged. Her disclosure suggests a positive therapeutic alliance with the interviewer, who observes that both she and Ernest are coping well.

MS. MONAHAN: But is there anybody that can help us? I just know that I'm not getting any information now.

INTERVIEWER: The point of this evaluation is to get to know something about everybody in the family, and I don't understand enough yet to start answering your questions.

MS. MONAHAN: OK.

As the theme broadens to "Who is the patient?", the informant's frustration turns toward the interviewer. However, she accepts this forthright explanation.

INTERVIEWER: Is your husband's health good?

MS. MONAHAN: He's a horse. He has his problem areas. He has terrible knees, because he was injured in the military when a piece of a helicopter door flew back on one. The other knee took a piece of a motorcycle through it.

INTERVIEWER: You've been married 6 years, so this was all before your time.

MS. MONAHAN: Previous history, yeah.

INTERVIEWER: But you said he was a college sweetheart?

MS. MONAHAN: We met while we were in college. Then he went into the Army—medics. He was slogging around with his unit for 33 months; he came back much more aware of his capabilities and limits. And he doesn't have any lingering nightmares or anything.

INTERVIEWER: Did he come back and finish college?

MS. MONAHAN: No.

INTERVIEWER: What does he do?

MS. MONAHAN: We are starting a software company. He's working full time on this, and I'm the primary support of the family.

INTERVIEWER: Where'd he learn that?

MS. MONAHAN: The Army. And he also taught physics and electronics.

The adoptive father has high aspirations and achievement, but no college degree. It is now evident that both parents have never achieved their academic goals. Is this the developmental path that Ernest is to follow? It is difficult for Ernest to succeed in an area in which both parents appear not to have reached their expectations.

INTERVIEWER: So everyone in this family is very bright.

MS. MONAHAN: Yeah.

INTERVIEWER: Can we just take a few minutes and go back another generation? You said that your father's alive and still healthy? How old is he, roughly?

MS. MONAHAN: My dad is 71, and my mom is 66. My dad was an active alcoholic for a number of years while I was growing up. And I was the truth-sayer of the family. I would scold my dad and say, "You're drinking too much. You need to see a doctor." I still have a very honest relationship with him.

INTERVIEWER: How many kids were there?

MS. MONAHAN: Four.

INTERVIEWER: Were you the oldest?

Another phrasing ("How far along were you in the birth order?") would be marginally better, but this casual phrasing gets the job done.

MS. MONAHAN: Third. Three girls and a boy. The boy's the oldest.

INTERVIEWER: What's he doing?

MS. MONAHAN: He's a professor of engineering.

INTERVIEWER: And your sister?

Ms. Monahan: I have an older sister who is a stockbroker. Strange person—she beds both the seller and the buyer to make a better deal.

Interviewer: She brokers the best deal for both parties?

Ms. Monahan: She takes them to bed as part of what she's doing in sales. She's done this for years.

Interviewer: I don't understand.

Ms. Monahan: I don't either. She's been married six times, was recently divorced because she was sleeping around. The lady has a lot of problems. My younger sister is very much the same way—compulsive liar and extremely self-destructive. She smokes like a chimney, weighs 320 pounds. Psychologically, and I think physically, she abuses her children. Ernest has seen her, what, twice?

A lot of family psychopathology is emerging. It seems to have struck everybody else in the family.

Ernest: She yells a lot.

Ms. Monahan: She's very unhappy, a very miserable person.

Ernest: She has a bad temper.

Interviewer: Really?

Ms. Monahan: My brother is a nice man. He's not mean, he doesn't lie, but he takes the absolute path of least resistance in all things.

[After some more discussion of details of Ms. Monahan's family of origin, the interviewer announces that they will have to stop for that session. There ensue a few minutes of wrapping up and arranging to see Ernest's father during the next session the following week.]

In the future course of this evaluation, decisions will need to be made about what further evaluation is necessary, whom it will involve, and when it should take place. Will treatment be necessary? Of whom? Of what sort? With what professional(s)? What will be its goals? How many sessions, over what period of time, are likely to be needed?

CHAPTER 10

The Written Report

Written reports constitute the standard medium for communicating the findings of mental health investigations to other practitioners, to insurance companies, to relatives, and sometimes even to patients themselves. A report offers a clinician the opportunity to organize the material about a patient into a logical narrative that concisely presents all of the evidence gathered thus far and supports the most likely diagnosis. Although many formats are possible for the written report, years of experience and tradition stand behind the one we use here. We illustrate each portion of the written report with portions taken from all available material about Casey, whose interview we have presented in Chapter 8.

IDENTIFYING DATA

A brief sentence or two of identifying data provides the description the reader needs to form a mental image of the patient. Include gender, race, occupation, religion, marital status (for late adolescent/young adult patients), and any other such information that may seem relevant. Previous experience with mental health treatment is often

> Of course, this scheme represents only one of myriad ways to write up an assessment. It depends almost entirely on DSM-5's categorical approach to diagnosis, which divides disorders into groups based on discrete signs and symptoms that are ascertained in the course of the evaluation. Other diagnostic systems measure degrees of variability; patients are therefore not compartmentalized, rather measured on various dimensions. DSM-5 allows for some dimensional ratings—such as when it asks for a number that corresponds to a general assessment of overall functioning, and in the severity ratings of mood disorders, intellectual disability, and some other disorders. However, some diagnosticians prefer to describe behavioral and emotional characteristics as points on continua, rather than assigning any patient—child, adolescent, or adult—to a compartment.

included, as is some statement about the quality of information provided by the informants (this is especially useful if reliability seems low).

> This is the second mental health inpatient evaluation of Casey P., a 14-year-old ninth grader referred by Dr. Z., his outpatient therapist. Casey and his mother are the principal informants. They were seen independently first and then for a brief session together. Mrs. P. is considered a good observer and reliable; Casey was minimally cooperative, but what information he provided seemed accurate.

THE CHIEF COMPLAINT

In the case of an older adolescent, the chief complaint is the patient's stated reason for entering treatment. For a child or a younger teenager, it will usually be the statement of the principal informant. In either case, it will usually be recorded as a direct quotation, though a statement that is complex, long, or vague is often better summarized. Recording the chief complaints from both patient and parent may sometimes be useful in demonstrating their different perspectives on the problem.

> Casey's mother states, "He's just changed since last year. I want him to be OK." Casey reports, "I just wanna get out of here."

HISTORY OF THE PRESENT ILLNESS

The principal focus of any report, the history of the present illness, is a chronological account of the reason or reasons the patient has come for treatment. Often it begins with a statement such as "The patient was well until age 7, when he suffered the first [episode of . . .]." However, for a disorder that has been present since birth, such as intellectual disability or cerebral palsy, the story might begin with a recounting of the mother's health during pregnancy or of any problems during delivery or the postnatal period.

Many life histories, even those of young children, contain multiple threads that must be disentangled. Sometimes this means presenting one strand at a time—for example, one paragraph devoted to behavior problems, another to learning disabilities. Alternatively, less relevant material may be reserved for later portions of the report. Regardless of approach, the history of the present illness should set forth all the pertinent positive data that help to support the preferred ("best") diagnosis, as well as any pertinent negative data that would help refute less likely or incorrect diagnoses. All of this should be presented as succinctly as possible in jargon-free language, beginning with first symptoms and flowing smoothly to the precipitant(s) for the present evaluation.

Ever since he was a toddler, Casey has had behavioral problems. Overly active from a very early age, he was distractible and had poor attention span in school. Throughout his childhood, he was defiant toward his parents and had repeated temper tantrums; since the age of 11, he has run away from home overnight on at least four occasions. Upon return, he would never tell where he had stayed, but at least once he was treated by the family physician for a sexually transmitted disease.

His mother thought that at one time there seemed to be a cyclic quality to his moods and behavior, with Casey behaving much better in the springtime. In the past year, however, there has been no discernible pattern, and his behavior has become progressively worse. His downward mood swings last only a few days and include feelings of depression, as well as some difficulty sleeping (initial and interval insomnia), but no stated suicidal ideas.

As a first grader, Casey was treated for hyperactivity. Old school records indicate that he frequently talked out in class, answered questions "almost before they were asked," interrupted teachers and other children, and would wander from his seat. Even his mother noted that he fidgeted and had trouble playing quietly. Nonetheless, because he is bright and has received help with homework from his engineer father, he has never failed a grade and is currently in the ninth grade at C— High. He responded well to Dexedrine, which he took from ages 6 through 13, stopping about a year ago when it seemed to lose its effectiveness. By that time, his overactivity in class had abated to the point that further treatment with medication did not seem warranted.

Casey has recently taken Zoloft (150 mg/day) and lithium (900 mg/day). Besides Dexedrine, he has previously tried Wellbutrin, Norpramin, Tofranil, Catapres, Mellaril, Tegretol, Depakote, and Ritalin. The last two of these reportedly increased his degree of violence, and the others either sedated him excessively or produced no benefit. He has had two seizures described as grand mal in nature, once in the second grade and once in the seventh grade. A seizure workup has reportedly found nonspecific, nonlocalizing slowing on his EEG; an MRI was negative.

In the past 6–8 months, Casey's behavioral problems have escalated. First he cut school; now he curses his teachers. He was recently arrested on burglary charges and placed on probation. On at least two occasions, he has physically assaulted and threatened to kill his father. The current hospitalization was precipitated when he responded to what he felt were unreasonable amounts of homework by spitting on his teacher and threatening his principal.

PERSONAL AND SOCIAL BACKGROUND

In a paragraph or so, relate details of the patient's birth, developmental milestones, schooling (including disciplinary as well as academic problems), physical health, friends and social life, hobbies and interests, and (when appropriate) dating and sexual history. Other types of information that are increasingly factors in young patients' lives include details of adoption, parental separations or divorces, and living arrangements such as shared custody and visitation schedules. Use of substances (drugs, alcohol, tobacco), to the extent that any of this material has already been covered in the history of the present illness, may be omitted here.

Casey's mother was 37 when he was born, in D—, Delaware. She is European American; his father is African American. She completed 1 year of college, then quit to support herself. He is a college graduate who is now employed as an electronics engineer. They were married when they were in their early 20s and intentionally delayed having children until they felt financially able to do so. Throughout the pregnancy, Mrs. P.'s emotional health was good. At birth, Casey weighed 7 pounds, 4 ounces and was 21 inches long. He remained in the hospital for several days due to mild jaundice, but did not require a transfusion. His developmental milestones occurred at the expected ages. He sat by 6 months, walked by 15 months, and began to speak words at 16 months. His fine motor skills appeared clumsy—he frequently dropped objects and tripped. He entered day care at about 6 weeks and continued there until age 3, when Mrs. P. quit work. His sister was born when Casey was 2; 3 years later, the family moved west and has lived in California ever since.

Casey began to use alcohol when he was 12 and has had some difficulties with it since. However, he has never had symptoms of alcohol use disorder. Although he has occasionally smoked cigarettes during the past year, he has had no symptoms of tobacco use disorder.

Although Casey can be induced to cooperate in a one-on-one situation, in a group setting he can be difficult to manage, showing off and demonstrating negative leadership talents. He often tests limits and is quick to alienate peers with rude, deliberately provocative comments.

FAMILY HISTORY

Mental disorders in both close and more distant family members, through biological or environmental means (or both), may have influenced the patient's development. Any noteworthy characteristics of personality or temperament in members of the patient's nuclear family should also be described.

About 4 years ago Mrs. P. had a several-month period of depression, for which she received Prozac. Casey's father has never been diagnosed with a mental disorder. There is no family history of substance use other than that of Casey's maternal grandfather, who was a heavy drinker until about 25 years ago, when he joined Alcoholics Anonymous.

MEDICAL HISTORY

The traditional medical history includes history of immunizations, childhood diseases, major illnesses, operations, hospitalizations, medications, and allergies. Where appropriate, a medical review of systems will include any positive responses to questions about past or current problems concerning any of the organ systems of the body.

Other than the apparent seizure disorder, Casey's physical health has been good. He has had no operations or nonmental hospitalizations. He takes only the medications mentioned above and has had no allergies. He has had careful pediatric care, and his immunizations are up to date. Physical examination revealed no abnormalities.

MENTAL STATUS EXAMINATION

For adults, adolescents, and many children, the report of the mental status examination will include appearance, speech and language, motor activity, sensory capacities, affect and mood, thinking, intelligence, attention, orientation, and relationship with the examiner. Of course, the emphasis will vary, depending on a patient's age and developmental stage. For adolescents, the information will vary little from that for adults; for preverbal children, the differences will be marked. For the majority of children, Table 1.1 offers a satisfactory outline, whereas the material in Table 3.1 provides a guide to behaviors expected at different developmental stages.

> Casey is a slightly built but well-nourished boy of mixed racial ancestry who appears small for his stated age of 14. He was dressed casually in baggy jeans, a sweatshirt with the hood pulled up, and flashy, name-brand basketball shoes. Initially his psychomotor activity was mildly slowed, though it quickened as the session progressed.
>
> At times he showed some irritability, but his predominant mood was mild to moderate depression with a somewhat constricted range of affect. At all times, his mood was appropriate to his content of thought. He was tearful several times during the initial interview and during subsequent interviews.
>
> Although Casey's rate of speech was normal, the volume and tone were subdued; only occasionally did he offer spontaneous comments. Speech was relevant and coherent. Content of thought largely concerned his desire to be released from the hospital and feelings that he had been unfairly blamed for his recent problems with his teachers and parents.
>
> Casey was fully oriented to person, place, and time. Despite the fact that he had some difficulty recalling all three of a short list of words after 5 minutes, his memory was felt to be unimpaired, because he put forth minimal effort. He could spell *world* backward, but was concrete in his interpretation of proverbs.
>
> He had little insight into how difficult it was for other people to tolerate his behavior, though he did appear to understand at a basic level that his own behavior was responsible for this hospitalization. His recent history reveals extremely poor judgment, though he said he "hoped" he would behave differently, given another chance.

FORMULATION

The case formulation attempts to synthesize from interviews, school reports, and reports of previous mental care all that a clinician has learned about a patient—symptoms, medical history, current living situation and environment, family history, mental status examination, and any other aspects that might help predict the future.* Although various formats have been used, we recommend two that are simple yet cover the important aspects of the child's history and presentation. Above all, the formulation should be brief. We briefly present the relevant sections, then present an example based on Casey's history.

The Classical Formulation

1. **Brief restatement of the material.** Here are stated a few bits of identifying data and a précis of core material about the symptoms and course of the illness, along with the most important mental status material.

2. **Differential diagnosis.** This lists the possible diagnoses for the patient that should be considered before treatment begins. Although all diagnoses (even those that are only remotely likely) should be included, obviously some will be more likely than others. At the top of the list will appear those diagnoses that, because they may be dangerous (for example, cognitive disorders) or more readily treatable (such as mood disorders), are most urgently in need of treatment or elimination from consideration. A detailed formulation will include arguments for and against each diagnosis on the list. Be sure to include any diagnoses suggesting that the difficulty may lie not with the identified patient, but with the family or within the patient's greater social milieu.

3. **Best diagnosis.** This is the diagnosis that, regardless of its place on the differential list, is considered most likely for the given patient.

4. **Contributing factors.** Here is described how the various hereditary and environmental factors promote the development of the patient's main problems. Specify the biological, psychological, and social contributing factors—the familiar *biopsychosocial model*. Depending on the availability of material, this section may be quite short, perhaps only a sentence. Statements as to significant strengths and the use of coping (defense) mechanisms should also be included here.

5. **Additional information needed.** What further records, interviews, or tests might confirm the diagnosis?

6. **Treatment plan.** An outline of treatment should include biological, psychological, and social methods.

7. **Prognosis.** Based to the extent possible on systematic follow-up and randomized, controlled treatment studies of similar patients, this last section should state the likely outcome for this particular patient.

---

*Some clinicians would also attempt to formulate the dynamics pertaining to a given clinical problem.

The Four P's Formulation

An alternative to the traditional biopsychosocial formulation uses *four P's*—those factors you consider to be *predisposing, precipitating, perpetuating,* and *protective,* given the patient's current presenting symptoms and the most likely diagnosis. Depending on the availability of material, this section may be quite short, perhaps only a sentence or two for each of the four parts. Statements as to significant strengths and the use of coping (defense) mechanisms are of obvious value here. We've included a reference for the four P's in Appendix 1.

Classical Formulation for Casey P.

The bracketed numbers would not ordinarily appear in a written formulation; we include them as a road map.

[1] Casey is a 14-year-old boy of mixed racial parentage who was hyperactive throughout his earlier childhood and has persistently defied and argued with adults, blamed others, and easily lost his temper. In the past few months he has used alcohol and tobacco, though no problems characteristic of a substance use disorder have resulted. He has been in physical conflict with his father, a teacher, and peers. He was recently arrested on burglary charges and admits to at least one episode of joy riding. Although his EEG has been reported as mildly abnormal and he has had two seizures, he has had no recent seizures.

[2] Differential diagnosis:

> Depressive disorder due to seizure disorder
> Alcohol-induced depressive disorder
> Rule out major depressive disorder
> Possible bipolar II disorder, depressive episode
> Unspecified depressive disorder
> Attention-deficit/hyperactivity disorder (by history)
> History of excessive alcohol use
> Oppositional defiant disorder
> Rule out conduct disorder

[3] Most likely diagnosis: oppositional defiant disorder in a child who clearly had attention-deficit/hyperactivity disorder when he was younger. Despite several symptoms of depression by history, no definite mood disorder diagnosis can be made now.

[4] Contributing biological factors include a depressive disorder (unspecified) in his mother and a history of apparent alcohol use disorder in a grandfather. Psycho-

logical contributors may include parental reactions to Casey's own violence in the home, whereas social factors could include an arrest and probation for burglary. There have been no obvious precipitating factors. His above-average intelligence is a significant personal strength.

[5] Further information should be sought from Casey's father, who has contributed only indirectly to the database; further exploration with Casey is needed about his sexual experience; additional neurological evaluation is indicated for his abnormal EEG.

[6] Treatment will focus on (a) further attempts at treating depression and preventing seizures with medication; (b) individual brief psychotherapy, possibly cognitive-behavioral therapy, to help Casey identify the origins of his anger toward adults and explore other behavioral responses; and (c) discussion with teachers to determine whether his school placement is optimal, even after several moves.

[7] Prognosis could be quite good if a biological basis for his mood symptoms can be found and treated. However, if his current downward spiral from ADHD through ODD continues to conduct disorder and beyond, the possibility of antisocial personality disorder is worrisome.

A preliminary diagnosis for Casey P. is as follows (a similar diagnostic summary is provided for each of the vignettes we present in Part II):

F91.3	Oppositional defiant disorder, severe
F90.1	Attention-deficit/hyperactivity disorder, predominantly hyperactive/impulsive presentation, in partial remission
F32.9	Unspecified depressive disorder
R56.9	Unspecified seizure disorder
CGAS	55 (upon admission)
CGAS	65 (upon discharge)

Four P's Formulation and Intervention Plan for Casey P.

Formulation

Casey is a 14-year-old boy of mixed racial parentage who was hyperactive throughout his earlier childhood and has persistently defied and argued with adults, blamed others, and easily lost his temper. In the past few months he has used alcohol and tobacco, though no problems characteristic of a substance use disorder have resulted. He has been in physical conflict with a teacher, his father, and peers. He was recently arrested on burglary charges and admits to at least one episode of joy riding. Although his EEG has been reported as mildly abnormal and he has had two seizures, he has had no recent seizures. The most likely diagnosis is oppositional defiant disorder in a child who clearly had attention-deficit/hyperactivity disorder when he was younger. Despite several symptoms of depression by history, no definite mood disorder diagnosis can be made now.

PREDISPOSING FACTORS

Casey's mother was depressed several years ago, and a grandfather apparently abused alcohol; each of these may have contributed to the genetic loading for Casey's difficulties. Psychological contributions may include parental reactions to Casey's own violence in the home. His mother stated that he and his father have had numerous altercations over Casey's deportment, and his father may have used harsh discipline when Casey was younger. Social factors could include an arrest and probation for burglary.

PRECIPITATING FACTORS

History obtained from his mother revealed that Casey's problems of feeling picked on by teachers and difficult behaviors in school were associated with the family's move from Delaware to his present home. His feelings of loneliness and sadness seem to have fluctuated since that time, further implicating family stress centered around the move and his poor adjustment to his new setting. A verbal fight just prior to the interview may explain Casey's initial surliness.

PERPETUATING FACTORS

Casey's former school situation (same teacher for 6 years, then a switch to high school) could have both caused and perpetuated his current difficulties. Other perpetuating factors could include an ongoing hostile relationship with his father and the influence of his peer group, as well as an unspecified seizure disorder, probation from the juvenile justice system, and (most recently) an inpatient stay.

PROTECTIVE FACTORS

In his attitude toward his sister, Casey shows a capacity for empathy, and he is able to relate a fondness for animals. (He was also able to warm up to the examiner, with whom he did develop a meaningful working relationship.) His family is intact; his father appears to have a stable job; and their living situation is stable (though his mother and sister would like to return to the area where Casey was born). He has support from his mother, who picks him up from school and apparently has time to devote to his needs. And Casey has friends—perhaps not the sort that his parents would desire (though not a gang), but he isn't a loner.

Intervention Plan

ADDRESSING PREDISPOSING FACTORS

Conduct a further search for a history of premature birth, birth complications, or early developmental problems (including central nervous system infections and head trauma).

Conduct psychological testing and serial interviews to further evaluate the possibility that Casey needs treatment for his symptoms of depression (though he does not currently meet criteria for major depressive disorder).

ADDRESSING PRECIPITATING FACTORS

Explore the possibility that racial discrimination at school has been a factor in Casey's slide into antisocial behavior.

Consider psychotherapy such as anger management training to address the problem of his short fuse.

ADDRESSING PERPETUATING FACTORS

Explore the stresses, conflicts, and dynamics within Casey's family.

Evaluate his relationship with his "homeboys."

Help both parents shape their responses to Casey's outbursts and other conduct problems (stealing, shoplifting at an early age, truancy, fighting).

Work with teachers and counselors in his new school, which Casey seems to like better than his former school, to facilitate more appropriate behavioral responses when he becomes frustrated.

Engage his physician in a discussion as to whether the control of his seizure disorder is optimal.

ADDRESSING PROTECTIVE FACTORS

Draw on Casey's feelings for his sister and for animals in an effort to engage him more positively with other people and in life-fulfilling activities.

Support his parents in their efforts to support Casey's rehabilitation from drugs and alcohol.

PART II

DSM-5 DIAGNOSES

APPLICABLE TO

CHILDREN AND ADOLESCENTS

Although the diagnostic manuals set apart those emotional and behavioral disorders usually first diagnosed prior to adulthood, this division is rather artificial and not a little deceptive. We say this because many of these diagnoses persist into the adult years, and so many "adult" diagnoses, which we discuss in Chapters 12–26, begin before a person is fully grown.

In 2009, a worldwide mental health survey underscored the second of these issues. In the words of Dr. Philip Wang, director of the National Institute of Mental Health Division of Services and International Research, "Mental disorders worldwide are basically disorders of the young." He noted, for example, that half of all anxiety disorders begin prior to age 11, and half of substance use disorders by age 20. Mood disorders begin in half the cases by age 25, making these relative latecomers. Add in the age of onset for schizophrenia—typically the late teens or early 20s—and these figures suggest that more thought and research must be given to the categorization of "adult" versus "child/adolescent" diagnoses in our current diagnostic system.

Nonetheless, to maintain compatibility with DSM-5 and to maintain the illusion of order in the world, Chapters 11–26 present all diagnoses in their current categories. The Quick Guides, however, include other disorders that may be considered as possibilities along with the disorders covered in that chapter.

CHAPTER 11

Neurodevelopmental Disorders

QUICK GUIDE TO THE NEURODEVELOPMENTAL DISORDERS

In this Quick Guide (and every other Quick Guide in Part II), the page number following each item indicates where in the text a discussion of the item begins. Remember, too, that the Quick Guide to each chapter includes some conditions that are actually discussed in other chapters.

Intellectual Disabilities and Autism

Intellectual disability. Beginning usually in infancy, this disorder involves low intelligence that causes people to need special help in coping with life (p. 164).

Borderline intellectual functioning. This category (an R-code) is used for persons nominally scoring in the IQ range of 71–84 who do not have the coping problems associated with intellectual disability (p. 444).

Global developmental delay. Use this diagnosis when a child under the age of 5 seems to be falling behind developmentally but you cannot reliably assess the degree (p. 172).

Unspecified intellectual disability. Use this category when a child 5 years or older cannot be reliably assessed, perhaps due to physical or mental impairment (p. 172).

Autism spectrum disorder. From early childhood, a patient has impaired social interactions and communications, and shows stereotyped behaviors and interests (p. 181).

Communication and Learning Disorders

Language disorder. A child's delay in using spoken and written language is characterized by small vocabulary, trouble forming sentences, and difficulty expressing ideas in sentences (p. 172).

Social (pragmatic) communication disorder. Despite adequate vocabulary and the ability to create sentences, these patients have trouble using language in social contexts; their conversational interactions tend to be inaccurate and inappropriate (p. 177).

Speech sound disorder. A patient has trouble producing the sounds needed for communication through speech (p. 175).

Childhood-onset fluency disorder (stuttering). The normal fluency of speech is frequently disrupted (p. 176).

Unspecified communication disorder. Use for communication problems where you haven't enough information to make a specific diagnosis (p. 179).

Selective mutism. A child chooses not to talk, except when alone or with select intimates. DSM-5 lists this as an anxiety disorder (p. 266).

Specific learning disorders. The patient has important problems with reading (p. 198), mathematics (p. 201), or written expression (p. 202).

Academic or educational problem. This Z-code is used when a scholastic problem (other than a learning disorder) is the focus of treatment (p. 444).

Motor Disorders

Developmental coordination disorder. The patient is slow to develop motor coordination; some also have ADHD or learning disorders (p. 203).

Stereotypic movement disorder. Without obvious cause, patients repeatedly rock, bang their heads, bite themselves, sway, or flap their hands (p. 207).

Tourette's disorder. Multiple vocal and motor tics occur frequently throughout the day in these patients (p. 209).

Persistent (chronic) motor or vocal tic disorder. A patient has either motor or vocal tics, but not both (p. 209).

Provisional tic disorder. Tics occur for no longer than 1 year (p. 209).

Other specified, or unspecified, tic disorder. Use one of these categories for tics that do not meet the criteria for any of the preceding (p. 214).

Attention-Deficit and Disruptive Behavior Disorders

Attention-deficit/hyperactivity disorder. In this common condition, almost always abbreviated as ADHD, patients are hyperactive, impulsive, or inattentive, and often all three (p. 192).

Other specified, or unspecified, attention-deficit/hyperactivity disorder. Use one of these categories for symptoms of hyperactivity, impulsivity, or inattention that do not meet full criteria for ADHD (p. 196).

Oppositional defiant disorder. Multiple examples of negativistic behavior persist for at least 6 months. DSM-5 groups this and conduct disorder with the disorders of impulse control (p. 386).

Conduct disorder. A child persistently violates rules or the rights of others (p. 389).

Disruptive mood dysregulation disorder. Between severe temper outbursts, a child's mood is persistently negative (p. 246).

Disorders of Eating, Sleeping, and Elimination

Pica. The patient eats material that is not food (p. 345).

Rumination disorder. There is persistent regurgitation and chewing of food already eaten (p. 347).

Encopresis. At age 4 years or later, the patient repeatedly passes feces into clothing or onto the floor (p. 361).

Enuresis. At age 5 years or later, there is repeated voiding of urine (it can be voluntary or involuntary) into bedding or clothing (p. 363).

Non-rapid eye movement sleep arousal disorder, sleep terror type. During the first part of the night, these patients cry out in apparent fear. Often they don't really wake up at all. This behavior is considered pathological only in adults, not children (p. 369).

Non-rapid eye movement sleep arousal disorder, sleepwalking type. Without awakening, the patient gets up and walks; this behavior can be interrupted only with difficulty (p. 371).

Other Disorders or Conditions That Begin in the Developmental Period

Parent–child relational problem. This Z-code is used when there is no mental disorder, but a child and parent have problems getting along (for example, overprotection or inconsistent discipline) (p. 437).

Sibling relational problem. This Z-code is used for difficulties between siblings (p. 438).

Problems related to abuse or neglect. A variety of Z-codes and other codes can be used to cover difficulties that arise from neglect or from physical or sexual abuse of children (p. 441).

Separation anxiety disorder. A patient becomes anxious when apart from parent or home (p. 262).

Posttraumatic stress disorder for children 6 years and younger. Children repeatedly relive a severely traumatic event, such as car accidents, natural disasters, or war (p. 303).

Gender dysphoria in children. An occasional boy or girl feels distress because birth gender and personal gender sense do not jibe (p. 377).

Reactive attachment disorder. There is evidence of pathogenic care in a child who habitually doesn't seek comfort from parents or surrogates (p. 297).

Disinhibited social engagement disorder. There is evidence of pathogenic care in a child who fails to show normal reticence in the company of strangers (p. 297).

Factitious disorder imposed on another. A caregiver induces symptoms in someone else, usually a child, with no intention of material gain (p. 338).

Other specified, or unspecified, neurodevelopmental disorder. These catch-all categories cover mental disorders that begin in early life but do not fulfill the descriptions set for any disorder described above (p. 215).

INTELLECTUAL DISABILITIES

Intellectual Disability

People with intellectual disability (ID), formerly called mental retardation, have difficulties in intellectual functioning—meaning that they have trouble with such activities as making plans, forming sound judgments, reasoning, thinking abstractly, and solving problems. The degree to which they have these difficulties roughly equates to a Full Scale intelligence quotient (IQ) of less than 70, though IQ per se is no longer a criterion for this diagnosis.

Instead, diagnosis requires difficulties in adaptive functioning, which is split into three domains:

- *Conceptual.* This includes executive functioning, reasoning, memory, and academic skills.
- *Social.* This comprises interpersonal relations, regulation of emotion, communication, empathy, and social judgment.
- *Practical.* By this we understand the age-adjusted ability to manage activities of daily living, organizing tasks, and choosing appropriate recreational activities.

These challenges do not result from a traumatic event or a new medical illness, and they must be present from the early developmental years of the patient's life. The deficits in adaptive functioning must also be present in at least two of the three different environments—school, home, and community. DSM-5 lists specific criteria for level of severity (mild, moderate, severe, profound); we've outlined these in the Essential Features below (p. 167).

The patient's success in coping can be enhanced (or diminished) by the effects of education, training, motivation, personality, and support from family members and other important associates—friends and caregivers. Depending on the level of ID severity, many of these children can go on to lead productive and satisfying lives. Even though they start behind their peers, most will experience an upward, if slow, developmental arc. Pointing this out to families and patients can help put fears and hopes into practical perspective.

Aside from functional cognitive impairment, children with ID may have additional problematic behaviors, including aggression, dependence, impulsiveness, passivity, self-injury, stubbornness, and poor tolerance for frustration. Low attention span and hyperactivity have frequently been noted, as have mood-related symptoms such as depression and low self-esteem. Between one-third and two-thirds of individuals with ID will have other diagnosable mental disorders. It is not clear whether these behavioral and emotional symptoms are primarily consequences of the ID syndrome or are due to an interaction between cognitive development and environmental stressors—for example, problems resulting from attempts to meet developmentally challenging expectations of family members or friends.

Causes of ID include genetic abnormalities, structural brain damage, inborn metabolic errors, toxic exposure (for example, lead exposure and the fetal alcohol syndrome), and childhood infectious disease (see Table 11.1). Some individuals experience more than one cause; for nearly a third, none can be identified. When no cause can be found, it is important to support the relatives who, fearful that they are to blame, may be desperate for an explanation. When you are informing relatives of your impressions, be mindful of their expressed or unexpressed grieving process, since this is not the child they dreamed of having.

ID affects approximately 1% of the general population. For reasons that are unclear (and still debated), males predominate by a 3:2 ratio. About 85% of individuals with ID are mildly affected (IQs in the range of 50–70); they can often attain at least sixth-grade academic skills. Schoolwork comes more slowly to them, so such individuals can profit from tutoring to augment their formal education. They can learn to read for pleasure, use computers, and have friends and intimate partners. With family and other social support, many hold jobs and live more or less independently in the community.

When still young, moderately affected individuals (IQs of about 45–55), who constitute about 10% of the population with ID, usually learn to speak well enough to communicate their basic needs; some will be able to hold simple conversations. Although they can learn social, job-related, and self-care skills and can work in sheltered workshops, they will probably never live independently.

TABLE 11.1. Common Causes of Intellectual Disability

Suspected etiological conditions	% of total	Examples
Early pregnancy	40	Down syndrome, maternal infections, maternal substance use (fetal alcohol syndrome)
Later pregnancy and perinatal period	10	Anoxia, birth trauma, fetal malnutrition, prematurity
Environmental and mental disorders	10	Cultural deprivation, early-onset schizophrenia
Hereditary conditions	5	Fragile X syndrome, tuberous sclerosis, Tay–Sachs disease
Acquired physical conditions	5	Anoxia (such as near-drowning), infections, lead poisoning, trauma
Unknown	30	

Another 5% of patients with ID are severely affected (IQs roughly in the 20–40 range). They may learn to talk, to perform simple jobs with appropriate supervision, and perhaps even to read a few words. The most severely affected individuals of all (those with profound ID) constitute 1–2% of all patients.

Mel

Mel was 10 years old when he was brought to the mental health clinic for evaluation. The foster mother in the home where he had been living for the past 4 months voiced the chief complaint: He had exhibited himself to other children at school.

Mel's biological mother was just 18 when he was born; he and his twin brother were her fourth and fifth babies. Although she received prenatal care, she was probably using cocaine during much of her pregnancy. Mel and his brother each weighed just under 5 pounds at birth; however, it was Mel whose jaundice required light therapy for a week before he could be discharged from the hospital. Three months later he was back, suffering from seizures that for a time were treated with phenobarbital.

Until he was a year old, Mel lived with his mother; after that, she paid more attention to her crack habit than to Mel and his siblings. According to records, at 7 months Mel still could not remain in a seated position when placed there, and didn't respond to sounds with alertness the way his twin did. During that first year of life, he had three hospitalizations— once when he stopped breathing, and twice for seizures. When the time came for his third hospital discharge, he went to the first of many foster homes, several of which eventually rejected him because of his slow development.

The foster mother with whom Mel lived the longest—from the time he was 6 until just before he turned 8—had noted how slowly he learned even the rudiments of self-care, such as tying his shoes and brushing his teeth. At the child guidance clinic, he received

ESSENTIAL FEATURES OF **INTELLECTUAL DISABILITY**

From their earliest years, these people struggle cognitively. Actually, it's trouble of two sorts. (1) As assessed clinically and with formal testing, they have difficulty with cognitive tasks such as reasoning, making plans, thinking abstractly, making judgments, and learning from formal studies or from life's experiences. Both clinical judgment and the results of one-on-one intelligence tests are required to assess intellectual functioning. Their cognitive impairment leads to (2) difficulty adapting their behavior so that they can become independent and socially accountable citizens. These problems occur in conceptual, social interaction, and practical living skills; to one degree or another, depending on severity, they affect a patient across multiple life areas—family, school, work, and social.

F70 Mild. As children, these individuals learn slowly and lag behind schoolmates, though they can be expected to attain roughly sixth-grade academic skills by the time they are grown. As they mature, deficiencies in judgment and solving problems cause them to require extra help managing everyday situations—and personal relationships may suffer. They usually need help with such tasks as paying their bills, shopping for groceries, and finding appropriate accommodations. However, many work independently, though at jobs that require relatively little cognitive involvement. Though memory and the ability to use language can be quite good, these patients become lost when confronted with metaphor or other examples of abstract thinking. The typical IQ range is 50–70. Persons with mild ID constitute 85% of all patients with ID.

F71 Moderate. As small children, these individuals' differences from nonaffected peers are marked and encompassing. Although they can learn to read, to do simple math, and to handle money, language use is slow to develop and relatively simple. Far more than is the case for individuals with mild ID, in early life they need help in learning to provide their own self-care and engage in household tasks. Relationships with others (even romantic ones) are possible, though they often don't recognize the cues that govern ordinary personal interaction. Although they require assistance making decisions, they may be able to work (with help from supervisors and coworkers) at relatively undemanding jobs, typically at a sheltered workshop. IQs will range from the high 30s to low 50s. Persons with moderate ID represent about 10% of all patients with ID.

F72 Severe. Though these people may learn simple commands or instructions, communication skills are rudimentary (single words, some phrases). Under supervision, they may be able to perform simple jobs. They can maintain personal relationships with relatives, but require supervision for all activities; they even need help dressing and with personal hygiene. IQs are in the low 20s to high 30s. They make up roughly 5% of all patients with ID.

F73 Profound. With limited speech and only rudimentary capacity for social interaction, much of what persons with ID communicate may be through gestures. They rely completely on other people for their needs, including activities of daily living, though they may help with simple chores. Profound ID usually results from a serious neurological disorder, which often carries with it sensory or motor disabilities. IQ ranges from the low 20s downward. About 1–2% of all patients with ID are so profoundly affected.

The Fine Print

The D's: • Duration (from early childhood) • Differential diagnosis (autism spectrum disorder, neurocognitive disorders, borderline intellectual functioning, learning disorders)

Coding Notes

Specify level of severity (and code numbers) according to descriptions above.

a Wechsler Intelligence Scale for Children—Revised (WISC-V) Full Scale IQ of 71, with identical Verbal and Performance scores. When he started first grade at the age of 6 years, 8 months, he was initially mainstreamed but quickly fell behind his younger classmates. Thereafter, he attended special education classes.

Throughout school, Mel's special education teachers regarded his progress as adequate, if unspectacular, for his developmental level. Although sometimes restless, Mel would mostly sit quietly in his seat unless disturbed. His attention span was normal, especially for the activities he enjoyed—drawing spaceships and coloring. When required to engage in activities he disliked, he sometimes lashed out verbally or physically. His progress cards noted that he generally spoke distinctly, but that his language skills lagged behind his age level by at least 2 years.

Mel's current teacher reported that he was easily led. On the playground and after school, he was often seen associating with Terry, a boy 2 years younger who was in a regular class. Terry's teacher described him as "sneaky and hyperactive." On several occasions he had persuaded Mel to implement some of his own plans, such as taking sandwiches from another child's lunch box. Once he even persuaded him to steal money from a teacher's desk drawer, but Mel cried about it afterward. The current evaluation was precipitated when Terry persuaded other children to applaud each time Mel removed an article of clothing, which he did, right down to the skin. He later repeated the performance at his foster home.

When evaluated in the clinic, Mel looked a lot like other 10-year-olds. His posture, gait, and psychomotor activity were completely normal. His grooming was passable, but his glasses had slipped far down on his nose and he didn't bother to adjust them; his runny nose also needed more attention than he gave it. However, he was attentive throughout the course of the interview. He spoke mainly in response to questions, which he answered mostly in a word or two. When he spoke at greater length, he didn't really have much to say. His sentence structure was simple, but betrayed no illogicalities or incoherence of thought.

Although Mel said that he felt "OK," he appeared somewhat sad during portions of the interview. However, after the session he was observed interacting with another child in the hallway, with an affect that appeared to be "about normal." He denied wanting to hurt himself or other people, or feeling that anyone was trying to harm or otherwise interfere with him.

Mel had considerable difficulty understanding the concept of hallucinations, which, after several minutes of repeated explanations (and often giggling responses), he finally denied having. His insight was evaluated as "limited": At first, he couldn't see any connection between taking his clothes off and the current interview. When asked the same question later on, he admitted that there might be a connection, adding, "Geez, I've told you a hundred times!" Because of his recent history, his judgment was regarded as poor.

Evaluation of Mel

Mel's deficits in intellectual functioning (Criterion A) are clear from his relative lack of academic progress and from the results of testing. (Earlier DSMs measured severity in IQ points, but IQ level per se is no longer the standard for a diagnosis of ID, as noted earlier.) Nonetheless, the Full Scale IQ score of 71 would place him on the arbitrary line dividing persons with ID from those with borderline intellectual functioning, and IQ historically has helped to establish the need for special educational and other services.

His problems with adaptive functioning (Criterion B) can be discussed with reference to each of the three domains specified by DSM-5. His conceptual difficulties are evident from, among other things, his delayed language skills (his language use lagged behind that of other children by 2 years; he required special education classes) and his difficulty in understanding the notion of hallucinations. His delayed language skills contributed to poor social relationships and an inability to explain his needs instead of acting aggressively. His social deficits are also demonstrated by poor judgment with regard to exposing himself and lack of age-expected insight about his interactions with others. He showed deficits in the practical domain when he didn't attend to his runny nose or wear his glasses where they would serve him best, as well as the fact that several foster homes had rejected him due to his slow progress in self-care (learning to tie his shoes and brushing his teeth). Although the vignette mainly describes Mel's school problems, they had clearly spilled over into other life areas.

Mel's difficulties preceded his school career, though often the first evaluation of a child is prompted by school problems. The clinician noted that his speech was impoverished, which could be taken as evidence of poor communication skills, but many typical children will respond to a stranger with apparent poverty of speech. In Mel's case, however, the observation was consistent with reports from his teachers. (We recommend using multiple sources to verify information about areas of impairment.)

In all, his intellectual impairment affected his adaptive functioning in at least two different environments (school and social life), adequately sustaining the diagnosis of ID. Had this not been the case, **borderline intellectual functioning** (R41.83) would be the appropriate diagnosis. His intellectual impairment had been noted from infancy (Criterion C), ruling out any of the **neurocognitive disorders** as a possible alternative diagnosis. **Autism spectrum disorder** requires repetitive behavioral patterns that Mel did not have, though many lower-functioning children with ASD will also be diagnosable as having ID. Patients with **learning disorders** may appear slow in certain areas but will function normally in many others.

Persons with ID can have nearly any other diagnosis found in DSM-5. In fact, the prevalence of such conditions as **mood disorders** and **psychotic disorders** may be several times that in individuals with normal intelligence. **Seizure disorders** are also more prevalent in individuals with ID than in age-equivalent peers. **Stereotypic movement disorder** should be diagnosed in addition to ID if body rocking, head banging, or other repetitive behavior is so severe that it would require treatment, regardless of intelligence level.

From his academic progress and his actual IQ score, we can derive Mel's level of ID severity. The physical condition responsible (such as Down syndrome), if known, should be recorded. Mel's full diagnosis would be as follows:

F70	Mild intellectual disability
CGAS	51 (current)

ASSESSING INTELLECTUAL DISABILITY

General Suggestions

A big challenge when interviewing children (and adults) with ID is to pitch the questions at just the right level—neither so complex as to confuse nor so simple as to insult. Here is an excellent reason to begin with an open-ended invitation to speak freely and at length: You will have time to judge how to tread that fine line. Generally, keep things simple: Brief sentences with short words and concrete concepts have the best chance of being understood. Avoid preambles and lengthy or complicated explanations that may divert attention from the focus of inquiry. Don't hesitate to repeat a question that goes unanswered; give examples if they appear needed. Remind yourself to "take it slow." These individuals often require time for mentally processing your questions before responding to them.

However, with increasing degrees of ID, open-ended questions are less and less likely to be productive. Although yes–no questions have the virtue of simplicity, they may encourage inaccurate information because persons with ID frequently tend to favor "yes" responses; multiple-choice questions are often better for this reason. Also, be careful not to use positive reinforcement excessively—this can also yield answers biased toward what a patient believes you want to hear.

Keep in mind several points about interviewing patients with ID:

- Some individuals "look" as if they have ID (for example, those with Down syndrome), but most whose ID is mild do not.

- Don't avoid discussing physical disabilities as you review the problems a child or adolescent with ID faces.

- Higher-functioning patients may have a sense of humor and will enjoy a joke, as long as they do not perceive it to be at their expense.

- Younger or less well-functioning patients will require questions that are relatively concrete, tightly structured, and simply phrased. Especially if an answer you obtain seems irrelevant, obscure, or bizarre, make sure the patient has understood the question by requesting a repetition of the question itself. Don't forget to determine whether the patient knows the meaning of a word important to the sense of the question.

- Some children and adolescents with ID may have rich fantasy lives that render them vulnerable to an inappropriate diagnosis of psychosis. It is vitally important to carefully evaluate material that is reported by caregivers as "hallucinations" (these might be fantasies) or "delusions" (children and adolescents with ID are often suspicious of the new or unknown).

- Self-esteem, which is often low in patients with ID, needs careful and repeated evaluation. Although these people can become depressed, poor self-image is more nearly universal.

- An initial evaluation will in all likelihood take extra time. The attention span of an individual with ID can be short, so the evaluation may require several sessions.

- Finally, many causes of ID (such as fragile X syndrome, phenylketonuria, and tuberous sclerosis) can be detected by means of laboratory studies, whose use is beyond the scope of this volume.

Developmental Factors

The tools appropriate to determine the developmental quotient (DQ) and IQ will vary, depending on the patient's chronological age. The WISC (now in its fifth edition, WISC-V) is appropriate for children ages 6 years, 0 months to 16 years, 11 months. Measurement of infants' DQ is more problematic. The Denver-II Developmental Screening Test, normed for ages 0–6, is often used by pediatricians. The Ages & Stages Questionnaires (ASQ) constitute another evidence-based battery for children ages 4–60 months. The Screening Test from the Bayley Scales of Infant and Toddler Development, Third Edition (Bayley-III), can be used to assess children ages 1–42 months. Except for the Denver-II Developmental Screening Test and the ASQ, these instruments are usually administered by clinical psychologists or by other clinicians who have had special training. Look for information about the WISC-V and the Bayley-III in Appendix 1. Of course, children with severe ID and those who have associated characteristic physical features (such as Down syndrome) are likely to be diagnosed at an earlier age.

F88 Global Developmental Delay

Use the category of global developmental delay for a patient under age 5 years—perhaps one with delayed developmental milestones—who has not yet been adequately evaluated.

F79 Unspecified Intellectual Disability

The category of unspecified intellectual disability is for someone age 5 years old or older who has one or more additional disabilities (such as a severe mental disorder or a sensory deficit) that are too severe to permit full evaluation of intellectual abilities.

COMMUNICATION DISORDERS

The disorders described in this section, which account for a large percentage of referrals for evaluation, impair the ability of children (and sometimes adults) to communicate with others. Problems with communication can be symptomatic of a broader developmental condition, such as autism spectrum disorder, but many children have stand-alone issues with speech and language. Despite their frequent occurrence (perhaps 5% of children overall), several of these disorders have not been well studied. Indeed, in DSM-5 they have been largely recast and renamed from DSM-IV. Childhood-onset fluency disorder is well known because stuttering is obvious and relatively common, but other communication disorders are less readily recognized and so may go undiagnosed.

F80.2 Language Disorder

Children with language disorder (LD) have trouble communicating, whether by speech or written material—or even by sign language. Their problems with language use are varied and broad, including having a small vocabulary, trouble constructing sentences from the rules of grammar, and trouble using words and sentences to exchange information or converse with another person. LD can occur despite normal intelligence. It subsumes the DSM-IV expressive and receptive language disorders; deficiency in both types of skill are inherent in LD, though one may be minimal.

The difficulty can show up in a variety of ways. It may be suspected in early infancy, when babbling fails to occur. These patients learn to speak late, and they speak little for their age. When they do speak, they use short sentences and simple grammar. They may have trouble learning new words, use words incorrectly, and omit important parts of sentences; they may even invent their own word order. As they grow older, they may fail to develop the varieties of grammatical structure (such as the use of different verb forms) and sentence type (such as the use of commands) that characterize the speech of their agemates. Their disability often renders these children shy; they may speak only with relatives, or may appear inattentive, perhaps responding inappropriately during a conversation.

LD runs in families and has a strong genetic basis. Although the prevalence of LD has not yet been ascertained, 3–7% of young children were said to have one of its DSM-IV predecessors, with a male preponderance. Most often, it persists through adolescence and into adult life. LD may be comorbid with other communication disorders and with ADHD.

Susan

On an Internet chat group, Mrs. Barrett discussed the development of her daughter, Susan:

"I just finished searching for 'Language Disorder,' and it brought me to this website. I think my 3-year-old daughter has this problem—at least, that's what the pediatrician said. She seems to understand everything we say, even tries to do little chores like her older

ESSENTIAL FEATURES OF **LANGUAGE DISORDER**

Beginning early in childhood, a patient's use of spoken and written language persistently lags behind age expectations. Compared to agemates, patients will have small vocabularies, impaired use of words to form sentences, and reduced ability to employ sentences to express ideas.

The Fine Print

The D's: • Duration and demographics (begins in early childhood; tends toward chronicity) • Disability (social, academic, occupational, or personal impairment) • Differential diagnosis (sensory impairment, autism spectrum disorder, intellectual disability, learning disorder—though each of these may coexist with language disorder)

brother. But she hardly speaks any words. She tries so hard to communicate with us, uses a lot of hand gestures to let us know what she wants or means. It's really heartbreaking! At first we thought it might be her hearing, but the audiometry was normal. We know she has a problem—her two older brothers both spoke early. Any advice?"

In a subsequent telephone interview, Mrs. Barrett expanded on Susan's symptoms. Although Susan's sentences were largely limited to one or two words ("I got," "You bed"), she could identify subtle shades of color (indigo, azure, aqua) by pointing. But when asked, "What color is this?", she would just laugh and point to it. She also lisped quite badly; she pronounced her own name as "Thuthan." She habitually mispronounced many words ("bul-lah" for *butter* and "ikeem" for *ice cream*).

"She's a dear, sweet, usually happy child," her mother concluded. "She adores TV, especially if there is a program about babies. She loves to curl up on my lap; she'll pull on my sleeve and hum a little, which means she wants me to sing to her. But she can't talk. She just can't talk."

On the Internet, another parent responded to this plea with the information that many school districts had testing programs for children as young as 2. This was the case where the Barretts lived. Susan had scored more than two standard deviations below expectations on the Carrow Elicited Language Inventory.

Evaluation of Susan

Susan's vocabulary was small, even for her age, and her sentence structure was rudimentary (Criteria A1, A2). Each of these qualities limited her ability to communicate (A3). (Some children, like Susan, have relatively little difficulty with receptive language but have a great deal of difficulty expressing themselves through language.)

Criterion B in DSM-5 is actually a two-parter. First, it requires the problems with communication to be quantifiably below what you would expect for the patient's age. This implies testing, as was done for Susan. But what if it had not? What about another child for whom only history was available? At least in Susan's case, the history obtained from her mother and the observations of her clinician seemed to be enough to warrant a tentative diagnosis.

The second part of Criterion B is the usual requirement, somewhat disguised, for an indication of distress or disability. Although Susan was too young for anything to interfere with her educational or occupational achievement, her language problem was an undeniable social impairment, even at her young age. Of course, her difficulties began early in the developmental period (Criterion C).

Testing had already verified that Susan did not have **intellectual disability** (Criterion D). The fact that she related well emotionally to her family in effect ruled out an **autism spectrum disorder**, though abnormal communication skills do figure prominently among the symptoms of ASD. Other conceivable problems include **impaired hearing** (already ruled out for Susan) and **environmental deprivation**, for which there wasn't a shred of evidence.

Like many other children with (and without) LD, Susan also had significant difficulty with pronunciation (**speech sound disorder**, Criteria A and B; see the next section). Her mother noted that she dropped certain sounds (the sibilant in *ice cream*) and substituted consonants (*l* for *t* in *butter*, for example). Her lisp even extended to the pronunciation of her own name. In defining the diagnosis of SSD, many of the same conditions must be identified (or ruled out) as for LD (D).

Susan had no known physical cause for either of her two communication disorders. Her complete diagnosis would be the following:

One cause of acquired language deficit is found in a rare neurological disorder called Landau–Kleffner syndrome. In this condition, a child's development is normal until about age 4, when progressive loss of the ability both to understand and to produce spoken language begins. The inability is so profound as to be called *acquired aphasia* by some writers. It is accompanied by seizure disorders or abnormal EEG. The pattern of normal development during the first few years of life has also led some clinicians to confuse this syndrome with autism spectrum disorder. Recognizing it is important: Some patients respond to anticonvulsants or even surgery.

F80.2	Language disorder
F80.0	Speech sound disorder
CGAS	65 (current)

F80.0 Speech Sound Disorder

Children with speech sound disorder (SSD) make speech errors not explainable by their age or dialect. They may omit certain sounds completely or substitute one sound for another (lisping is a common example). Consonants are most often affected. In milder cases, the effect may be only quaint, even cute; more severely affected individuals may be difficult to understand or even unintelligible. Obvious physical causes include hearing impairment, cerebral palsy, cleft palate, and intellectual disability, but in most cases the actual cause is unknown.

Clinically important and therefore diagnosable SSD (in DSM-III-R it was called developmental articulation disorder; in DSM-IV it was phonological disorder) can be found in 2–3% of preschool children, with boys predominating. Although these children interact and communicate normally at home, with peers or in the classroom, frustration and embarrassment may lead to withdrawal. However, spontaneous improvement often occurs, so that by the late teens the prevalence has declined to about 1 in 200.

SSD runs in families and is often associated with other communication disorders and with reading disorder; anxiety disorders and ADHD are often comorbid. For a clinical vignette and evaluation, see the case of Susan, presented above to illustrate LD.

ESSENTIAL FEATURES OF **SPEECH SOUND DISORDER**

The patient has problems producing the sounds of speech, compromising communication.

The Fine Print

The D's: • Duration (beginning in early childhood) • Disability (social, academic, or occupational impairment) • Differential diagnosis (physical disorders such as cleft palate or neurological disorders; sensory impairment such as hearing impairment; selective mutism)

F80.81 Childhood–Onset Fluency Disorder (Stuttering)

The speech pattern of an individual who stutters is marked by an often agonizing loss of fluency and rhythm that any layperson can recognize. Less familiar may be some of the person's accessory, or secondary, sensations when grappling with the burdens of sound production. These individuals often experience a sense of momentary loss of control; they may take extreme measures to avoid difficult sounds or situations (such as using a telephone) that exacerbate their misery. They typically feel anxiety or frustration; many report actual physical tension. Head jerks, clenching of fists, blinking, or raising an upper lip may be encountered even in a child of 4.

Depending on age and a host of other factors, a person with typical speech may speak up to 220 words per minute and will be dysfluent on 2% of words; a person who stutters speaks roughly 25% slower and will be dysfluent about five times as often. Stuttering is especially likely with consonants; initial sounds of words; the first word of a sentence; and words that are accented, long, or infrequently used. It may be provoked by telling jokes, saying one's own name, talking to strangers, or speaking to an authority figure or to someone who is perceived as critical. People who stutter often achieve fluency when singing or swearing, or speaking to the steady beat of a metronome.

Stuttering typically begins in early childhood, sometimes as early as the age of 2, but typically by age 5. Of course, it is quite usual for tiny children to have nonfluencies of speech, so early stuttering may not signify anything. Onset may be either gradual or sudden; the latter may correlate with greater severity. As in so many other childhood mental disorders, there is a high male-to-female ratio—in this case, about 3:1. Data do not support the notion that children who stutter are likely to have a preexisting tendency to emotional reactivity, shyness, or social anxiety. However, a subgroup may have traits of inattention and hyperactivity/impulsivity.

Based on supposed cause, three types of stuttering have been identified: *developmental* (the most common); *neurogenic* (following physical brain insults such as traumatic brain injury or stroke); and the rarely encountered *psychogenic*, which usually occurs in adults with a history of emotional trauma or other psychological disorder. In the developmental type, stuttering occurs especially at the beginning of words, and secondary behaviors are prominent. Twin studies suggest that 70% of the variance is genetic; even the tendency to chronicity or spontaneous recovery may be genetically determined.

Although tension worsens stuttering (public speaking is a notorious example), it does not account for the tendency to stutter in the first place. In fact, apart from other communication disorders and ADHD, children who stutter may have fewer emotional ills than you might encounter in the general population. With maturity, however, many patients develop symptoms of social anxiety disorder.

As many as 3% of young children stutter; the percentage is higher for children who suffer brain damage or intellectual disability. About 75% of cases remit within 4 years; resolution by adulthood is more common among females. Nonetheless, early intervention may be indicated for a child who is bullied, taunted, or excluded by peers. Although opinions vary, the prevalence rate of stuttering in adults is on the order of 0.1%, of whom about 80% are male.

Because of the general awareness of symptoms, we've provided no vignette for this disorder.

F80.89 Social (Pragmatic) Communication Disorder

Social communication disorder (SCD) describes patients who, despite adequate vocabulary and ability to form sentences, still have problems with the everyday practical use of lan-

ESSENTIAL FEATURES OF
CHILDHOOD-ONSET FLUENCY DISORDER (STUTTERING)

A patient has problems speaking smoothly, most notably with sounds that are drawn out or repeated; pauses occur in the middle of words. The individual experiences marked tension while speaking, and will repeat entire words or substitute easier words for those that are difficult to produce. The result: anxiety about the act of speaking.

The Fine Print

The D's: • Duration (beginning in early childhood) • Distress or disability (social, academic, or occupational impairment) • Differential diagnosis (speech motor deficits; neurological conditions such as stroke; other mental disorders)

Coding Note

Stuttering that begins later in life should be recorded as adult-onset fluency disorder and coded F98.5.

A tangential note on cluttering is in order here. In cluttering, abnormalities of both rate and rhythm of speech create dysfluency, impairing intelligibility. Whereas persons who stutter repeat only a single sound, individuals who clutter may repeat syllables, words, or even short phrases, often backtracking and substituting words or ideas in speech that comes too rapidly, before their thoughts are adequately organized.

Stuttering: "I've got to g-g-g-g-go to the store to buy some muh-muh-muh-muh-milk."

Cluttering: "I've got to go-go-go to the st-, to the, uh, sto-sto, to the market to buy, uh, to get some, um, some m-m-m-, some ice cream."

Pure cluttering is rare; it is found in perhaps only 5% of patients with disorders of fluency. However, many persons who stutter also clutter at times. Barely mentioned in DSM-III, cluttering shared stuttering's code number in DSM-III-R, wherein it enjoyed a full-page write-up. As of DSM-IV, it disappeared completely as a diagnosable entity. Its demise can be traced to a paucity of research and lack of advocates, along with the belief of some that cluttering is really a problem of expression, not speech.

guage. The world of communications calls this *pragmatics*, and it involves several principal skills:

- Using language to pursue different tasks, such as welcoming someone; communicating facts; or making a demand, promise, or a request

- Adapting language to the needs of a particular situation or individual, such as speaking differently to children than to adults or in class versus at home

- Adhering to the conventions of conversation, such as taking turns; staying on topic; using nonverbal (eye contact, facial expressions) as well as verbal signals; allowing adequate physical space between speaker and listener; and restating something that's been misinterpreted

- Understanding implied communications, such as metaphors, idioms, and humor

Whether they are children or adults, patients with SCD have difficulty understanding and using the pragmatic aspects of social communication, to the point that their conversations can be socially inappropriate. Yet they do not have the restricted interests and repetitive behaviors that would qualify them for a diagnosis of autism spectrum disorder. SCD can occur by itself or with other diagnoses, such as speech sound disorder, learning disorders, or intellectual disability.

Demographics are not known for this new (as of DSM-5) disorder.

ESSENTIAL FEATURES OF
SOCIAL (PRAGMATIC) COMMUNICATION DISORDER

From early childhood, a patient has difficulty with each of these features: using language for social purposes, adapting communication to fit the context, following the conventions (rules) of conversation, *and* understanding implied communications.

The Fine Print

The D's: • Disability (social, academic, occupational, or personal impairment) • Duration (usually first identified by age 4–5) • Differential diagnosis (physical or neurological conditions, autism spectrum disorder, intellectual disability, social anxiety disorder, attention-deficit/hyperactivity disorder)

F80.9 Unspecified Communication Disorder

Use unspecified communication disorder for patients whose disorders of communication don't fit the criteria for any more specific disorder—including other types of neurodevelopmental disorders. DSM-IV gave examples of abnormalities in the pitch, loudness, quality, tone, or resonance of the voice. However, this category might also apply to the occasional child who appears to comprehend language poorly, yet can produce it relatively well.

ASSESSING COMMUNICATION DISORDERS

General Suggestions

Because these disorders manifest themselves as childhood speech problems, you would think that casual conversation would suffice for their identification. But any of them can be mild to the point of being missed in the brief responses a child may make to an interviewer, especially one who relies on closed-ended questions.

Encouraging a child to talk at length and without interruption may be the best way to obtain samples of speech that will demonstrate problems with rate, repetition, lack of prosody, dropped sounds, and other possible deficits of speech perception and speech production. Asking the patient to tell a story or recount an event is one way to accomplish this objective—for example, "Tell me how you get to school in the morning," or "Can you finish this story? Once upon a time, in a land far away, there lived a. . . . " Some patients with LD may speak in one- or two-word sentences; leave sentences incomplete; and have trouble coming up with the right words in describing their experiences, feelings, and needs. Others may respond inappropriately or appear not to understand. Still others may seem inattentive, ask many questions before comprehending, or appear to forget easily what they have been told.

An audio recording of the evaluation (made with parental permission) can facilitate speech analysis after the child has left the office; a video recording may help discern signs of tension (eye blinking, fist clenching, facial grimacing) that often accompany stuttering. Pursue responses that seem inappropriate by asking the child, "What did I just ask?" Also watch for shyness, aloofness, or withdrawal, any of which may indicate a communication disorder.

Apart from listening to the child produce language, assess the following:

- Use of symbols—for example, does the child let a paper cup represent a house, or a stick stand for a car?
- Ability to comprehend language—can the child follow a command that is given without the use of gestures?

A rule of thumb for stuttering is to obtain formal evaluations of children who show dysfluencies that are frequent (3% of speech or more) or long (half a second or more of repeated short words or syllables). Also watch for associated physical signs of distress, such as blinking, clenching of fists, or glancing sideways.

Developmental Factors

As with so many other childhood disorders, early identification of communication disorders often occurs in severely affected patients. A mild case of LD may go unnoticed until a patient's teens, the age at which language normally begins to develop the rich complexity characteristic of adult speech. However, you will find instances where problems with language reception become evident by the grade school years. Rarely, very young children may have so much difficulty comprehending speech that they appear deaf when spoken to; older children may seem only confused.

In older children, a deficit in vocabulary may only affect certain word types—nouns, for example, or personal pronouns. However, younger children affected to a similar degree may commit vocabulary errors for a variety of word types.

Older children and those with less severe SSD will have trouble with the more difficult consonant sounds, such as *s, z, sh,* and *ch.* Younger children may also have problems with the easier consonants that are learned earlier—*h, m, t, d, n, h,*—and are especially likely to omit sounds, such as at the beginning and end of words. Stuttering usually begins in early childhood, between the ages of 2 and 7; onset after the age of 10 is rare. Because individuals who stutter often avoid words that they know will cause them trouble, asking older children to read from a text may help in identifying the stuttering.

F84.0 AUTISM SPECTRUM DISORDER

If ever a diagnostic category could be said to be in flux, it is the one we now call autism spectrum disorder (ASD). Early in the lifetimes of some clinicians still working today, it wasn't even known. It achieved official status with DSM-III in 1980, and was split into several parts in DSM-IV; in DSM-5, those parts were joined in a unitary concept that encompassed patients with a variety of symptoms and disabilities. Throughout its history, the descriptions and definitions (and debate as to causation) of ASD have been in almost constant ferment.

Relevant still today are the clinical observations of Leo Kanner, a child psychiatrist at Johns Hopkins University who in 1943 first described 11 children with the syndrome. His patients shared a fundamental inability to interact socially and to use language appropriately. All manifested a range of limited, odd, stereotypic behaviors. Kanner believed that the condition was congenital and familial, though because the children appeared normal at birth, their parents weren't immediately alarmed.

Concern often arises during the second 6 months of life, when parents note problems with socialization. An infant does not make eye-to-eye contact, smile, or nuzzle into a parent's neck and chest when being held, preferring instead to arch away and stare into space. During early visits to the pediatrician, parents may be told, "Everything will be OK—your baby is doing well." Pediatricians may show their concern when language is late in appearing, most often after 3 years of age. By then, a range of symptoms will probably be evident.

The symptom spectrum of these individuals is currently divided into two principal groups.

1. Social interaction and communication:

   ● They don't understand relationships, as shown by a relative lack of interest in making friends or sharing in fantasy play; they don't cuddle; toddlers may not extend their arms in anticipation of being picked up.

   ● They don't communicate well by nonverbal means such as eye contact, facial expression, body language, and hand gestures (they don't point to things).

   ● They have trouble with what's called *social–emotional reciprocity*—the sort of shared interest that people normally experience with one another; they don't initiate (or even participate in) social interactions such as ordinary conversation.

2. Restricted or repetitive behaviors that manifest in abnormal patterns of interests and activities:

   ● Play may be repetitive and nonsymbolic; toys are objects to suck or twirl; these individuals may use peculiar speech phrases, echolalia, or other stereotypies. Some will show compulsive rocking, hand flapping, head banging, or maintenance of posture oddly reminiscent of catatonic behavior.

- They cling to routine, insisting on the same patterns of both verbal and nonverbal behavior, perhaps becoming distraught when forced to deviate from what is usual for them. This is especially relevant for adequate nutrition, because children with ASD often refuse new foods and insist on a range of foods that is too narrow.

- They tend to be preoccupied with a tiny selection of sometimes unusual objects or interests, to the exclusion of all else.

- Some children are exquisitely sensitive to sensory input. They hate bright lights or loud sounds, and even the prickly feel of certain types of cloth or other surfaces may bother them to an extreme degree. Alternatively, some appear insensitive to pain or extremes of temperature.

Children with ASD may not bond normally (such as following a parent from room to room). Calling a toddler's name may elicit no response; normal fear of strangers or anxiety at separation from parents may be absent. Although younger children with ASD are often hyperactive, as teenagers they tend to slow down and may even become less active than is usual for adolescents. Their sleep may be compromised by initial insomnia or early morning awakening; rarely, children may experience a complete reversal of the night–day patterns of sleeping.

More seriously affected patients will have impaired use of language, ranging from peculiar speech patterns to absence of speech (in nearly half) to failure to use even nonverbal communication, such as head nods or facial expressions appropriate to mood or situation. Those who do speak may be unable to comprehend humor; communication may suffer because children with ASD do not understand that words can have multiple or abstract meanings. Their speech may lack prosody, the normal lilt that makes it musical. They may talk to themselves or hold forth at great length on subjects that interest no one else; others may be unable to begin or sustain normal conversation.

Although many children with ASD have some degree of intellectual impairment, about one-fourth register IQs of greater than 70; some patients are actually quite bright. Seizure disorders are especially likely to develop in those who also have significant intellectual impairment. Sometimes present are so-called *cognitive splinter skills*, including abilities in computation, music, or rote memory that far exceed an ordinary person's capabilities (*savantism*).*

In general, social development takes place much more slowly than normal, and in phases that occur out of the expected sequence. Although the degree of disability varies

---

*The 1988 film *Rain Man* features Dustin Hoffman playing a man with ASD who has the savant ability to count objects very rapidly. The film won four Academy Awards, including best picture and best actor for Hoffman.

widely, the effect upon the lives of most patients and their families is profound and permanent.

Not too long ago, ASD was thought to occur relatively infrequently; prevalence rates
of 4 children in 10,000 were reported. Over the past several decades, however, rates as high
as 1 in 68 have been observed—in part as a result of more complete ascertainment. The
disorder affects all socioeconomic and cultural groups. Boys strongly outnumber girls (4:1 or
5:1), but a girl with ASD is likely to be more severely affected and to have comorbid intellectual disability.

The etiologies of ASD are unknown, but most experts believe that genetic vulnerabil-
ity and biological failures in neuronal development during gestation are responsible. Family
pedigree and twin studies suggest that genetics (multiple genes) account for perhaps half
the variance. ASD is associated with several medical illnesses: congenital rubella, phenylketonuria, tuberous sclerosis, and a history of perinatal distress. The age of both mothers and
fathers is directly proportional to the risk for having a child with ASD.

During adolescence, seizures develop in up to one-fourth of patients. Minor physical
abnormalities (such as a high-arched palate) are often discovered on examination. Cerebral
ventricular enlargement with increased head circumference at birth has been reported, as
has high platelet serotonin level (an abnormality also noted in many children who have
intellectual disability *without* features of autism).

Jonathan

Because his mother's concerns about Jonathan's peculiar behavior had been dismissed as
trivial by their family physician, he was almost 5 when she first brought him to the specialty
clinic. Now many aspects of his behavior worried her. He had gradually become unmanage-
able in public places. He wouldn't follow directions and rejected the structure of school;
when confronted, he boisterously disrupted those about him. Yet, when left alone, he would
watch television by the hour, preferring to view the same videos over and over. He had no
friends and did not seem to want any; for long stretches he played alone in his room, often
with objects that he could twirl. Sometimes he would spin himself, as though he enjoyed
becoming dizzy. If these routines were interrupted, he'd become angry. Then he might hit,
kick, or bite the person who interfered.

Jonathan was a sturdy, handsome youngster—neatly dressed and groomed—who
appeared his stated age. When he and his mother entered the playroom, he didn't acknowledge the presence of the examiner, whom he seemed to gaze right through with a nearly
blank, somehow distressingly pleasant expression on his immobile face.

Jonathan went directly to a toy car on the table and began sniffing it. Next he ran it
back and forth across his chest, while swaying and humming quietly to himself. He refused
to speak with the examiner and avoided eye contact. Yet his hearing was not impaired; he
looked up whenever there was a noise outside the playroom. While his mother related his

ESSENTIAL FEATURES OF **AUTISM SPECTRUM DISORDER**

From early childhood, contact with others affects (to some extent) nearly every aspect of how these patients function. Social relationships vary from mild impairment to almost complete lack of interaction. There may be just a reduced sharing of interests and experiences, though some patients fail utterly to initiate or respond to the approach of others. They tend to speak with few of the usual physical signals most people use—eye contact, hand gestures, smiles, and nods. Relationships with other people founder, so that patients with ASD have trouble adapting their behavior to different social situations; they may lack general interest in other people and make few, if any, friends.

Repetition and narrow focus characterize these individuals' activities and interests. They resist even small changes in their routines (perhaps demanding exactly the same menu every lunchtime, or endlessly repeating already answered questions). They may be fascinated with movement (such as spinning) or small parts of objects. The reaction to stimuli (pain, loud sounds, extremes of temperature) may be either feeble or excessive. Some are unusually preoccupied with sensory experiences: They are fascinated by visual movement or particular smells, or they sometimes fear or reject certain sounds or the feel of certain fabrics. They may use peculiar speech, or show stereotypies of behavior such as hand flapping, body rocking, or echolalia.

The Fine Print

Note that there are varying degrees of ASD. What DSM-IV called Asperger's disorder is relatively milder; many of these people communicate verbally quite well, yet still lack the other skills needed to form social bonds with others.

The D's: • Duration (from early childhood, though symptoms may appear only later, in response to the demands of socialization) • Distress or disability (social, educational, occupational, or personal impairment) • Differential diagnosis (ordinary children can have strong preferences and enjoy repetition; intellectual disability; stereotypic movement disorder; obsessive–compulsive disorder; social anxiety disorder; language disorder)

Coding Notes

Specify:

   {With} {Without} accompanying intellectual impairment
   {With} {Without} accompanying language impairment
   Associated with a known medical or genetic condition or environmental factor
   Associated with another neurodevelopmental, mental, or behavioral disorder
   With catatonia (sidebar, p. 220)

Specify severity (separate ratings are required for social communication and restricted, repetitive behavior).

Social Communication

Level 1 (mild). The patient has trouble starting conversations or may seem less interested in them than most people. Code as "Requiring support."

Level 2 (moderate). There are pronounced deficits in both verbal and nonverbal communication. Code as "Requiring substantial support."

Level 3 (severe). Little response to the approach of others markedly limits functioning. Speech is limited, perhaps to just a few words. Code as "Requiring very substantial support."

Restricted, Repetitive Behaviors

Level 1 (mild). Change provokes some problems in at least one area of activity. Code as "Requiring support."

Level 2 (moderate). Problems coping with change are readily apparent and interfere with functioning in various areas of activity. Code as "Requiring substantial support."

Level 3 (severe). Change is exceptionally hard; all areas of activity are influenced by behavioral rigidity. Causes severe distress. Code as "Requiring very substantial support."

history, he occupied himself by rubbing the car along his leg. Occasionally he returned to his mother and, without speaking, took her hand and guided it toward an object that he could not reach.

At one point during the interview, Jonathan noticed the light switch and began turning it on and off. Later, he flapped his arms repeatedly while walking on his toes around the room, and could not be persuaded to stop. During much of the interview he showed little change in facial expression. Even as he screeched loudly while his mother led him away from the light switch, his mouth was fixed in a smile, rather than an expression more appropriate to pain, anger, or defiance. Results of the Peabody Picture Vocabulary Test suggested an IQ of 75.

When the examiner sat on the floor and began parallel play with a toy car, Jonathan sat nearby and copied the behavior. To the question "What's your name?", Jonathan replied, using exactly the same intonation, "What's your name?" When the examiner tried (with the mother's permission) to hug him, Jonathan froze and arched away. "He's reacted like that since before he was a year old," his mother commented. At one point when his mother left the room, Jonathan hardly seemed to notice her absence, and he ignored her when she returned. At the end of the session, he first resisted leaving. Then suddenly, without saying goodbye, he darted from the playroom, his mother in rapid pursuit.

Evaluation of Jonathan

The criteria for ASD are among the more complicated DSM-5 has to offer in child and adolescent mental health. In part, this is because they need to reflect the way this disorder pervades all areas of a patient's (and family's) life. Here is how Jonathan fulfilled these criteria.

From an early age (Criterion C), his communication and social interactions had been abnormal. His symptoms included multiple impairments of nonverbal behavior (A2: refusal to cuddle, avoidance of eye contact, blank or inappropriate facial expressions) and lack of peer relationships (A3: no apparent interest in making friends). As for social reciprocity (A1), there was no evidence of sharing of interests, and he neither initiated nor responded to social interactions. Note that all three of these A criteria must be met.

Next, we must evaluate Jonathan's behavioral patterns (DSM-5 requires two of four possible types of abnormality). His speech was stereotyped (echolalia as he exactly repeated the examiner's questions), and he twirled and flapped his arms (Criterion B1 for both). By history, he demonstrated a marked preference for sameness (B2: watching the same movie over and over), and his sniffing behavior is an example of hyperactive response to sensory input (B4); a hypoactive response to or interest in sensory stimuli would also fulfill this criterion. We probably need to interview further to learn whether he also showed highly restricted interests (B3), but given the rest of the history, it seems likely.

His symptoms caused impairment both socially and with his schooling (Criterion D). Although his intellectual abilities were below average, his social communication behaviors went far beyond those we'd expect from someone whose sole diagnosis was intellectual disability (Criterion E). Jonathan would qualify for the specifiers *with accompanying intellectual impairment* and *with accompanying language impairment*. Although a number of his physical behaviors were peculiar, they were not of the types (see sidebar, p. 220) that would justify a specifier of *with catatonia*.

In addition, Jonathan showed some other symptoms that were at one time considered emblematic of what we now call ASD, but no longer serve as core symptoms: He seemed to use his mother as a "part object" (guiding her by the hand to obtain a toy), and he used a toy car as an object for self-stimulation, rather than as the symbolic representation of an actual vehicle. Other behavioral features included resisting physical comfort from the examiner and failure to acknowledge his mother's disappearance from the room.

Several additional disorders belong in the differential diagnosis. Note that ASD doesn't protect against the development of **schizophrenia**, which occasionally begins in childhood; the (rare) co-occurrence of these two conditions can lead to diagnostic chaos. Some symptoms of youngsters with ASD can look like prodromal or residual symptoms of schizophrenia—isolation, disorganized behavior, blunted affect, peculiar beliefs or interests. However, patients with schizophrenia almost always appear normal for the first 12 or more years of life, and certainly during the first 3–4 years. For the two diagnoses to be made in a single individual, DSM-5 requires the presence of prominent delusions *and* hallucinations for 1 month—perhaps less, if treatment is rapidly successful. In Jonathan's case, this differential diagnosis was easy: Although he had a notable lack of affect and odd motor behavior, there were no delusions or hallucinations.

Children with **stereotypic movement disorder** have repetitive movements but not the social and language abnormalities that characterize ASD; the two diagnoses can be made simultaneously, but the movement symptoms have to be so pronounced as to be a focus of treatment (not the case for Jonathan). **ADHD** did not seem a likely diagnosis for Jonathan, but up to half of children with ASD also have enough symptoms of hyperactivity or attention deficit to receive that diagnosis. Although Jonathan had significant language delays in both verbal and nonverbal (pragmatics) domains, DSM-5 requires us to choose between ASD and **social (pragmatic) communication disorder.** His parents were supportive and sensitive to his needs, which effectively eliminated **severe psychosocial deprivation** as a competing etiology.

Of course, Johnathan's restricted and repetitive behavior and patterns of interest as well as his impoverished communication skills and social interactions far exceed what we'd expect for a person whose sole diagnosis was (relatively mild) intellectual disability. But should we diagnose concomitant **intellectual disability?** Even though his *measured* IQ was 75 (borderline range), the limits of error could place his *actual* IQ lower than that. We would make the additional diagnosis were he severely or profoundly intellectually disabled, but that is not the case with Jonathan. His intellectual level is low enough, however, that DSM-5 asks us to add a specifier.

Two tasks remain in diagnosing any patient with ASD—the description of severity and the application of descriptive specifiers. DSM-5 asks us to judge not the overall severity of Jonathan's ASD, but to break it down into social communication and restricted, repetitive behaviors. Each is described in terms of the degree of support that will be required (see the Essential Features, p. 185). Jonathan's clinician judged each of these severity levels as requiring very substantial support; however, this is not to say that other patients will not be even more impaired than he was. Jonathan's full diagnosis would thus be as follows:

F84.0	Autism spectrum disorder, with accompanying intellectual impairment, with accompanying language impairment, requiring very substantial support for social communication and for restricted, repetitive behaviors
CGAS	35 (current)

Asperger Syndrome

Although Asperger syndrome (DSM-IV called it Asperger's disorder) was first described at the same time (1944) as classic autism and affects more patients, until the last few years it has been less well known. This is related partly to the obvious, devastating psychopathology of so many children with the broader disease, and partly to the ease with which patients who have Asperger syndrome may be misdiagnosed as having other major mental conditions.

People with this syndrome share the social impairments and idiosyncratic, stereotypic behaviors of other patients with ASD, but their verbal language skills and cognitive functioning are intact. Unlike many other children with ASD, these children do not show delays in language development. Not only may early growth and development appear completely unremarkable, but in many cases intelligence remains normal throughout life (some individuals suffer from mild intellectual disability).

Although they usually like the company and conversation of other people, individuals with Asperger syndrome lack a sense of "social intelligence," making them appear insensitive to the feelings of others. As a result, they often become solitary, perhaps desiring friends but lacking the skills necessary to acquire them. Young adults with this form of ASD may produce words and sentences that seem perfectly normal when written on paper, but their speech is marked by repetition, mild circumstantiality, and absence of the usual prosody and body language that accompany speech in normal persons. Although less physically impaired than is typical of other patients with ASD, these individuals are often notably clumsy as children. Some writers note that the clinical picture is similar to that of schizotypal personality disorder.

Along with childhood disintegrative disorder and Rett's disorder, Asperger's disorder was a new diagnosis in DSM-IV. Like those other diagnoses, it has now been eliminated from the diagnostic nomenclature.* Because it presents a picture so different from many other cases of ASD, we have retained the following illustrative vignette.

Arthur

When Arthur was born, his mother expressed relief. Her first baby, a premature boy, had died when he was only 2 weeks old. But pink, chubby Arthur had been the picture of health, as his milestones attested. He spoke words at 14 months and sentences at 18 months. He was toilet-trained when he was 28 months old. Although he stood alone at 10 months and walked at 1 year, he fell down a good deal and walked with a rolling gait; his mother called him her "little sailor."

After only a few weeks of nursery school, the teacher requested a conference with Arthur's parents. She said that Arthur seemed to enjoy the company of other children, but pointed out that his approach to them—screaming or punching to get their attention—was self-defeating in the extreme. She also noted that whenever she tried to talk to him, he

---

* At about the time that DSM-5 was published in 2013, many patients with DSM-IV diagnoses of Asperger's disorder protested the loss of a diagnosis that affords them identity.

would turn his gaze away from her. When he spoke, his voice had a certain steady quality to it she couldn't quite define—"like he was singing, only just on one note."

Nevertheless, with above-average intelligence (Full Scale WISC-V IQ = 116), Arthur made good progress throughout school. He was referred for evaluation when he was in the sixth grade, only because he seemed have no friends outside his own family. Instead, he had two consuming interests: telephone systems and his CD collection. Arthur had memorized huge quantities of information about the history, construction, maintenance, and even financing of telephone systems. His room was strewn with parts of numerous old telephones, and in the basement he had assembled a manual switchboard with plugs that actually worked. His CD collection was highly specialized—nothing but original-cast musicals. According to his mother, if anyone disturbed the precise order in which he had arranged his collection, he would fly into a rage. Even then, his voice showed little modulation, though his speech was clear and coherent, and he could express complex ideas.

During the interview, Arthur spoke clearly but monotonously about telephone line repair, ignoring the examiner's attempts to change the subject.

Evaluation of Arthur

Arthur's social communication deficits caused him obvious difficulties. He had no friends other than within his family (Criterion A3), and his approach to other children was obviously abnormal (A1). His lack of eye contact was just one example of deficient nonverbal communication (A2); speaking in a monotone was another.

What about his behavior? We don't know of any actual stereotypies, but his interests were highly restricted to his telephone equipment (B3). Furthermore, he became irate whenever the exact order of his CD collection was disturbed (B2). These two characteristics would be enough to enable us to label his behavior as restrictive/repetitive.

Arthur's symptoms had begun early in his life (C); the impairment they caused him was manifested in the conversation his parents had with his teacher (D). **Intellectual disability** was not an issue (E).

Had Arthur been referred for evaluation when he was a few years older, someone not alerted by his early history might have thought he had **schizoid personality disorder.** However, that condition usually becomes apparent later in life and impairs social interaction to a lesser extent than was true of Arthur. Although his highly circumscribed interests superficially resembled the obsessions of **obsessive–compulsive disorder,** OCD doesn't usually restrict a child's interests so severely as with Arthur. OCD does often begin in childhood, however.

Of course, the degree of impairment for any patient is a matter of clinical judgment. For Arthur, we could make a case for either "Requiring support" or "Requiring substantial support" for both social communication and restricted, repetitive behaviors. Arthur's clinician chose the least severe category because many other children are much more seriously

Whatever happened to Rett's disorder? DSM-IV's *pervasive developmental disorders*, the umbrella classification for the spectrum encompassing classic autism and its cousins, included a subtype called Rett's disorder. First described in 1966, Rett's disorder didn't achieve worldwide recognition until the first English-language publication describing it appeared in 1983.

After the first few months of life, about 1 in 10,000 girls lose already acquired purposeful hand movements and begin making stereotyped hand-washing movements. They may also grind their teeth and have trouble with chewing, as well as breathing difficulties (hyperventilation, air swallowing, or apnea). Those who can walk at all have a stiff-legged gait. These children lose already acquired language abilities and show little or no interest in objects or other people; three-fourths or more have seizures. Their intellectual disability is often severe or profound. With capacity for self-care often completely lost, the effects upon a child and family are devastating, though the child may ultimately regain some ability to communicate (chiefly by visual contact).

In 1999, the responsible factor was found to be a new mutation of a gene located on the X chromosome; because in any given patient the mutation has just occurred, the disease is not inherited from either parent, and siblings are not affected. Affected boys usually do not survive.

So whatever happened to Rett's disorder? Now called Rett syndrome, it's still around—though it is better defined and better understood, and is no longer considered a major subgroup of ASD. This change reflects its proven monogenetic etiology and the fact that autistic features are usually prominent only during years 1–4 of a child's life. In DSM-5, if autistic symptoms warrant an ASD diagnosis, you add the specifier *associated with Rett syndrome.*

affected than he was; other clinicians might choose differently. Arthur's full diagnosis would be as follows:

F84.0	Autism spectrum disorder, without accompanying language or intellectual impairment, requiring support for social communication and for restricted, repetitive behaviors
CGAS	45 (current)

ASSESSING AUTISM SPECTRUM DISORDER

General Suggestions

Perhaps more than any other diagnosis, ASD will tax your ability to evaluate a differential diagnosis. This is because aspects of these disorders overlap with so many others; you may need to rule out neurological disorders, many other major mental disorders, and (when a patient has reached young adulthood) schizotypal or schizoid personality disorder. Children with ASD may be clumsy or have other voluntary motor problems, so you must pay careful attention to gross and fine motor coordination; a child may even be diagnosable as also having developmental coordination disorder.

Some children with ASD don't speak, and those who do may use language inappropriately. They may ask overly personal questions. (An appropriate response to a personal question is often some variation of "I can't tell you that, but I can let you look to see what's in this toy box.") As in the evaluation of other young patients, following a child's own favorite interests or pastimes and demonstrating willingness to enter into the child's activities may help you to form some relationship with the child. And as it often is for children who have intellectual disability, the default answer for children with ASD to questions they don't completely understand is "yes."

When you are evaluating a child for ASD, it is critical to note how readily the child interacts verbally and affectively with you. Does this child appear indifferent? Refuse physical contact? Even fail to make eye contact? You may sometimes find it helpful to rock or sway, mirroring (but being careful not to mock) the child's own behavior. After a time, the child may be willing to follow your motions, thus establishing a connection at some level and helping you assess how far the child is willing/able to relate to others, even on an entirely nonverbal level.

About 30% of these children are also cognitively impaired; performance on nonverbal IQ subtests is usually better than that on verbal subtests. Like those with intellectual disability, people with ASD can have such widely varying abilities that it is a good idea to put aside any preconceived notions about a patient's capabilities. Such a child can challenge your interactional skills and experience as an interviewer, perhaps more so than one with any other severe disability. Several sessions may be needed to complete an evaluation.

Developmental Factors

There is considerable individual variation in age of onset. Recognition of Asperger-like symptoms may not occur until well into toddlerhood, when expected degrees of socialization fail to develop. (Home videos can sometimes help establish whether there was early normal development.) But the diagnosis of ASD may be suspected in children as young as 1 year by their stiff resistance to cuddling, failure to raise their arms to be lifted, inconsistent social smile, and resistance to new experiences (especially new foods). In the second year, their social aloofness may become apparent in their lack of shared attention, failure to point, or unwillingness to hold the gaze of an adult. Later, the delay in spoken language will become apparent.

ATTENTION-DEFICIT/HYPERACTIVITY DISORDER

Through multiple changes in criteria and even more changes of name, attention-deficit/hyperactivity disorder (almost always abbreviated ADHD) remains one of the most frequently diagnosed mental health conditions of childhood. When evaluated over a series of studies, it is found in about 7% of school-age children—and it may be increasing. It affects boys over twice as often as it does girls (to a degree, girls may be underidentified); the gender disparity disappears with maturity. It is less commonly diagnosed by Europeans, who think that North Americans often mislabel children who "only" have a disorder of conduct.

Symptoms usually begin before a child goes to school; the definition requires some symptoms before age 12, though the diagnosis is usually made several years into elementary school. Mothers sometimes report that their children with ADHD cried more than their other babies, or that they were colicky, irritable, or wakeful (or even kicked excessively before they were born).

ADHD has long been noted to run in families, and a genetic basis is now generally accepted; indeed, heritability may be around 75%. Evidence for environmental influence has been found for maternal smoking and alcohol consumption, and for childhood exposure to toxins such as lead. Putative factors that have *not* held up to scientific scrutiny include television viewing and a diet rich in carbohydrates or artificial coloring.

Although some children may show only symptoms of hyperactivity/impulsiveness, the vast majority also (some, exclusively) have symptoms of inattention. The hyperactive/impulsive presentation is especially encountered in younger children. But the presentations (DSM-IV called them *types*) are unstable. Disruptiveness, poor-quality schoolwork, clumsiness, and impulsive comments often make these children unpopular with peers and adults alike. For a full evaluation, behavior should be assessed in the various environments inhabited by a child or adolescent—home, school, social relationships, possibly work. The environment can itself affect symptoms; it has been noted that children with ADHD control themselves better when in a clinician's office—and when their fathers are present. Performance is better early in the day, and with simpler tasks.

Oppositional defiant disorder and, to a lesser extent, conduct disorder are often comorbid with ADHD, with the latter commonly developing first. Persistent depressive disorder (dysthymia) and anxiety disorders are comorbid in 25–30% of children with ADHD. The distinction is important, because children who have comorbid disorders may benefit from medication plus psychosocial treatments, whereas children who have only ADHD are likely to do well with medication alone.

With adolescence, the symptoms of ADHD usually tail off, though aspects of the disorder itself sometimes persist into adult life. ADHD is also a risk factor for later depressive and anxiety disorders, and many such children are at risk for substance or alcohol abuse.

ESSENTIAL FEATURES OF
ATTENTION-DEFICIT/HYPERACTIVITY DISORDER

Teachers notice and refer for evaluation these children, who are forever in motion, disrupting class by their restlessness or fidgeting, jumping out of their seats, talking endlessly, interrupting others, seeming unable to take turns or to play quietly.

In fact, hyperactivity is only half the story. These children may also have difficulty paying attention and maintaining focus on their work *or* play—the inattentive bit. Readily distracted (and therefore disliking and avoiding sustained mental effort such as homework), they neglect details and therefore make careless errors. Their poor organization skills result in lost assignments or other materials and an inability to follow through with chores or appointments.

These behaviors invade many aspects of their lives, including school, family relations, and social life away from home. Somewhat modified, these behaviors may accompany them through the teen years and beyond.

The Fine Print

The D's: • Duration and demographics (6+ months; onset before age 12) • Disability (social, educational, occupational, or personal impairment) • Differential diagnosis (intellectual disability; anxiety and mood disorders; autism spectrum disorder; conduct or oppositional defiant disorder; intermittent explosive disorder; specific learning disorders; disruptive mood dysregulation disorder; psychotic or other mental or personality disorders)

Coding Notes

Specify (for the past 6 months):

> **F90.0 Predominantly inattentive presentation.** Inattentive criteria are met, but not hyperactive/impulsive.
> **F90.1 Predominantly hyperactive/impulsive presentation.** The reverse.
> **F90.2 Combined presentation**. Both criteria sets are met.
> **In partial remission.** When the condition persists (perhaps into adulthood), enough symptoms may be lost that the full criteria are no longer met but impairment persists.

Specify current severity:

> **Mild.** Relatively few symptoms are found.
> **Moderate.** Intermediate.
> **Severe.** Many symptoms are experienced, far more than required for diagnosis.

Randy

Her experience with his two placid brothers left his mother ill prepared for 8-year-old Randy. "He never did learn to walk—when he was 10 months old, he started to run. He's been running ever since," she told the interviewer.

"Even before he went to school, I knew he was different. His brothers could sit and color or build with blocks by the hour, but Randy would only last a few minutes. And every evening I'd have to remind him to feed the dog. But he was very quick to learn even complicated things, if you could just get his interest."

In the first grade Randy did quite well. It was a small "demonstration" class, and there was a student teacher who redirected his obvious, persistent overactivity enough to keep him out of trouble. But this year the class size had grown, and complaining notes from his new teacher accompanied Randy home in a steady stream. One read in part: " . . . and he answers questions I've asked other children. He often interrupts me, even before I've finished asking. It doesn't help that he's often right." He would talk during "quiet period," and he *never* stayed in his seat longer than 5 minutes, unless the teacher stood directly over him. Then Randy would wriggle, squirm, tap his fingers, or make popping sounds with his mouth until no one near him could concentrate any better than he could.

His mother had noted many of the same problem behaviors at home. He wouldn't finish his homework unless she or his father stood over him; he would be distracted by his brothers, the TV, the cat, or a spider spinning a web in the corner. The work he completed was hurried and "filled with mistakes that he shouldn't have made, he's so bright."

"His father was like that when he was a kid—he's a research chemist now, but he still has trouble concentrating. But Randy must have gotten his disposition from my side of the family; he's pretty happy-go-lucky and positive. Even his brothers like him, though they complain that he's always butting in."

During the first interview, Randy sat at the art table and cheerfully drew a crayon picture of a child drawing a picture with crayons. He was a freckle-faced redhead who admitted that sometimes he didn't behave very well. "I can't seem to help it," he said, then added brightly, "Maybe I'll learn how next year." He said that his teacher didn't seem to like him much. "Miss Rucker says I'm careless and lose my things, like my pencil and my books. And when she lifted up my desk top and showed the class how my stuff looked inside, the kids all laughed."

Later, commenting on Randy's quiet behavior during the interview, his mother said, "He was that way when we took him to the pediatrician, too. It's like trying to get your TV fixed—it always works fine in the shop."

Evaluation of Randy

ADHD can be diagnosed with relatively few symptoms, but there must be at least six in either the inattention or the hyperactivity–impulsiveness group. Randy had symptoms in both of these groups. In the inattention group, he often made careless mistakes (Criterion A1a), did not sustain attention (A1b), seemed not to listen (A1c), didn't complete chores (A1d), had trouble organizing things (A1e: messy desk), lost school supplies (A1g), and was easily distractible (A1h). In the hyperactivity–impulsiveness group, he squirmed (A2a), roamed the classroom (A2b), talked during quiet period (A2d), was excessively on the go (A2e), talked far too much (A2f), and answered questions for the other children in the classroom (A2g). Even his brothers found him intrusive (A2i).

Some of Randy's symptoms had been present from youngest child-

A couple of generations ago, the hallmark of ADHD was considered to be fidgety behavior, which determined one of its former names: *hyperactive child syndrome*. These children were described as "motorically driven," as always running, and as having trouble sitting quietly. In the last decade or two, problems maintaining attention became a new focus for this disorder, now somewhat clumsily renamed attention-deficit/hyperactivity disorder (no wonder the abbreviation ADHD has become popular!). More recent work suggests yet another theory: namely, that it results from delayed development of brain mechanisms responsible for self-control and the inhibition of impulses. If support for this construct continues to accumulate, a future edition of the diagnostic manuals may confer yet another name on this puzzling, widely prevalent condition.

hood (B), and the problems that resulted from his behavior were evident both at school and home (C); his teacher's note makes it clear that his symptoms did interfere with his academic success. But to judge from the exclusions listed (E), DSM-5 seems to regard ADHD as something of a diagnosis of late (though not last) choice. Therefore, could any other disorder explain Randy's symptoms? Children with **autism spectrum disorder** do not communicate as well as Randy. **Intellectual disability** could be ruled out by the fact that he learned quickly, once his attention was captured. Patients with **mood disorders** (especially bipolar disorders) may be agitated or have a poor attention span; although Randy's demeanor was cheerful, more information would have to be obtained from his parents about depressive and manic symptoms, as well as symptoms of **anxiety disorders**. Of course, there was no evidence whatsoever for a **psychotic disorder** such as **schizophrenia**. Many patients with **Tourette's disorder** are also hyperactive; the vignette includes no evidence for **motor or vocal tics**, and his parents would have to be asked about these. Although DSM-5 advises ruling out **personality disorders**, such a diagnosis would be hard to sustain in a child so young.

Children reared in a **chaotic social environment** can be hyperactive or inattentive; as far as our information goes, Randy's home life was stable and supportive. The vignette contains no evidence of willful misbehavior that would suggest other **behavior disorders**, such as **oppositional defiant disorder** or **conduct disorder**, both of which often accompany ADHD. In fact, Randy seemed to feel bad that he could not control himself. **Specific learning disorders** can also be comorbid with ADHD and the disruptive behavior disorders, and should be considered in the differential diagnosis of any child who acts out in school.

Because Randy exhibited symptoms sufficient for diagnosis in both the hyperactivity–impulsiveness and inattention groups, his subtype diagnosis would be *combined presentation*. In fact, this is the most common subtype in older children (small children most commonly qualify for the *predominantly hyperactive/impulsive presentation*). Randy's diagnosis, pending a further interview with his parents, would be as follows:

F90.2	Attention-deficit/hyperactivity disorder, combined presentation
CGAS	65 (current)

F90.8 Other Specified Attention–Deficit/Hyperactivity Disorder

F90.9 Unspecified Attention–Deficit/Hyperactivity Disorder

Children who are hyperactive or who have problems maintaining attention but who do not fulfill the criteria for ADHD may be coded as having either other specified or unspecified ADHD. The former diagnosis may be used for cases in which you wish to specify why a child does not meet the criteria for ADHD or any other particular neurodevelopmental disorder.

ASSESSING ATTENTION-DEFICIT/HYPERACTIVITY DISORDER

General Suggestions

Evaluating behavior that is hyperactive, inattentive, oppositional, disruptive, or otherwise difficult to control can pose a challenge to any interviewer, no matter how experienced. Though many children who come for evaluation of hyperactivity or oppositional behavior may fidget and squirm, significant hyperactivity is often not evident when such a child is being interviewed. New situations or environments, such as a first office visit, sometimes act to suppress activity. Serial observations over several visits may bring disruptive behaviors to the fore. Negativism may only become manifest with adults a child knows well. However, even a single meeting may be enough to reveal inattention to conversation, disorganized play with dolls and toys, or inability to wait for turns when playing a game.

In no other area of child mental health is it more important to seek out and use multiple resources; the combination of unknowing parents with an unreliable child—children don't become dependable observers of their own problem behaviors until around age 9—is a setup for diagnostic confusion. As the child ages, it becomes more and more important to assess the effects of behaviors in school.

Developmental Factors

In toddlers and preschool children, ADHD can be difficult to discriminate from inattentiveness resulting from the normal drive for exploration. Then you must place even greater emphasis than usual on the histories from parents *and* teachers. (DSM-5 requires these behaviors to be reported in at least two settings.) Older children may be self-aware enough to report feeling inner restlessness. Younger children tend to be more hyperactive/impulsive; older ones more often tend to have the combined presentation of ADHD. Adolescents (and adults) experience problems with attention and organization, and are far less likely than younger children to show signs of frank motor hyperactivity.

Although the DSM-5 criteria for ADHD specify only a 6-month duration, it may be safer to consider symptoms that have lasted 12 months or longer, especially in young children.

SPECIFIC LEARNING DISORDER

A specific learning disorder (SLD) is a specific problem in acquiring or using a basic academic skill (reading, writing, or arithmetic). This problem must be out of proportion to a child's age and cannot be explained by factors such as culture, another mental disorder, sensory deficit (such as a vision or hearing impairment),* socioeconomic status, or exposure to teaching. These exclusions are important, for they help to define a set of problems in which there is a discrepancy between the child's actual academic achievement and theoretical ability to learn—an inconsistency that some have called *unexpected* because it is not predicted by the person's intelligence or exposure to teaching methods.

Although the presence of an SLD will be suspected from the history given by a parent, making the diagnosis requires an individually administered, standardized test. Of course, to be valid, any such instrument must be culturally appropriate and sensitive. Like almost all other disorders in DSM-5, SLDs cannot be diagnosed unless they have consequences for scholastic, work, or social life. Because of differing standards and methods of ascertainment, the epidemiology of SLDs remains highly speculative. The lifetime general population prevalence of any form of SLD is probably 10% or even higher. SLD with impairment in reading is by far the most common type; the others are probably highly correlated with it.

The magnitude of a learning disorder's behavioral and social consequences is directly related to the severity of the impairment and to the educational remediation and social

---

*Actually, the child *can* have a sensory deficit or intellectual disability, but the SLD must be worse than what you'd expect as a result.

The *specific* part of the name *specific learning disorder* refers, oddly, to the fact that in diagnosing learning disorders, we must rule *out* several specific causes. That is, the ability to read, write, or do math is not impeded by a sensory problem, such as dim vision or being hard of hearing; nor is it what you might expect from a person with intellectual disability or other mental disorder; nor from any other medical disorder (such as a neurological problem). Nor can the SLD be due to lack of opportunity to learn (poverty, failure to attend school). The fact that it may be limited to one facet of an academic skill (such as accurate spelling) is given as yet another reason to regard these disorders as specific. The best reason of all, in our opinion, to label these deficits as *specific*: They are presumed to have a biological basis that includes genetic and environmental factors that affect brain development.

support available. About three-quarters of children with SLDs have social problems with peers; low self-esteem is also a frequent consequence. Over 30% of children formally diagnosed with SLDs never receive a regular high school diploma, as compared with the national average of under 20%. Associated childhood behavioral disorders include conduct disorder, oppositional defiant disorder, ADHD, and various communication disorders. In fact, some authorities believe that communication disorders and learning disorders belong on a continuum, rather than being separate entities. DSM-5 does not take this approach, however.

F81.0 SLD with Impairment in Reading

Called reading disorder in earlier DSMs, and also often called dyslexia, SLD with impairment in reading is the best studied of the SLDs. It occurs when a child (or adult, should it persist) has any of these three problems related to reading: (1) reads words inaccurately, (2) reads slowly or haltingly, or (3) has difficulty understanding what's meant by the text (comprehension). Fluency of reading is the main issue. Comprehension and poor vocabulary may result, due to insufficient reading. Difficulties with reading can present as disruption in the classroom or noncompliance with homework assignments.

SLD with impairment in reading probably affects about 5% of school-age children, and the percentage affected would probably be higher than that if reading comprehension were routinely considered. Boys are usually overrepresented by 3:1 to 4:1, though in populations carefully defined by research criteria, the male-to-female ratio may be closer to unity. These findings suggest that boys are only more likely to be referred; perhaps other factors (activity level?) cause parents or teachers to decide that they need evaluation.

SLD with impairment in reading has been attributed to a variety of causes. Unless treated, it doesn't improve with time, so it cannot be viewed as just a lag in maturation. Some studies suggest that approximately half the risk for this disorder may have a genetic basis: Many patients have a parent with dyslexia, and in monozygotic twin pairs where one twin has dyslexia, two-thirds of the co-twins are also affected. Phonological skills are important to the development of reading ability, and speech sound disorder is often found

ESSENTIAL FEATURES OF **SPECIFIC LEARNING DISORDER**

The patient has important problems with reading, writing, or arithmetic, *to wit*:

Reading is slow or requires inordinate effort, or the patient has marked difficulty grasping the meaning.

There are problems with writing content (not the physical aspects of writing): grammatical errors, ideas that are expressed in an unclear manner or poorly organized, or unusually creative spelling.

The patient experiences unusual difficulty with math facts, calculation, or mathematical reasoning.

Whichever skill is affected, standardized tests reveal scores markedly lower than those expected for a child's age.

The Fine Print

School records of impairment can be used instead of testing for someone 17+ years of age.

The D's: • Demographics (beginning in early school years, though full manifestation may come only when demands exceed patient's abilities) • Disability (social, academic, occupational impairment) • Differential diagnosis (physical disorders such as vision, hearing, or motor performance; intellectual disability; ADHD; lack of adequate instruction; poor language ability)

Coding Notes

Code by area of impairment:

F81.0 With impairment in reading. Specify word reading accuracy, reading rate or fluency, or reading comprehension.

F81.81 With impairment of written expression. Specify spelling accuracy, grammar and punctuation accuracy, or clarity or organization of written expression.

F81.2 With impairment of mathematics. Specify number sense, memorization of arithmetic facts, accurate or fluent calculations, or accurate math reasoning.

For each affected discipline (and subset), specify severity:

Mild. There are some problems, but (often with support) the patient can compensate well enough to succeed.

Moderate. There are marked difficulties will require considerable remediation for proficiency. Some accommodation may be needed.

Severe. Critical problems will be difficult to overcome without intensive remediation. Even extensive support services may not promote adequate compensation.

in the families of patients with dyslexia. Neuroimaging studies have found abnormalities in brain regions (left posterior fusiform cortex) responsible for language functions such as word recognition. Because early stimulation is so important to early development, socially disadvantaged children are especially at risk. Indeed, both behavioral and pharmacological interventions for attention defects have been reported to help patients with dyslexia.

As with so many other childhood disorders, prognosis depends on a number of factors. Foremost among them is severity: Reading at two standard deviations below the mean carries an especially poor outlook. Other factors that suggest a poor prognosis are parents who are poorly educated and a child's lower overall intellectual capabilities (though we know of one child with Down syndrome and an IQ of barely 70 who learned to read sentences phonetically by age 3½). In one follow-up study of 7-year-olds after treatment, 40% were reading normally at age 14. Prognosis in this group was not related to gender, the presence of phonological problems, or ADHD (which is comorbid in about a third of cases).

Tad

Tad Lincoln, the youngest son of Abraham Lincoln, provides an example of how several childhood disorders may occur in a single individual. Tad (his real name was Thomas, but his father thought that his squirming as an infant resembled the motions of a tadpole) probably had what today we'd call ADHD. At that time, his always spirited, often frenetic behavior earned him a variety of epithets, including "spoiled brat" and "the madam's wildcat."

As one biographer put it, "Tad's mind teemed with plans and his body never rested." Even his doting mother, Mary Todd Lincoln, who herself almost certainly had something like somatic symptom disorder, referred to him as "my troublesome Sunshine." White House staff members of the era related tales of Tad's energetic mischief. He ate the strawberries the cook had cultivated out of season for a state dinner; he kicked a chess board balanced across the knees of his father and a visiting judge; he whittled on the White House furniture; he drove goats through the East Room, riding a kitchen chair behind them. He fired a gun from an upstairs window and waved a Confederate flag when his father was reviewing Union troops.

Besides his conduct and activity level, Tad had other developmental problems. Among them was difficulty with pronunciation. Following his father's assassination, 12-year-old Tad was reported to have said, "Papa's tot," meaning that his father had been shot. Another story from about the same time described Tad's efforts to read. His mother showed him a picture of a primate with the word *ape* printed below it. "Monkey," pronounced Tad.

Not long after his father died, Tad was reportedly behaving better. "I am not a President's son now," he was quoted as saying. "I won't have many presents anymore. Well, I will try and be a good boy . . . " He began to study in earnest and drew abreast his agemates in both learning and ambition by age 18, when he died of tuberculosis.

Evaluation of Tad

Was Tad's delay in learning to read better explained by the fact that he abhorred books and study, or was the cause–effect relationship the reverse? Tad's subsequent history argues against physical causes such as **impaired vision or hearing**, and other mental disorders such as **autism spectrum disorder** or **intellectual disability**—though all of these conditions figure in the differential diagnosis of any SLD. One can argue that word substitution (*monkey* for *ape*) is evidence for dyslexia. And what about Tad's difficulty with pronunciation? Of course, a diagnosis of **speech sound disorder** would require a much larger sample of speech than has come down to us by report, as well as evidence that his problems with speech production independently contributed to Tad's difficulties at home, at work, or with studies. At least one observer claimed that Tad had a cleft palate, which is one of the structural defects commonly associated with speech sound disorder. **Cultural factors** should sometimes be considered, as in cases where there is inadequate exposure to the native language.

In the opinion of contemporary observers and some biographers, Tad's developmental delays and undisciplined behavior stemmed from pampering and laziness. A modern diagnosis of ADHD (found in up to 20% of children with an SLD) would require additional symptoms of overactivity, impulsiveness, distractibility, and inattentiveness in a variety of school and social situations.

Without the benefits of modern-day observation and testing, Tad's diagnosis remains uncertain . . . and so we will give no overall diagnosis for Tad Lincoln.

F81.2 SLD with Impairment in Mathematics

Far less is known about SLD with impairment in mathematics than about its counterpart for reading. It may be found in 5–6% of schoolchildren worldwide, with the ratio of boys to girls approximately 1:1. Obviously, it cannot appear until children begin to *do* mathematics—as early as kindergarten, but in most cases by the beginning of second grade. These children may have difficulty performing mathematical operations, ranging from the elementary to the complex: counting, recognizing mathematical symbols, learning math facts (such as multiplication tables), performing simple addition or other operations, comprehending mathematical terms, and understanding story problems.

Perhaps half of such children also have SLD with impairment in reading, which can exacerbate the difficulties with math (consider story problems), and many also qualify for a diagnosis of ADHD. SLD with impairment in mathematics must be discriminated from so-called "math anxiety," which causes some people to avoid math classes and careers that require computation. Recent work suggests that developmental *dyscalculia* (a sometimes-used synonym) results from a brain abnormality in the intraparietal sulcus that is at least partly genetic. Many people continue to have difficulty with mathematics into their adult years, when it can cause them trouble in understanding the risks and benefits commonly encountered in daily life.

F81.81 SLD with Impairment in Written Expression

SLD with impairment in written expression has been explored even less well than the other two SLDs. In part, this is because it is both hard to define and hard to test objectively. It involves copying and putting ideas on paper; mechanical aspects of writing, such as spelling, grammar, and punctuation; and organizing information for flow and sequencing to construct a clear presentation. Difficulties are usually apparent by second grade, when the child begins to make mistakes in grammar, spelling, punctuation, and paragraph organization. In later years, taking lecture notes may be particularly problematic. These children may also have indecipherable handwriting, but don't make the diagnosis if the *only* problem is penmanship. The diagnosis is generally not appropriate if a patient is only poorly coordinated, as in developmental coordination disorder.

The epidemiology of SLD with impairment in writing is murky. Although 1–3% of all school children are stated to be affected with this disorder in the early grades, the prevalence is variously estimated at 6–22% in middle school. It is often comorbid with dyslexia.

ASSESSING SPECIFIC LEARNING DISORDER

General Suggestions

The diagnosis of each type of SLD (aside from the minor qualification for written expression) requires standardized, individually administered tests. Of course, before an evaluation ever gets this far, in nearly every case there will be information from parents and teachers that points the way. For that reason, an interview of a patient with, say, SLD with impairment in reading might best be spent looking for accompanying disorders, such as another SLD, a communication disorder, or ADHD. Learning, motor, and communication disorders are seldom found in isolation.

An effective screen for dyslexia is often to have a child read an age-appropriate selection while you observe for the cardinal three features: slow reading, inaccurate reading, and poor comprehension of the material just read. Don't forget to assess the child's strengths, which may prove to be the "leg-up" for remediation.

Developmental Factors

Obviously, an SLD is unlikely to be diagnosed until a child reaches school age. But even earlier than that, symptoms suggested of later trouble may be apparent. We have tried to condense some of the earlier (and later) symptoms into Table 11.2.

TABLE 11.2. Development of Specific Learning Disorders

Age (years)	Reading	Math	Writing
3–5	Delay in speaking; difficulty pronouncing certain sounds Problems with fine motor control Trouble rhyming, learning nursery rhymes Mispronounces words; uses baby talk Difficulty following directions	Trouble reading numbers, learning to count	Trouble writing own name, copying words, cutting with scissors, coloring within the times
5–6	Can't recognize words that rhyme (*day, way, hay*)	Trouble associating symbols (Arabic numerals) with quantity; trouble counting	Odd positions of hand or arm when writing can occur
7–8	Can't read one-syllable words; trouble with nonphonetic words Substitutes words	Trouble learning basic number facts—addition, subtraction	Fingers cramp when writing; excessive erasures, poor legibility
9–11	When reading aloud: mispronounces words; skips parts of hard words Reads slowly Dislikes reading and doesn't complete assignments	Can't count, handle money, use calendar Doesn't pay attention to sign (+, –); forgets to carry; misplaces digits Trouble retrieving math facts (multiplication tables), remembering dates Avoids activities that involve math	Letters inconsistent in size or unfinished; inattentive to detail when writing
Adolescent–adult	Slow reading; poor comprehension Must read more than once to get sense Doesn't read for pleasure	Poor problem solving	Poor spelling

F82 DEVELOPMENTAL COORDINATION DISORDER

Developmental coordination disorder (DCD) has been a focus of controversy ever since it first appeared in DSM-III-R in 1987. Does DCD deserve to be called a mental disorder, any more than does any physical condition that produces social, educational, or occupational disability? Can it be differentiated from neurological conditions such as dyspraxia? (At times, the two terms have been regarded as more or less synonymous; either is preferable to the old pejorative term, *clumsy child syndrome*.)

Whatever the eventual answers to these questions, the current notion of such a child— one whose motor coordination is seriously below expectation for intelligence and age—may apply to 5% of children ages 5–10 years, with perhaps 2% severely affected. Boys appear to be affected twice as often as girls, though this could be an artifact of discrepant referral; some studies find approximately equal gender representation. Very young children may have delayed milestones, whereas older children may have difficulty with sports or handwork skills that involve fine motor coordination.

The cause of DCD is unknown and does not appear to be anything so simple as a problem with vision. With some studies showing as many as five different patterns of dysfunction, the ultimate "cause" will probably turn out to be a heterogeneous array, including physiological, genetic, neurological, and other contributions. At that point, a name change may be in order.

Tripper

Tripper (his family's nickname for him) was referred for evaluation at the age of 9, with the sole complaint that he was poorly coordinated for his age. "Preternaturally clumsy" was how his father explained it.

Tripper's dad was a professor of early English literature. As a child, he had himself been "locally famous" for poor coordination. "I could stumble on a bare wood floor," he told the interviewing clinician. But by the time he was 16, he had improved enough to play on his school's junior varsity tennis team.

It didn't seem that Tripper would excel at organized sports any time soon. "I couldn't even make the walking team," he said morosely. "Everyone laughs at me and says I'm the clumsiest guy in the galaxy." When he played at all, he was always chosen last for team

ESSENTIAL FEATURES OF
DEVELOPMENTAL COORDINATION DISORDER

Motor skills are so much less well developed than you'd expect, given a child's age, that they get in the way of progress in school, sports, or other activities. The specific motor behaviors involved include general awkwardness; problems with balance; delayed developmental milestones; and slow achievement of basic skills such as jumping, throwing or catching a ball, and handwriting.

The Fine Print

The D's: • Disability (social, academic, occupational, or personal impairment) • Differential diagnosis (physical conditions such as cerebral palsy, intellectual disability, autism spectrum disorder, ADHD)

sports; for the past couple of years, he had spent lunch and recess in the classroom, reading. He did well in classes such as math and English, but his handwriting was nearly illegible. At a time when he should be developing some fluency, his letters tilted and careened into one another—even when he painstakingly drew each character, lifting his pencil several times in the course of a single word. Homework "took forever," and his badly smeared pages often ended up crumpled in a wastebasket.

The product of a full-term, normal delivery, Tripper had had no allergies or unusual diseases. He sat up at 7 months and took his first steps at 13 months; he spoke words and sentences at the developmentally expected ages. His mother remembered that he had required much longer than his siblings to learn to manipulate a spoon, however.

On neurological examination, Tripper attended to the tasks well and appeared to respond normally except when asked to perform motor tasks, such as copying a diamond. "This is going to be tough," he said, then drew a shaky figure with five sides. His WISC-V Verbal IQ was 123, but his Performance IQ was only 79. On the Beery Developmental Test of Visual–Motor Integration, he scored a borderline 77; however, when the motor component was ignored, his Visual–Spatial Integration score was a normal 105.

Evaluation of Tripper

Although Tripper's developmental milestones (sitting, walking) occurred within the normal range, he was particularly clumsy (even demonstrating it on standardized testing, though this is not required for diagnosis). The second half of Criterion A—that there be slowness of execution—was apparent from watching him trying to write with a pencil. His sociability and schoolwork both suffered from it (B). He did not have **intellectual disability** (which can co-occur with DCD, so long as the motor difficulties exceed what you'd expect under the circumstances), and there was no known medical or neurological disorder that could better account for his symptoms (D). He had had these symptoms since he was tiny (C).

His ability to attend to tasks suggested that he did not have **ADHD**; children with ADHD often have accidents or bump into things because their attention is on other matters. (However, ADHD is often comorbid with DCD.) Children with **autism spectrum disorder** are sometimes clumsy, but we can discount this diagnosis on the basis of Tripper's ability to relate to others, including the examiner. The normal physical exam rendered unlikely such **neurological conditions** as cerebellar, peripheral neuromuscular, or connective tissue disorders. Only if his tortured handwriting had been accompanied by mistakes in grammar, spelling, punctuation, or paragraph organization would we make the additional diagnosis of **specific learning disorder with impairment in written expression**. Other learning, mental, or congenital disorders may accompany DCD and should be sought.

As things stand, however, Tripper's full diagnosis would be this:

| F82 | Developmental coordination disorder |
| CGAS | 75 (current) |

ASSESSING DEVELOPMENTAL COORDINATION DISORDER

General Suggestions

Unlike the communication and learning disorders, DCD does not require standardized tests for diagnosis. Rather, you need to be familiar enough with norms for physical ability in children of all ages to recognize deviations. (A toddler learning to walk is naturally wobbly; a 4-year-old who wobbles may have DCD.) Table 3.1 provides approximate ages for some of these milestones. If it seems difficult to draw these children into discussion of their symptoms, focus first on areas where they excel; this may bolster their self-esteem enough to enable them to talk about the areas of deficiency. It is also important to learn the norms for an individual child's playmates and classmates. Ask, "What is your class doing in gym? How do you spend recess?"

Obtain a firsthand demonstration of physical abilities by asking the child to hop on one foot, climb stairs, tie a shoe, catch and throw a ball; to copy symbols such as a diamond, a triangle, and intersecting polygons; to rotate the hands rapidly back and forth at the wrists; and to touch a finger first to the child's own nose, then to your finger. Instead of asking the child to perform these tasks directly, it is often helpful to play the game "Simon Says." Then you can also test the child's ability to concentrate and follow instructions while assessing coordination. Begin with easy tasks and make them progressively more complicated. Join in and have fun. Make testing enjoyable.

Children whose development has regressed (that is, their balance, coordination, or skill has deteriorated from previously achieved landmarks) *must* be assessed for possible medical or neurological disorders with a physical examination and any appropriate lab tests.

Developmental Factors

Of course, because symptoms change with age, assessment depends heavily on the appropriateness of the task in relation to a child's chronological age. Indeed, normal variability in developmental progress argues against diagnosis of DCD before age 5. Many children seem to outgrow their immaturity spontaneously; yet in one study, nearly half of those diagnosed as having DCD when they were 5 were still demonstrably different from an age-matched comparison group by the age of 15. Note that assessment may depend as much on history (delayed developmental milestones) as on a cross-sectional evaluation of the child in an office setting.

F98.4 STEREOTYPIC MOVEMENT DISORDER

Stereotypic movements (or *stereotypies*) are behaviors that an individual seems compelled to repeat over and over without having any particular goal in mind. Early in life, stereotypies are common and normal. Babies often rock themselves and put things into their mouths; they apparently derive comfort or information from these behaviors. But when stereotypies create problems well into later childhood, they may constitute stereotypic movement disorder (SMD). In addition to the more benign behaviors (for example, hand flapping or nail biting), they may include self-injurious acts such as head banging, biting of lips or fingers, picking at places on the skin, and hitting of the child's own body. At the extreme, all this hitting, biting, and even tooth grinding (bruxism) can cause chronic tissue damage.

SMD affects as many as 3% of young children. No one knows how many adults may be affected, though it is probably uncommon except among those with intellectual disability. Body rocking has been reported in some with generalized anxiety disorder. It has been said that head bangers tend to be boys, whereas self-biters are more often girls. In a study of 20 adults with SMD, only 6 were males; many also had a mood or anxiety disorder. Its causes are unknown, though boredom, frustration, or stress may increase the behaviors.

Claudia

At the age of 14, Claudia continued to suck her thumb and rock. When she was 4, her parents had tried behavior modification to break her of the habit. For 2 weeks she gladly accepted the treat (extra dessert at supper), but reverted to thumb sucking when the bribe was no longer forthcoming.

The behavior had persisted throughout her childhood, though by the time she was 10 she had learned to suppress it most of the time when she was in school. At other times it would recur—when she was doing her homework, while she was falling asleep, and even occasionally when she was eating supper. Because of the merciless ribbing she took, especially from the boys in her neighborhood, she had formed few friendships. She had never spent the night at another child's house.

"Nobody much likes me," she said. After this speech, she popped her thumb back into her mouth and curled her index finger across the bridge of her nose as from the waist up she gently rocked, back and forth.

Claudia weighed 8 pounds, 4 ounces when she was born. According to her mother, her developmental milestones occurred at the expected times, and there had been no history of tics or hair pulling. Despite her isolated existence, she enjoyed the company of others and got along well with her two older sisters. Other than a red thumb and slightly protuberant front teeth, her physical examination was completely normal.

"I don't *have* to do it," Claudia said of her thumb sucking. "I just like it."

ESSENTIAL FEATURES OF **STEREOTYPIC MOVEMENT DISORDER**

You can't find another physical or mental cause for the patient's pointless, repeated movements, such as head banging, swaying, biting (of self), or hand flapping.

The Fine Print

The D's: • Demographics (begins in early childhood) • Distress or disability (social, educational, occupational, or personal impairment; self-injury can occur) • Differential diagnosis (obsessive–compulsive disorder, autism spectrum disorder, trichotillomania, tic disorders, excoriation disorder, intellectual disability, substance use disorders, physical disorders)

Coding Notes

Specify:

> **{With} {Without} self-injurious behavior**

Specify current severity:

> **Mild.** Symptoms are readily suppressed behaviorally
> **Moderate.** Symptoms require behavior modification and specific protective measures.
> **Severe.** Symptoms require continuous watching to avert possible injury.

Specify if: Associated with a known medical or genetic condition, neurodevelopmental disorder, or environmental factor (such as intellectual disability or fetal alcohol syndrome)

Evaluation of Claudia

Although thumb sucking isn't usually considered pathological, it was one of the stereotypies reported in 1 of the 20 adults in the study mentioned in the introduction to SMD. DSM-5 specifically mentions body rocking. Neither behavior would qualify at all had it not begun when Claudia was tiny (Criterion C), persisted (A), and interfered with her social development (B). There is no information that would suggest **intellectual disability** or **autism spectrum disorder,** and she specifically denied any compulsive quality to the behavior, as would be the case with **obsessive–compulsive disorder.** Her mother's report ruled out **trichotillomania** and **tic disorders.** Her physical examination was normal, suggesting that no **other medical condition** (especially a neurological disorder, such as Huntington's disease) could explain her behavior. Therefore, no other disorder would seem to explain the behavior better (D).

Claudia required no special protective measures for the sake of her physical health, earning her the specifier *without self-injurious behavior.* Although her behavior wasn't extinguished by behavioral means, she could voluntarily suppress it and she didn't require special protective measures; therefore, her clinician assigned her a *mild* level of severity.

F98.4   Stereotypic movement disorder, without self-injurious behavior, mild
CGAS   65 (current)

ASSESSING STEREOTYPIC MOVEMENT DISORDER

General Suggestions

SMD is one of the few DSM-5 diagnoses that can be made solely by observation. Even so, ask whether stress worsens the abnormal movements. Also, note whether you can distract the patient from the behaviors by directing attention elsewhere (this will be the case with children who do not have SMD). A complete physical exam is strongly indicated; observe for evidence of chronic tissue damage (one preteen girl developed massive bumps on her forearms from repeatedly banging them on the edges of table tops). Ask about other such behaviors as compulsions, hair pulling, and tics.

Developmental Factors

These movements typically begin in the first several years of life, peak during adolescence, and then decrease in frequency. Nearly all children whose movement disorders persist beyond adolescence begin to have symptoms before age 12. Note that the vast majority of adult patients reported with SMD have intellectual disability.

TIC DISORDERS

F95.2 Tourette's Disorder

F95.1 Persistent (Chronic) Motor or Vocal Tic Disorder

F95.0 Provisional Tic Disorder

Tics can be motor or vocal, simple or complex, transient or chronic. These dimensions define the three main members of the tic disorder family. Simple motor tics include grimaces; eye muscle twitches; abdominal tensing; and jerks of shoulder, head, or distal extremities. Simple vocal tics may include barks, coughs, throat clearing, sniffs, and single syllables that may be muttered or called out. Complex tics are more organized patterns of speech or motor movement, such as touching things or imitating the behavior of others.

Tics are rapid and recurrent; they begin suddenly and occur without special rhythm, often in clusters. Although tics are generally involuntary, patients can often temporarily suppress them; they usually disappear during sleep. Under conditions of stress, fatigue, or illness, they may increase in frequency and intensity.

Motor tics first appear during childhood, sometimes in a child as young as 2, and classically involve the upper part of the face (especially eye blinking). Vocal tics begin somewhat later. It is clear, however, that affected children present with a wide range of symptoms. On one end of the continuum is the simple, occasional eye blinking tic when a child is fatigued or under stress. On the other end are the multiple motor and vocal tics so extreme that they preclude participation in a traditional classroom.

Tics leave children feeling out of control of their own bodies and mental processes—an experience that is especially true of Tourette's disorder (TD), which was first described in 1895 by the French neurologist Georges Gilles de la Tourette. These patients have not only multiple motor tics, but also vocal tics; a few (perhaps 10%) eventually utter coarse language (*coprolalia*) at socially inappropriate times. It is still not clear whether there is a developmental progression from transient tics to chronic tics to TD. About 80% of patients with TD and other tic disorders report an intrusive premonitory urge—a feeling of discomfort somewhat similar to an itch or the need to sneeze that comes on just before and is relieved by the tic. Obsessions and compulsions are also common among people with tics or TD.

Tics are common among children; community surveys find them in perhaps 10% of boys and 5% of girls (the range is wide, depending on the study). Of course, these are predominantly transient motor tics, many of which never cause enough concern to warrant an evaluation. Lifetime prevalence of chronic tics is about 1.6%, with boys and girls about equal. Estimates of TD prevalence have recently been revised upward to nearly 1% of the general child population, with boys outnumbering girls 4:1. It may be less common among African American children; only rarely has it been reported in black people living in Africa. The severity of both tics and TD tends to diminish as a child progresses through adolescence.

The perceived frequency and severity of tics in any child are complicated by the social context in which they occur. Family studies suggest that TD is strongly genetic. What is inherited seems to be a genotype not for TD, but for a broadly defined spectrum of disorders that includes tics, TD, and obsessive–compulsive disorder. Other factors possibly associated with the development of TD include stress, maternal smoking during pregnancy, and low birth weight. The underlying pathology is thought to relate to increased dopamine signaling to and from the striatum and basal ganglia.

Although several effective pharmacological (and, more recently, behavioral) treatments exist, TD tends to persist throughout life once it is diagnosed. Some families (and classrooms) are better able than others to mitigate the shame, embarrassment, and guilt that attend the vocal outbursts. The presence of a compassionate, understanding, supportive environment greatly increases the likelihood of enhanced self-esteem and improved social relationships.

The prognosis for other tic disorders is far better. Of course, by definition, transient tics disappear within months. Even "chronic" motor or vocal tics usually wane and disappear within a few years. Motor tics rarely persist into young adulthood and beyond.

Because a tic is defined the same way, regardless of which of the three DSM-5 tic disorders it occurs in, we present only one vignette.

Neal

When Neal was 5, he was referred to a day treatment program because of his hyperactivity and motor tics. Though he could express himself quite well, he had difficulty listening to his kindergarten teacher, who reported that he was impulsive and had a short attention span. These difficulties were first noted at about the time of his parents' divorce. Then Neal often cried, which progressed to temper tantrums and aggressive acting out in the classroom. At the request of the teacher, the family physician started him on Ritalin. He was referred to the day treatment program largely because the Ritalin did not manage his aggression and impulsiveness.

Although Neal's mother hadn't thought he'd been especially hyperactive, she *had* become concerned when the tics began, a few months before that first evaluation. First there was a barely perceptible blinking of his eyes, which occurred many times each day. These minor facial twitches were later coupled with a drawing down of the corners of his mouth. Over

> Let's scrutinize the bare definition of a tic. A *tic* is a movement or vocalization that is all of the following:
>
> *Nonrhythmic.* It occurs without apparent periodicity.
>
> *Rapid.* An individual, simple tic lasts less than a second—it occurs in the blink of an eye, so to speak.
>
> *Repeated.* It's persistent, occurring over and over.
>
> *Sudden.* An individual tic occurs without warning.

ESSENTIAL FEATURES OF **TOURETTE'S DISORDER**

The first tics of patients with this disorder are often eye blinks that appear when the children are age 6 or thereabouts. These are joined by vocal tics, which may initially be grunts or throat clearings. Eventually, patients with TD have multiple motor tics and at least one vocal tic. The best-known tic of all, coprolalia—swear words and other socially unacceptable speech—is relatively uncommon.

The Fine Print

The D's: • Duration and demographics (1+ years; beginning before age 18, though typically by age 4–6) • Differential diagnosis (OCD, other tic disorders, substance use disorders, medical disorders)

ESSENTIAL FEATURES OF **TIC DISORDERS (COMPARED)**

	Tourette's disorder (F95.2)	Persistent (chronic) motor or vocal tic disorder (F95.1)	Provisional tic disorder (F95.0)
Specific tic type	1+ vocal tics and 2+ motor tics	Motor or vocal tics, but *not* both	Motor or vocal tics, or both, in any quantity
Duration	Longer than 1 year		Less than 1 year
Differential diagnosis	No other medical condition or substance use	No other medical condition or substance use; not Tourette's	No other medical condition or substance use; not Tourette's; not chronic motor or vocal tic disorder
Demographics	Must begin by age 18		
Specify if:	—	Motor tics only or Vocal tics only	—
Tic definition	Abrupt, nonrhythmic, quick, repeated		

The Fine Print

In TD, motor and vocal tics need not occur in the same time frame.

a 6-month period, these single motor tics became ever more frequent and developed into a complex series of muscle twitches in patterns that involved his face, neck, arms, and hands. The treatment center staff discontinued the Ritalin when his tics became obvious, but their intensity and severity continued to increase. Sometimes Neal's tics seemed almost to yank him from his chair onto the floor. All the while, the gentler facial grimacing continued as well.

Then, when Neal was nearly 7, the vocal tics appeared. They started as soft, grunting sounds he would make whenever his shoulder twitched, but within a few months he was uttering barks, sniffs, and grunts that gradually became louder. Most of these verbal outbursts were unintelligible; soon, however, clearly audible, sexually explicit words crept into his output.

As the treatment team came to know him better, it was apparent that Neal was also beset with compulsive rituals. He organized his desk at school into small compartments and carefully placed his possessions into specific sectors. He also repetitively counted the ceiling tiles in his bedroom.

On close examination, his mother was noted to have occasional facial grimaces and mild motor head-jerking tics, which she suppressed most of the time, unless she was under stress.

Evaluation of Neal

A diagnostician who met Neal during the first few months that he had only the motor tics might have struggled to make any diagnosis at all. Tics are common in childhood and may cause no distress or impaired functioning. (Indeed, the criteria set for tic disorders is the only one in DSM-5's chapter on neurodevelopmental disorders that includes no requirement at all for distress or impaired functioning.)

During the first year, Neal could only have qualified for a diagnosis of provisional tic disorder, which can be assigned when motor tics, vocal tics, or both are present for 1 year or less. After the first year, chronic motor or vocal tic disorder would have been appropriate if Neal had had only motor *or* vocal tics. When we first met Neal, neither of the foregoing diagnoses was appropriate—one because of the time span (TD Criterion B), the other because of two types of tics were involved (A).

Of course, for any of these diagnoses, **other medical conditions** must be ruled out (D), including neurological movement disorders such as dystonia. Abnormal movements can sometimes be found in substance-induced toxicity, such as with amphetamine. Neal's prescription for Ritalin might have precipitated his tics; if that were the only cause of his symptoms, no tic disorder diagnosis would be needed (or, indeed, possible). Then a code describing the medication's effect could be indicated—**other medication-induced movement disorder** (see p. 445). Other conditions in which abnormal movements (such as hand flapping and other stereotypies) can occur include **autism spectrum disorder**, which did not apply to Neal. Neither did he have a history or other symptoms necessary for **schizophrenia with catatonia**.

With a more complete history, a diagnosis of **ADHD**, which is commonly (50% or more) comorbid with TD and other tic disorders, might be warranted except for one fact: Neal's symptoms seemed to be present only at school, not at home. Of course, this could have been due to selective reporting on his mother's part; however, with the information provided and adherence to ADHD Criterion C, only a diagnosis of **other specified ADHD** (in which his clinician would specify the reason why full diagnostic criteria were not fulfilled) would be warranted. His clinician would also need to watch for symptoms of **obsessive–compulsive disorder**, which might not become evident until Neal was older; anxiety and mood disorders are also commonly comorbid. As matters stand, Neal's complete diagnosis would be the following:

F95.2	Tourette's disorder
F90.8	Other specified attention-deficit/hyperactivity disorder, with symptoms in only one setting
CGAS	60 (current)

F95.8 Other Specified Tic Disorder

F95.9 Unspecified Tic Disorder

Use other specified tic disorder, or unspecified tic disorder, to indicate tics that don't fulfill criteria for another tic disorder. The former diagnosis may be used for cases in which you wish to specify why a child does not meet the criteria for another tic disorder or any other particular neurodevelopmental disorder.

ASSESSING TIC DISORDERS

General Suggestions

Although seizures can enter into the differential diagnosis of tics, an EEG is only rarely necessary. With no positive laboratory or imaging findings, the diagnosis of tics relies primarily upon observation. And because even moderately severe tics can be suppressed (with effort) for a time, extensive observation may be needed—sometimes over a period of hours. Ask about the experience of urges and itches that can precede an actual tic.

Don't forget the important role that historical information can play in diagnosing tics. Do the tics disappear during sleep or increase with anxiety, fatigue, or stress? Behavior initiated to prevent or relieve anxiety suggests the diagnosis of obsessive–compulsive disorder rather than a tic disorder. Some patients may require extended evaluation, involving a diary of times, places, and situations in which the tics occur. And ask about a premonitory urge to tic.

Watch for rapid contractions in related muscle groups, producing quick blinks or grimaces of the face or twitching of other body parts (simple motor tics). Complex motor tics, such as touching or smelling, are slower and may appear to be performed on purpose. Although the upper face is most often involved, the shoulder girdle and arms are sometimes affected.

Repetition is key to the identification of vocal tics. A lone, simple vocal tic can be passed off as a cough or a sneeze; repeated grunts, snorts, sniffs, or throat clearings confirm the diagnosis. Complex vocal tics include words or phrases that a patient utters or imitates from the speech of others. Vocal tics are especially likely to occur at natural pauses in speech, such as at the end of a phrase or sentence.

Developmental Factors

Tics are quite common in younger children. Motor tics begin at an average age of 7 and usually precede the onset of vocal tics. In patients with TD, severe symptoms such as coprolalia develop last of all (if ever). A parent often notices tics before the child does.

Why do only some children who inherit the tendency for TD develop symptoms? Although recent research has thrown cool (if not cold) water on it, the possibility remains that a streptococcal infection may in some way sensitize their brains. However, the associations between pediatric acute-onset neuropsychiatric syndrome (PANS) and TD is at this time best described as tenuous. Even should future research refute the association, such possibilities underscore the importance of asking about a history of physical illnesses, including one as seemingly minor as strep throat.

F88 OTHER SPECIFIED NEURODEVELOPMENTAL DISORDER

F89 UNSPECIFIED NEURODEVELOPMENTAL DISORDER

You would use the diagnosis of either other specified neurodevelopmental disorder or unspecified neurodevelopmental disorder for any patient whose disorder appears to have begun before adulthood and is not better defined elsewhere. For those in the first group, specify a reason, such as "neurodevelopmental disorder associated with the ingestion of lead." The second category is often used when you lack adequate information.

CHAPTER 12

Schizophrenia Spectrum
and Other Psychotic Disorders

QUICK GUIDE TO THE SCHIZOPHRENIA SPECTRUM AND OTHER PSYCHOTIC DISORDERS

Schizophrenia and Schizophrenia-Like Disorders

Schizophrenia. Patients with schizophrenia have been ill for at least 6 months with symptoms from at least two of these five groups: delusions, hallucinations, disorganized speech, disorganized behavior, and negative symptoms. (At least one must be from the first three groups.) These patients do not have significant manic or depressive symptoms, and both substance use and general medical conditions have been ruled out (p. 218).

Schizophreniform disorder. This category is for patients who have all the symptoms of schizophrenia, but who have been ill for only 1 to 6 months—less than the time specified for schizophrenia (p. 223).

Schizoaffective disorder. For at least 1 month, these patients have had symptoms of schizophrenia; at the same time, they have prominent symptoms of mania or depression. This condition is hard to diagnose (for one thing, the criteria keep changing), and it is rarely diagnosed in children, though it may occasionally be encountered in adolescents and young adults (p. 223).

Brief psychotic disorder. These patients will have had at least one of the basic psychotic symptoms for less than 1 month (p. 223).

Catatonia associated with another mental disorder (catatonia specifier). These patients have two or more of several behavioral characteristics (defined in the sidebar on p. 220): relative motor immobility or hyperactivity, mutism or marked negativism, peculiar voluntary movements, and echolalia or echopraxia. The specifier can be applied to disorders that include psychosis, mood disorders, autism spectrum disorder, and mental disorders due to other medical conditions.

Other Psychotic Disorders

Delusional disorder. These patients have had delusions for at least a month, but they have never fulfilled criteria for schizophrenia. Such a diagnosis is unusual in children and adolescents, but it is not unheard of (p. 223).

Psychotic disorder due to another medical condition. A variety of medical and neurological conditions can produce psychotic symptoms that may not meet criteria for any of the conditions above (p. 224).

Substance/medication-induced psychotic disorder. Alcohol or other substances (intoxication or withdrawal) can cause psychotic symptoms that may not meet criteria for any of the conditions above (p. 225).

Other specified, or unspecified, psychotic disorder. Use one of these categories for patients whose psychotic symptoms do not meet criteria for any of the disorders listed above (p. 225).

Other Disorders with Psychosis as a Symptom

Some patients have psychosis as a symptom of mental disorders that we discuss in other chapters. These disorders include mood disorders (either severe major depressive episode or manic episode), cognitive disorders (dementias or deliriums), and personality disorders (patients with borderline personality disorder may have transient periods of minutes or hours when they appear delusional).

Disorders That May Masquerade as Psychosis

Specific phobia. Some phobic avoidance behaviors can appear quite strange without being psychotic (p. 270).

Intellectual disability. These patients may at times speak or act bizarrely (p. 164).

Somatic symptom disorder. Sometimes these patients will report pseudohallucinations or pseudodelusions (p. 328).

Factitious disorder. A patient (or caregiver, in the case of factitious disorder imposed on another) may feign delusions or hallucinations in order to obtain hospital or other medical care (p. 338).

F20.9 SCHIZOPHRENIA

In the mental health literature, schizophrenia that begins in childhood or adolescence is termed *early-onset*; symptoms prior to age 13 are sometimes called *very-early-onset*. Note that puberty, which can occur at markedly varying ages, is no longer used as a point of reference for the beginning of a psychotic illness, though onset of schizophrenia before puberty appears to be rare. As in adults, the onset of schizophrenia symptoms is most often gradual; an insidious onset is especially likely for children with very early onset of symptoms. Symptoms usually occur earlier in boys than in girls, so the ratio of younger boys to girls is about 2:1. In contrast, the sex ratio for adults and adolescents approaches unity.

A patient with early-onset schizophrenia will probably pass through a premorbid phase that can include problems with thinking, learning, mood, and anxiety, as well as attention-deficit and behavioral disorders. Older children may have issues with substance misuse. Troubled relationships and withdrawal from family and friends may herald the move into the active phase. Negative symptoms are especially likely in the case of patients with early-onset schizophrenia, who are also at considerable risk for an incomplete recovery that leads to chronic impairment.

The causes of schizophrenia are varied, headed by genetic mutation (often recent and sporadic, and possibly linked to having a father who is older than average). Other risk factors include prenatal issues such as infection and complications of delivery; the use of marijuana; and immigrant status.

Because schizophrenia usually begins in late adolescence or young adulthood, children and young adolescents are likely to exhibit only precursor symptoms such as social withdrawal, acting out behavior, language and speech delays, and academic problems. Though few studies exist, the actual prevalence of schizophrenia in children and adolescents is probably only 1/20th of the 1% rate for the population as a whole.

However, DSM-5's schizophrenia criteria are far more important for children than numbers alone would suggest: They serve as a bulwark against an unwarranted diagnosis that, by suggesting a dismal prognosis and encouraging unwarranted therapy, can cause a lifetime of harm. The prognosis for children and adolescents validly diagnosed as having schizophrenia appears to be even poorer than that for patients who fall ill when they are older, though this may be due to the fact that males—who constitute the bulk of patients with early-onset schizophrenia—typically fare worse than females.

The Essence of Schizophrenia: The Principal Symptoms

The criteria for early-onset and very-early-onset schizophrenia are identical to those for adults. At the core of the diagnosis is the requirement that a spectrum (two or more) of psychotic symptoms must be present for at least 1 month for the diagnosis to be considered at all. The spectrum comprises psychotic symptoms of five types, each of which identifies a patient as being out of touch with reality. DSM-5 lists these in Criterion A by the numbers we give below, and we'll refer to them that way. Using the full criteria set identifies a population of juvenile patients whose diagnoses are about as stable as those of adult-onset patients: at follow-up, 80% retain the same diagnosis.

1. Hallucinations

Hallucinations are false sensory perceptions; an individual perceives something in the absence of any actual sensory stimulus. Hallucinations are the commonest symptom in early-onset schizophrenia. In adults, the hallucinations of schizophrenia are usually auditory; although DSM-5 notes that visual hallucinations may occur more often in children than in adults, conclusive data have not yet been reported. It is especially important to differentiate hallucinations from *illusions*, which are misinterpretations of actual sensory stimuli. Here is an example of an illusion: Upon entering a darkened bedroom, a child misperceives a high-backed chair as a giraffe, but realizes the mistake once the light comes on.

2. Delusions

A *delusion* is a fixed, false belief not explained by a patient's education or cultural beliefs. Even when presented with evidence to the contrary, delusional patients cannot be persuaded that their beliefs are wrong. Although many types are possible, children's delusions are usually persecutory in nature: They complain of being followed, observed, or otherwise interfered with. Delusional children may also fear abduction by a relative or experience unusual changes occur-

> Nonpsychotic hallucinations (especially hearing voices that no one else can hear) are reported by, on average, 17% of children ages 9–12 and 7.5% of adolescents. Of course, these percentages are vastly greater than the overall rates for psychotic illness. Many of these young people move into adult life without experiencing mental illness. However, their early psychotic symptoms may be risk markers for other forms of psychopathology, including mood, behavior, and anxiety disorders. Many are at special risk for multiple future diagnoses. And, at follow-up, their risk of actual psychotic illnesses is likely to be several times that of a person in the general population.

ring inside them. The evaluation of delusions is no longer based on whether they are bizarre (that is, improbable, incomprehensible, not based on real-world experiences).

Delusions must be distinguished from *overvalued ideas*—beliefs that, though not obviously false, cannot be proven to be correct. Usually learned from parents or peer groups, overvalued ideas include such concepts as racial superiority and gang allegiance. In young children, it is especially important not to mistake fantasies or play (an obvious example: imaginary playmates) for true delusions.

3. Disorganized Speech

The thinking of a patient with schizophrenia is often marked by peculiar associations that impede communication. These are sometimes called *loose associations,* and they usually affect the patient's ability to communicate (for example, disconnected syntax, incoherence). Children with schizophrenia are especially likely to have illogical thinking and thus disorganized speech. However, these may be hard to identify in a very young child or in any child with a communication disorder or autism spectrum disorder.

4. Disorganized Behavior

Any non-goal-directed behavior (such as making hand signals with no apparent purpose) may indicate psychosis, as may some behaviors that, though goal-directed, are grossly inappropriate for the situation (taking off one's clothes in public, smearing feces). Especially in children, however, great care must be taken to evaluate competing explanations—the diagnosis of intellectual disability provides ready examples. Always, the emphasis is on deterioration from a previous, more "normal" mode of functioning.

Catatonia constitutes a special example of disorganized behavior in which behaviors tend to be repeated without evident purpose:

Catalepsy—maintaining an uncomfortable posture, even when told it is not necessary to do so

Echopraxia—imitating another person's physical behavior, even when asked not to do so

Exaggerated compliance—at the slightest touch, moving in the direction indicated by another person; termed *mitgehen* in the older literature

Posturing—voluntarily assuming an unnatural or uncomfortable pose

Waxy flexibility—active resistance when an examiner tries to change the patient's position.

5. Negative Symptoms

The types of symptoms described to this point are *positive symptoms,* in the sense that each can be observed as the presence of something. *Negative symptoms* involve the absence of the customary aspects of interactive behavior; their occurrence suggests that something has been taken away. They include flattened or blunted affect (reduced range of emotional expression); lack of initiative (termed *avolition*); and reduced speech production, which can progress to the point of muteness.

Making the Diagnosis

A principal contribution of the DSMs has been to promote the careful discrimination of schizophrenia from other causes of psychosis. The Essential Features of Schizophrenia

(p. 222) clearly set forth several conditions that must be considered in a differential diagnosis of psychotic children and adolescents. We consider these further in the discussion that follows the single case vignette in this chapter.

Although the diagnostic criteria for children, adolescents, and adults are identical, their emphasis differs somewhat. Compared to patients with adult onset, young patients are more likely to have impaired premorbid personalities, and their measured IQs tend to be 10–15 points lower. Social, language, and motor functions are often delayed, perhaps shading into premonitory symptoms such as withdrawal from friends, peculiar behavior, and worsening performance in school. From this starting point, the actual psychosis begins gradually, characterized especially by negative symptoms and disorganized thinking.

In addition to the time factors and required symptoms, no diagnosis of a psychotic illness (or, for that matter, of any illness) can be entertained without evidence that it has caused some form of disability for the child or adolescent patient. In older children, this may take the form of regression from former levels of socialization (family or peers); especially in younger children, there may be inadequate development in social or academic life.

There are also several other medical and mental conditions that form the differential diagnosis for schizophrenia. We mention some of them in our discussion of Christa, below.

Course

Until 1 year after the onset of schizophrenia, you cannot assign any course specifier. After that, classify its course as set forth in the Essential Features. Most children who experience an episode of schizophrenia will recover to the extent that their acute psychotic symptoms improve, but most will have some residual symptoms. A patient encountered during the residual phase may display attenuated negative symptoms, such as a comparative lack of interest in age-appropriate activities, or affect that is bland compared with siblings or other children. As adults, they attain less education, have few if any friends and few interpersonal contacts other than with health care professionals, and tend not to live independently.

PSYCHOTIC DIAGNOSES OTHER THAN SCHIZOPHRENIA

The DSM-5 criteria for schizophrenia have intentionally been made strict to prevent misdiagnosis. A number of other diagnoses in this chapter offer options for patients who have psychotic symptoms but do not fully meet the DSM-5 criteria for schizophrenia. Because several of these disorders are encountered in young patients even less often than is schizophrenia itself, we provide Essential Features only for schizophreniform disorder. James Morrison's *DSM-5 Made Easy* (see Appendix 1 for the reference) provides information about the other disorders.

ESSENTIAL FEATURES OF **SCHIZOPHRENIA**

The classic picture of schizophrenia is a young person (at least age 5, but more often in the late teens or 20s) who has had (1) delusions (especially persecutory) and (2) hallucinations (especially auditory). However, some patients will have (3) speech that is incoherent or otherwise disorganized, (4) severely abnormal psychomotor behavior (catatonic symptoms), or (5) negative symptoms such as restricted affect or lack of volition (they don't feel motivated to do work, maintain family life). Diagnosis requires at least two of these five types of psychotic symptoms, at least one of which must be delusions, hallucinations, or disorganized speech (this requirement constitutes Criterion A for schizophrenia). The patient is likely to have some mood symptoms, but they will be relatively brief. Illness usually begins gradually, perhaps almost imperceptibly, and builds across at least 6 months in a crescendo of misery and chaos.

The Fine Print

The D's: • Duration (6+ months, with Criterion A symptoms for at least a month) • Disability (social, educational, occupational, or personal impairment) • Differential diagnosis (other psychotic disorders; mood or neurocognitive disorders; physical and substance/medication-induced psychotic disorders; peculiar ideas—often political or religious—shared by a community)

Coding Notes

Specify:

> **With catatonia** (see sidebar, p. 220)

Course. If the disorder has lasted at least 1 year, specify:

> **First episode, currently in acute episode**
> **First episode, currently in partial remission**
> **First episode, currently in full remission**
> **Multiple episodes, currently in acute episode**
> **Multiple episodes, currently in partial remission**
> **Multiple episodes, currently in full remission**
> **Continuous**
> **Unspecified**

Disorders That Are Similar to Schizophrenia

F20.81 Schizophreniform Disorder

For many decades, clinicians have observed that patients whose psychotic illnesses begin gradually often do not recover; those whose illnesses begin abruptly are more likely to recover completely. So patients who meet all the criteria for schizophrenia except time—they have been ill longer than a month but under half a year—should be given the diagnosis of schizophreniform disorder. This category, intended as a place holder, keeps a clinician thinking about such a patient until more time reveals the eventual outcome, which is usually either schizophrenia or a mood disorder. This diagnosis is probably used far too seldom for children and adults alike.

F23 Brief Psychotic Disorder

Patients with brief psychotic disorder have had at least one symptom of delusions, hallucinations, or disorganized speech, but they have been ill less than a month. As with schizophreniform disorder, time is required to see whether they recover or go on to develop schizophrenia or another disorder.

F25.0 or F25.1 Schizoaffective Disorder

In schizoaffective disorder, a manic episode or a major depressive episode lasts at least half of the total illness; for at least 2 weeks during the same continuous period, the patient fulfills Criterion A for schizophrenia *without* having symptoms of a mood episode. This diagnosis would rarely be justified in children, but DSM-5 notes that its onset can occur in adolescence.

F06.1 Catatonia Associated with Another Mental Disorder (Catatonia Specifier).

Patients with catatonia have two or more of several behavioral characteristics (defined in the sidebar on p. 220). The specifier can be applied to disorders that include the psychoses (especially schizophrenia), mood disorders, autism spectrum disorder, and other medical conditions.

Other Psychotic Disorders

F22 Delusional Disorder

As the name suggests, patients with delusional disorder have only one "A" list symptom: delusions. Delusional disorder is typically diagnosed in middle to late adult life, but it has

ESSENTIAL FEATURES OF **SCHIZOPHRENIFORM DISORDER**

Relatively rapid onset and offset characterize schizophreniform disorder. The term usually indicates a young person (at least age 5, but more often in the late teens or 20s) who for 30 days to 6 months has (1) delusions (especially persecutory) and (2) hallucinations (especially auditory). However, some patients will have (3) speech that is incoherent or otherwise disorganized, (4) severely abnormal psychomotor behavior (catatonic symptoms), or (5) negative symptoms such as restricted affect or lack of volition (they don't feel motivated to do work, maintain family life). Diagnosis requires at least two of these five types of psychotic symptoms, at least one of which must be delusions, hallucinations, or disorganized speech. The patient recovers fully within 6 months.

The Fine Print

The D's: • Duration (30 days to 6 months) • Differential diagnosis (physical and substance/medication-induced psychotic disorders; schizophrenia; mood or neurocognitive disorders)

Coding Notes

Specify:

> **{With} {Without} good prognostic features**, which include: (1) psychotic symptoms that begin early (in the first month of illness); (2) confusion or perplexity at the peak of psychosis; (3) good premorbid functioning; (4) affect not blunted. From 2 to 4 of these = With good prognostic features; 0 or 1 = Without.
> **With catatonia** (p. 220)

If it's within 6 months and the patient is still ill, use the specifier **(provisional)**. Once the patient has fully recovered, remove the specifier.

If the patient is still ill after 6 months, schizophreniform disorder can no longer apply. Change the diagnosis to schizophrenia or some other disorder.

occasionally been encountered in younger patients. Adolescents with delusional disorder have rarely been reported.

Psychotic Disorder Due to Another Medical Condition

Many medical and neurological illnesses can cause psychotic symptoms; those with relevance for children or adolescents include infectious disease, head trauma, vitamin deficiencies, autoimmune disease, neoplasms, and seizure disorders.

Substance/Medication–Induced Psychotic Disorder

During either intoxication or withdrawal, a variety of substances can cause psychotic symptoms. In children and adolescents, it is important always to consider the possibility that psychotic symptoms have been caused by one or more substances of misuse (which can include prescribed medications), especially when the symptoms begin suddenly in an otherwise normal young person. For symptoms, see the Essential Features of Substance Intoxication and Substance Withdrawal (pp. 403 and 404) and the Essential Features of Four Substance/Medication-Induced Disorders (p. 405) in Chapter 24. Table 24.1 can help with wording and code numbers.

298.8 Other Specified Schizophrenia Spectrum and Other Psychotic Disorder

298.9 Unspecified Schizophrenia Spectrum and Other Psychotic Disorder

A strong minority of psychotic children and adolescents may fit none of the above-described DSM-5 categories. They should be provisionally diagnosed with either other specified or unspecified schizophrenia spectrum and other psychotic disorder, and should be carefully observed for further developments. (As usual, the former diagnosis should be used if you wish to communicate the particular reason why a presentation does not meet the criteria for any other psychotic disorder.)

DIFFERENTIAL DIAGNOSIS OF PSYCHOTIC DISORDERS IN YOUNG PATIENTS

Even the best criteria currently available cannot always prevent misdiagnosis. Longitudinal studies reveal that a large minority of children who later turn out to have schizophrenia have been misdiagnosed as having a mood disorder; conversely, many children identified as having schizophrenia later develop mood disorders. When a child falls ill with psychosis, the clinical task is to obtain the relevant information necessary to allow a differential diagnosis. This information then provides the baseline for later follow-up and reevaluation, as in the case of Christa.

Christa

"She's always reminded me of her Aunt Pat, my other daughter." Christa's grandmother had given this history to the clinician. "Pat's still institutionalized, and Christa's mother is in jail."

Like her Aunt Pat, Christa had been a difficult child. As a baby she had been fussy and irritable, often crying with colic until late in the evening. When at the age of 18 months she still had not spoken her first word, she was taken for evaluation. With an intelligence level estimated to be in the normal range, she was diagnosed as having DSM-IV pervasive developmental disorder not otherwise specified.* Her condition improved with remediation, and by her third year she was speaking sentences.

Even before she talked much, Christa appeared to socialize well; she enjoyed playing with other children and began kindergarten just after she turned 6. Because she was small for her age, she did not appear out of place, and she progressed normally through the first five grades. Her grades, though only average, required effort. On her report card, her fifth-grade teacher observed: "Christa works hard and takes pride in producing the best work she can."

When Christa was 11½, her menses began; shortly after that, she complained to her grandmother of anxiety. She didn't know why she felt bad—only that her heart beat too hard and she felt "skittery." After 2 months, she started skipping classes. Several weeks of hit-or-miss attendance earned her an appointment with the guidance counselor, to whom she confided that she was frightened of a man she had seen lurking near the campus. The assistant principal investigated the story, but could not corroborate it: No one else had seen the man. Despite reassurance, and despite, several mornings, her teacher meeting her a block away to walk her safely onto the school grounds, Christa would not be comforted. She complained of aches and pains; her grandmother took her to the pediatrician, who diagnosed school refusal and reassured them that she would be fine.

But Christa was not fine. Her anxiety attacks continued, and she insisted even more strongly that she was being followed. One morning, about 4 months after her first anxiety attack, she matter-of-factly told her grandmother that her face in the bathroom mirror seemed to have melted; that afternoon she was admitted to the hospital.

The admission workup revealed a thin, slightly built girl with rather scraggly hair whose physical exam, despite her sallow complexion, was completely normal. She denied feeling depressed and showed little emotion as she retold the stories of the melting reflection and the man who followed her. She felt "sure" that these events were real and not imagined. Moreover, she now admitted that for several weeks she had heard a sound just behind her ear, "like crickets chirping." She thought it was trying to tell her something, but she couldn't work out the message.

Christa remained hospitalized for 3 months while being given trials of several antipsychotic drugs. None eliminated her symptoms, but a moderate dose of haloperidol relieved all but the faintest chirping remnants of her auditory hallucination. Although she no longer complained spontaneously of a lurking stranger, when questioned closely she would admit that he still might be there. Throughout her stay, as upon admission, she remained able to convey her thoughts in clear, goal-directed sentences. In the hospital classroom, she sat in one corner and spent much of her time staring out the window at a deserted bird feeder; her grades drifted into the C– and D range.

---

*In DSM-5, the equivalent diagnosis would be some variant of autism spectrum disorder.

Evaluation of Christa

The first step would be to determine whether Christa met the principal requirement—two of the five Criterion A symptoms (see the Essential Features of Schizophrenia and of Schizophreniform Disorder). If we consider her illness to have begun when she first complained of anxiety, she had been ill for about 4 months when she was hospitalized. For at least 2 months she had been delusional (A1: a persistent idea of a man lurking about outside). For several weeks she had been having hallucinations (A2)—the chirping (auditory) and, more recently, the melting of her reflection (visual). The clinician carefully determined that Christa's false beliefs and perceptions were held firmly enough to qualify as delusions and hallucinations, not illusions or fantasies. In addition, she probably also qualified for the negative symptom of flat affect (A5: she showed little emotion).

Although she had been ill for less than the 6 months required for a diagnosis of schizophrenia, the duration was just right for **schizophreniform disorder** (B). Christa had no prominent symptoms suggestive of a **major depressive episode** (C); if anything, as noted above, her affect was bland as she described her face melting. (However, mood symptoms are common, even usual, in children with schizophrenia.) Her physical health was evidently good; there was no evidence of **another medical condition** (D) that could account for her symptoms. There is no mention of **substance use** in the vignette, though her clinician would need to press the point in additional interviews (also D).

When schizophreniform disorder is diagnosed, we should make a statement of prognosis, based on four pieces of historical information and current symptoms (see the Essential Features). Of the good prognostic features, Christa had only one: Her premorbid functioning in school had been reasonably good. During this episode, however, her affect was blunted; she was never described as being confused or perplexed; and her psychotic features (delusions) apparently did not begin until she had had anxiety attacks for 2 months. Until such time as she recovered (or subsequent course necessitated a change of diagnosis), the diagnosis would have to be stated as *provisional*. Her main working diagnosis at admission would therefore be this:

F20.81   Schizophreniform disorder, without good prognostic features (provisional)

For 3 months after her admission, Christa was treated with a variety of medications. Despite the best efforts of her treatment team, her psychotic symptoms persisted, even at discharge. (Had she recovered within 6 months of onset, the diagnosis would have remained as above, with the "provisional" designation removed.) But once she passed the 6-month mark unrecovered, a change of diagnosis became necessary. To determine whether she would qualify for a discharge diagnosis of schizophrenia, let us reexamine the basic criteria.

- *Symptoms.* Of course, the fact that she once met Criterion A would not change.

- *Duration.* She had now been ill for longer than 6 months. (Christa was still having psychotic symptoms at discharge, but another patient might qualify for the 6-month duration criterion by having only residual, nonpsychotic symptoms of schizophrenia, such as the negative symptom of flat affect.)

- *Dysfunction.* For children, the statement of dysfunction requires only a failure to achieve at expected scholastic levels. From the vignette, Christa's school attendance had been markedly affected, and her grades declined during her 3 months in the hospital. The dysfunction must last for a "significant portion" of the time since onset.

- *Mood, substance use, and general medical condition exclusions.* These have been discussed above.

- *Autism spectrum disorder exclusion.* When small, Christa had been diagnosed as having DSM-IV pervasive developmental disorder not otherwise specified, but her current symptoms could not reasonably be explained by it.

So, at her discharge from the hospital, Christa fully met the criteria for schizophrenia. Until DSM-5, we would have been asked to name the subtype. But those hoary terms (paranoid, catatonic, disorganized, undifferentiated) have been discarded now, mainly because they never really predicted much of anything. Even at her discharge, Christa had been ill too briefly to qualify for any statement as to the course of her psychosis. But after another 5–6 months, if we assume that her symptoms persisted, she could be given a course specifier of *continuous.* With improvement, this specifier could change again later. Although many patients with psychosis have long-standing personality problems, none of the evidence cited suggests that this was the case with Christa, so she would not rate any personality disorder diagnosis.

Her complete diagnosis at discharge would be as follows:

F20.9   Schizophrenia
CGAS   35 (on admission to hospital)
CGAS   60 (on discharge)

ASSESSING PSYCHOTIC DISORDERS

General Suggestions

Even when they cooperate, children with psychosis present a special challenge. For one thing, childhood-onset schizophrenia is so uncommon that clinicians are unlikely to suspect it unless the symptoms are florid. Especially when it is early in the course of illness, such a diagnosis is likely to be confounded by symptoms that may seem more typical of other conditions—mood disorders, ADHD, anxiety disorders, accidental or intentional drug ingestion, febrile illnesses, and others.

All of this underscores the importance of a twofold approach to assessing psychosis. Begin by allowing the patient plenty of time to broach and freely discuss any topics that may be causing stress, anxiety, confusion, or mere curiosity. Later in the interview, specifically request information about unusual experiences or content of thought: "Have you ever heard [seen] things other kids couldn't? What sort of things?" (This question, or one like it, has been shown to have especially good specificity and sensitivity at picking up psychotic symptoms in general.) "Have you had thoughts that scare you or worry you?" The answers, combined with information derived from direct observation, will reveal a picture of psychosis in children that is not so very different from that in adults.

Hallucinations

Auditory hallucinations tend to be brief words or phrases. Children may mention hearing whispers rather than voices. As is true with adults, the hallucinations may be either friendly (such as the voice of God, Jesus, or the Virgin Mary) or hostile (for example, a devil "says bad words"). The voices may give orders: A refrigerator tells the patient to "take a drink"; the voice of a dead baby sister says, "Come to Heaven"; an angel suggests that the child go play outside. When visual hallucinations are identified, they may take the form of monsters; tactile hallucinations may be reported as being "touched by the devil."

Attributes of hallucinations to pursue in the interview include source, location, clarity, cause, number, identity ("Whose voices are they?"), subject ("Do they talk about you?"), and effect on the patient ("How does this make you feel?"). Similar questions will apply to hallucinations of the other senses. Remember that many young children, especially those who are socially deprived, have imaginary playmates who keep them company. Although about three-fourths of children with schizophrenia have hallucinations, it is crucial to differentiate between a child with an active imagination (or a different mental disorder) and one who is truly psychotic.

Delusions

Though delusions are usually less well organized (systematized) in children and adolescents than in adults, they are of the same varieties: persecutory (a boy felt commanded by the devil to jump off a cliff, a girl's bowl of Wheaties was poisoned); grandiose (an eighth grader was "the homeboy Jesus Christ"); referential (a seventh grader felt that classmates pointed and laughed at her); and bizarre (a boy believed that the growth of body hair meant that he was becoming a German shepherd). By definition, a delusion can only be diagnosed if it is firmly held and is contrary to the beliefs of a patient's culture. Assess a delusion by asking how long it has been held, what actions have been taken or are contemplated as a result, how the patient interprets its meaning, and whether it is mood-congruent (for instance, a depressed boy believes he is being deservedly punished).

Thought Disorder

Although complete incoherence is unusual, children with psychosis may become distractible, dropping words from sentences or leaving sentences unfinished. Speech may appear pressured. Identifying aspects of formal thought disorder, such as reduced amount of speech, illogical speech, or neologisms, may be facilitated by getting a patient to tell a story.

Behavior

Although frank catatonia is rare, all manner of unusual and even bizarre actions may be noted—mannerisms, poor hygiene, sleeping in strange places (such as under the bed). Many authorities have noted that children who will later develop schizophrenia have more behavioral (especially antisocial) symptoms than do other children.

Affect

Although psychotic children may react with fear to delusions or hallucinations, affect is more often blunted or flat. Expression may be blank, or an unwavering gaze; there is an absence of normal lilt (prosody) to the voice. Relatives may provide valuable historical information about these and other negative symptoms, such as loss of motivation.

Developmental Factors

Younger (school-age) children with schizophrenia tend to develop pretty much the same symptoms as do adolescents and adults. Of course, as noted above, the content of their delusions and hallucinations will depend on the child's developmental stage. The prognosis for recovery tends to be worse for those patients who develop psychotic symptoms when they are very young. Because children with very-early-onset schizophrenia grow up with their symptoms, they may come to regard them as egosyntonic. If so, they may not voluntarily discuss them with parents or teachers, thus limiting collateral information available to interviewers.

Studies have consistently shown abnormalities in the premorbid development of children who later are diagnosed with schizophrenia (especially in very-early-onset cases). Nearly every area of development is involved: Such children have significantly delayed acquisition of motor and speech skills; they have language deficits and abnormalities of social interaction. (Some are initially given a diagnosis of autism spectrum disorder.) Nearly half begin school when they are older than their classmates, or need to repeat a year of schooling. These findings offer an important opportunity for clinicians to identify behaviors early in the course of what may turn out to be the childhood onset of schizophrenia. On the other hand, they represent a challenge not to overinterpret behavior that may presage a less dire course of later illness.

At the core of the DSM-5 definition of schizophrenia lie two features: symptoms and time. Countless studies of adult patients have shown that chronic illness (so-called "real schizophrenia") is predicted by having serious symptoms and by having symptoms for a long period of time. Some writers complain that in the space of two generations, American criteria for schizophrenia have gone from the most relaxed in the world to the most stringent. We acknowledge the truth of this assertion and applaud its intent to protect patients. However, just as some data suggest that early diagnosis and treatment are associated with a better prognosis in autism spectrum disorder, early identification of schizophrenia precursors, with subsequent appropriate treatment, may presage a similar improved outcome for children with psychotic symptoms. Some clinicians worry that our zeal to diagnose only those children who are unquestionably ill may result in withholding treatment that could ameliorate the course in others who are in the early stages of their illness. Although this possibility exists and must be considered, we feel that the risks from casual diagnostic standards are greater by far.

CHAPTER 13

Mood Disorders

QUICK GUIDE TO THE MOOD DISORDERS

DSM-5 uses three groups of criteria sets to diagnose mental problems related to mood: (1) mood episodes, (2) mood disorders, and (3) specifiers describing most recent episode and recurrent course.

Mood Episodes

A *mood episode* refers to any period of time when a patient feels abnormally happy or sad. Mood episodes are the building blocks from which many of the codable mood disorders are constructed. By itself, no mood episode is a codable diagnosis. Most patients with mood disorders will have one or more of these three types of episodes (see Essential Features of Mood Episodes, p. 236):

Major depressive episode. For at least 2 weeks, the patient feels depressed (or cannot enjoy life) and has problems with eating and sleeping, guilt feelings, loss of energy, trouble concentrating, and thoughts about death.

Manic episode. For at least 1 week, the patient feels elated (sometimes, only irritable) and may be grandiose, talkative, hyperactive, and distractible. Bad judgment leads to marked social, educational or work impairment; patients must often be hospitalized.

Hypomanic episode. This is similar to a manic episode, but it is milder, does not require hospitalization, and can be briefer.

Mood Disorders

A *mood disorder* is an illness the principal feature of which is abnormal mood. Nearly every child or adolescent with a mood disorder experiences depression at some time, but some also have highs of mood. Many, but not all, mood disorders are diagnosed on the basis of a mood episode. Note that DSM-5 now covers depressive and bipolar disorders in separate chapters; for practical reasons, we cover these two groups of disorders together, and we continue to refer to them in the aggregate by the DSM-IV term *mood disorders*.

Depressive Disorders

Major depressive disorder. This disorder consists of one or more major depressive episodes, but no manic or hypomanic episodes (Table 13.1 and p. 239).

Disruptive mood dysregulation disorder. A child's mood is persistently negative between frequent, severe explosions of temper (p. 246).

Persistent depressive disorder (dysthymia). This type of depression is usually less severe than an episode of major depression. Symptoms must be present for 2 years or more in adults, 1 year in children. There are no high phases (p. 242).

Premenstrual dysphoric disorder. A few days before her menses, a patient experiences symptoms of depression and anxiety (p. 249).

Other specified, or unspecified, depressive disorder. Use one of these categories only when a patient has depressive symptoms that do not meet the criteria for the depressive diagnoses above or for any other diagnosis in which depression is a feature (p. 251).

Bipolar and Related Disorders

Bipolar I disorder. There must be at least one manic episode; most patients with bipolar I disorder have also had a major depressive episode (Table 13.1 and p. 253).

Bipolar II disorder. This diagnosis requires at least one hypomanic episode and one major depressive episode (Table 13.1 and p. 253).

Cyclothymic disorder. This disorder involves repeated mood swings, but none are severe enough to be called major depressive episodes or manic episodes (p. 254).

Other specified, or unspecified, bipolar and related disorder. Use one of these categories only when a patient has bipolar symptoms that do not fulfill the criteria for the bipolar diagnoses just mentioned (p. 257).

Other Mood Disorders

Depressive or bipolar and related disorder due to another medical condition. Either highs or lows of mood can be caused by various types of physical ailments (p. 258).

Substance/medication-induced depressive or bipolar and related disorder. Alcohol or other psychoactive substances can cause highs or lows of mood that do not meet criteria for any of the above-listed episodes or disorders (p. 258).

Other Causes of Depressive and Manic Symptoms

Mood symptoms are specifically mentioned in the DSM-5 criteria for the behavioral disturbances that can accompany dementia (major neurocognitive disorder with behavioral disturbances), adjustment disorder with depressed mood, personality disorders, and the Z-code for uncomplicated bereavement. Mood symptoms can affect patients with many other mental disorders, including schizophrenia, the eating disorders, somatic symptom disorder, and gender dysphoria. Mood symptoms are also encountered in patients with posttraumatic stress disorder and the personality disorders.

Specifiers

Once a mood disorder diagnosis has been made, two sets of specifiers can be added to describe (1) the most recent episode (with anxious distress, with atypical features, with catatonic features, with psychotic features, with melancholic features, with mixed features, with peripartum onset), and (2) the overall course of the mood disorder (with rapid cycling, with seasonal pattern). Their Essential Features are given on page 240.

INTRODUCTION

Although there are many impediments to the diagnosis of mood disorders in children, we have finally overcome the biggest of them—the once-held myth that childhood, happy and inviolate, cannot sustain depression or mania. Even so, there remain other obstacles to evaluation, most notably the difficulty of assessing the feelings of patients who may communicate poorly. Infants, of course, can only be observed. Even in preschoolers, mood must largely be inferred from behavior. Very young children, for whom depression and anxiety are not well differentiated, may express depression through irritability, somatic symptoms (aches and pains), or school refusal. Manic symptoms may be mistaken for other disorders, such as ADHD. As children mature, their mood symptoms increasingly resemble those of adult patients. While awaiting studies that will better discriminate the symptoms of mood disorders in early life, we can continue to be guided by these features:

■ When you suspect either depression or mania in young patients, look for mood disorders in close relatives. (A strong family history is even more likely in depressed juveniles than in depressed adults.)

■ Keep an open mind about causation. What we know now suggests that depression in early life is multifactorial, so watch out for events that could serve as environmental precipitants.

■ Even more than for adults, recurrence is the rule; most children and adolescents who are so severely ill that they need inpatient care will return to the hospital within 2 years.

■ Although the mood disorders are highly heritable (40–60% across many studies), episodes of major depressive disorder especially can be triggered by such events as loss of a loved one, abuse (sexual or physical), and other stressors.

DSM-5 adopts a building-block approach to the diagnosis of mood disorders. With three types of mood episodes (major depressive, manic, and hypomanic), each of which can have a variety of modifiers based on symptoms and course of illness, dozens of mood disorders are possible. No one knows how many of these actually occur in children and adolescents, and only a handful have received much attention in the mental health literature. These include major depressive disorder (single episode or recurrent), bipolar I disorder (current or most recent episode manic or depressive), and persistent depressive disorder (dysthymia). In addition, two syndromes with mood symptoms that are not mood disorders per se sometimes require our attention: adjustment disorder with depressed mood, and the Z-coded uncomplicated bereavement.

Clearly, the various mood episodes, disorders, and diagnoses constitute a complex set of diagnostic possibilities. To provide a guide to this complexity, we begin by outlining a step-by-step approach to diagnosing and coding the mood disorders, together with three sets of Essential Features (one for the mood episodes, one for the mood disorders based on the mood episodes, and one for the specifiers) and two tables (Tables 13.1 and 13.2). We then discuss the depressive disorders, the bipolar and related disorders, and (briefly) the other mood syndromes, with case vignettes illustrating the process of differential diagnosis and coding in the first two disorder groups.

A STEP-BY-STEP APPROACH TO DIAGNOSING AND CODING MOOD DISORDERS

The following steps provide a logical approach to the diagnosis of mood disorders in children and adolescents.

1. Using the Essential Features of Mood Episodes (p. 236), identify the current and any past mood episodes: major depressive, manic, and hypomanic. Mood episodes are not themselves codable; they serve as building blocks for most actual mood disorder diagnoses. If your patient's symptoms do not fulfill the requirements for a mood episode, skip to step 7.

ESSENTIAL FEATURES OF **MOOD EPISODES**

Episode	Major depressive	Manic	Hypomanic
Symptoms	Children feel sad, down, depressed, or sometimes only irritable. However, some instead insist that they've just lost interest in nearly all their once-loved activities. Other symptoms include fatigue, inability to concentrate, feeling worthless or guilty, and wishes for death or thoughts of suicide. Three symptom areas may show either an increase or a decrease from normal: sleep, appetite/weight, and psychomotor activity. (For each of these, the classic picture is a decrease from normal, but some patients with atypical major depression will report an increase.)	Children feel euphoric (though sometimes irritable), with high energy and frenetic activity. They are full of plans, which they may be too distractible to carry through. They may talk fast, often with flight of ideas. They need less sleep than usual. Grandiosity is sometimes so exaggerated that they become psychotic, believing that they are exalted persons (a king, a rock star) or that they have superpowers. With deteriorating judgment, functioning becomes impaired, often to the point they must be hospitalized for treatment or for their own protection or that of others.	Children have many manic-like, though less extreme symptoms. They feel euphoric or irritable, with high energy or activity. They are full of plans which, despite some distractibility, they may actually implement. Excessive speech reflects racing thoughts; they may have flight of ideas. Judgment may be impaired, but they don't need hospitalization. Grandiosity and self-importance never reach the point of delusion. You would notice the change in such a person, but it doesn't impair functioning—indeed, sometimes these kids get quite a lot done!
Intensity	Most of nearly every day		
Duration	2+ weeks	1+ weeks	4+ days
Impairment	Distress or disability (social, school/work, personal)		Functioning *not* impaired
Rule out	Substance use and physical disorders		
Differential diagnosis	Eating disorder, reaction to loss or trauma, sleep habits	Cyclothymic, bipolar II, cognitive, psychotic disorders	Other bipolar disorders

TABLE 13.1. ICD-10 Coding for Bipolar I and Major Depressive Disorders

Severity	Bipolar I, current or most recent episode			Major depressive, current or most recent episode	
	Manic	Hypomanic[h]	Depressed	Single	Recurrent
Mild[a]	F31.11		F31.31	F32.0	F33.0
Moderate[b]	F31.12		F31.32	F32.1	F33.1
Severe[c]	F31.13		F31.4	F32.2	F33.2
With psychotic features[d]	F31.2	—	F31.5	F32.3	F33.3
In partial remission[e]	F31.73	F31.71	F31.75	F32.4	F33.41
In full remission[f]	F31.74	F31.72	F31.76	F32.5	F33.42
Unspecified[g]	F31.9		F31.9	F32.9	F33.9

Note. Here are two examples of how you put it together: Bipolar I disorder, manic, severe with psychotic features with mixed features. Major depressive disorder, recurrent, in partial remission, with seasonal pattern. Note the order: name → episode type → severity/psychotic/remission → other specifiers.

[a]Mild. Meets the minimum of symptoms, which are distressing but interfere minimally with functionality.

[b]Moderate. Intermediate between mild and severe.

[c]Severe. Many serious symptoms that profoundly impede patient's functioning.

[d]If psychotic features are present, use these code numbers regardless of severity (it will almost always be severe, anyway). Record them as mood-congruent or mood-incongruent (p. 241).

[e]Partial remission. Symptoms are no longer sufficient to meet criteria.

[f]Full remission. For 2 months, the patient has been essentially free of symptoms.

[g]If the episode type isn't specified, code as noted, regardless of severity.

[h]Hypomanic episode has no severity level, so F31.0 always applies.

2. Use the building blocks to select the appropriate mood disorder from the Essential Features of Mood Disorders Based on the Mood Episodes (p. 239). If the diagnosis is bipolar II disorder (at least one hypomanic episode and no manic episodes), there is no severity, so skip to step 5.

3. If step 2 has yielded a diagnosis of bipolar I disorder or major depressive disorder, examine the course of your patient's illness to select the appropriate type. Major depressive disorder will be either single episode or recurrent. Bipolar I disorder will be most recent episode manic, depressed, hypomanic, or unspecified.

4. When the current or most recent episode is major depressive or manic, choose the severity level from Table 13.1. (Because hypomanic episode is inherently mild, it requires no special severity criteria.) When a major depressive episode has lasted continuously for 2 years or more, go to step 7 and consider a diagnosis of persistent depressive disorder (dysthymia).

5. Although episode specifiers are not often applicable to children, add here the word-

ing of any that apply (see the Essential Features of Mood Specifiers, p. 240). No special numbers apply; the verbiage is simply strung out after the main diagnosis, separated by commas.

6. Many children have a recurrence of a mood disorder within a year or two of the index episode. Therefore, check the Essential Features of Mood Specifiers again to see whether the specifiers for rapid cycling or seasonal pattern apply.

7. If your patient does not meet criteria for any mood episode, consider the following: persistent depressive disorder (dysthymia), cyclothymic disorder, depressive or bipolar and related disorder due to another medical condition, or substance/medication-induced depressive or bipolar and related disorder. Each of them has its own set of criteria independent of any mood episode, but only dysthymia has been often described in children. Its Essential Features are given on page 242; a number of specifiers can be applied (Table 13.2).

8. If none of the categories above seems appropriate, consider other specified, or unspecified, depressive or bipolar and related disorder.

TABLE 13.2. Descriptors and Specifiers That Can Apply to Mood Disorders

	Severity / remission	Mixed features	Anxious distress	Catatonia	Atypical features	Melancholia	Peripartum onset	Rapid cycling	Psychotic features	Seasonal pattern
Major depression										
Single episode	×	×	×	×	×	×	×		×	
Recurrent	×	×	×	×	×	×	×		×	×
Bipolar I										
Recent manic	×	×	×	×			×	×	×	×
Recent depressed	×	×	×	×	×	×	×	×	×	×
Recent hypomanic	×	×	×				×	×		×
Recent unspecified										
Bipolar II										
Recent hypomanic	×	×	×				×	×		×
Recent depressed	×	×	×	×	×	×	×	×	×	×
Cyclothymia			×							
Persistent depressive (dysthymia)	×	×	×		×	×	×			

Note. Table 13.1 presents the descriptors for severity/remission. All specifiers are described in the Essential Features of Mood Specifiers (p. 240).

DEPRESSIVE DISORDERS

The Diagnosis of Depressive Disorders in Young Patients

Although children, adolescents, and adults may experience mood disorders differently, their core depressive symptoms are so similar that, with slight modifications, the same DSM-5 criteria are used to diagnose depressive disorders at all ages. However, the core symptom that may be expressed differently from adults in children or adolescents is an important one, for it helps describe the mood abnormality itself. An adult must feel *depressed* (or express loss of pleasure), whereas a child or adolescent may express or demonstrate a mood that is either *depressed or irritable*.

For a major depressive episode, a patient must experience either low or irritable mood or loss of interest for most of at least 2 consecutive weeks. In addition, the patient must have four other symptoms from a list that includes appetite or weight change (for children, it could be a failure to gain weight), problems with sleep (too little *or* too much), speeded or slowed psychomotor activity, low energy, worthlessness or guilt, trouble thinking or concentrating, and thoughts of death or suicide. Two types of major depressive disorder (MDD) can be diagnosed (Essential Features of Mood Disorders Based on the Mood Episodes, below): single episode or recurrent. The one you choose depends on whether this is the patient's first major depressive episode or a subsequent one.

ESSENTIAL FEATURES OF
MOOD DISORDERS BASED ON THE MOOD EPISODES

	Major depressive disorder		Bipolar I disorder				Bipolar II disorder
	Single depressed	Recurrent	Manic	Depressed	Hypomanic	Unspecified	Depressed or hypomanic
Most recent episode	Single depressed	Recurrent	Manic	Depressed	Hypomanic	Unspecified	Depressed or hypomanic
Previous episodes	None	1+ major depressive	1+ mania				1+ hypomanic *or* major depressive
Exclusions	No manic or hypomanic episodes				No psychotic episodes		No manic episodes
	Symptoms are not caused by a general medical condition or by use of substances						
	Not better explained by a psychotic disorder						
Distress/ impairment	Symptoms cause distress or impairment						Only with depression

ESSENTIAL FEATURES OF **MOOD SPECIFIERS**

With Anxious Distress

During an episode of major depression, or dysthymia, the patient feels markedly edgy or tense and may be extra restless. Typically, it is hard to focus attention due to worries—"Something terrible could happen," or "I could lose control and [fill in the awful consequence]."

Specify severity: **mild** (2 symptoms of anxious distress), **moderate** (3 symptoms), **moderate to severe** (4–5 symptoms), **severe** (4–5 symptoms plus physical agitation).

With Atypical Features

A depressed patient feels better when something good happens ("mood reactivity," which is experienced during both depressed and well times). The patient has additional atypical symptoms: an *increase* in appetite or weight, *excessive* sleeping, feeling sluggish or paralyzed, and long-standing sensitivity to rejection, whether or not depressed.

Cannot be diagnosed with melancholia or catatonic features.

With Catatonia

The patient has prominent symptoms of catatonia, such as catalepsy, negativism, posturing, stupor, stereotypy, grimacing, echolalia, and others (see sidebar, p. 220, for definitions).

With Melancholic Features

When depressed, the patient cannot find pleasure in accustomed activities *or* feels no better if something good happens (both could be true). In addition, some of the following: a mood more profoundly depressed than you'd expect of bereavement; diurnal variation (more depressed in the morning), terminal insomnia (awakening at least 2 hours early), slowed (more usual) or agitated psychomotor activity, marked loss of appetite or weight, and unwarranted or excessive guilt feelings. Melancholia is extremely severe and can border on psychosis.

With Mixed Features

There are two ways mixed features can happen: (1) A patient with a manic or hypomanic episode most days also has some noticeable symptoms of depression (depressed mood, low interest or pleasure in activities, slowed or speeded activity level, feeling tired, feeling worthless or guilty, repeated thoughts about death or suicide). (2) A patient with major depressive episode most days also has some noticeable symptoms of mania (elevated mood, grandiosity, increased talkativeness, flight of ideas, increased energy level, poor judgment, and reduced need for sleep).

Record a patient who fully qualifies for *both* manic and depressive episodes as manic episode, with mixed features.

With Peripartum Onset

A female patient's mood disorder starts during pregnancy or within a month of giving birth.

With Psychotic Features

The patient has delusions or hallucinations.

If you can, note whether the psychotic features are **mood-congruent** (they match what you'd expect from the basic manic or depressive mood) or **mood-incongruent**.

With Rapid Cycling

A patient has several episodes per year of major depression, mania, or hypomania. Count as a separate episode one that is marked by remission (part or full) for 2+ months or by a change in polarity (such as from manic to major depressive episode).

With Seasonal Pattern

The patient's mood episodes repeatedly begin (and end) at about the same time of year.

Two caveats: (1) Seasonal episodes must have been the only ones for at least the past two years, and lifelong, seasonal episodes must materially outnumber nonseasonal ones. (2) Disregard examples where there is a clear seasonal cause, such as being laid off every summer.

The symptoms required for persistent depressive disorder (dysthymia) (see its Essential Features, p. 242) are fewer and generally milder than those for a major depressive episode. Early onset of dysthymia predicts a longer duration of depression and the eventual co-occurrence of MDD. Although children tend to recover faster from dysthymia than do adults, they're more likely to develop MDD subsequently.

Research on the ascertainment of depressive disorders in juveniles is still in its early stages, and the figures given by various investigators vary widely; overall, rates may be increasing with time. It should come as no surprise that these disorders are found more frequently in adolescents than in school-age children, and hardly at all in preschoolers. For what they are worth, then, our best estimate for prevalence of dysthymia in adolescents is 3–6%, and far less frequent in young children. The prevalence of MDD in adolescents is about 8%; in about one-third of these, it is severe. For school-age children, it is 2%; for toddlers, it is essentially nil. Until puberty, the boy–girl ratio of depressive disease approximates 1:1; subsequently, females predominate, as is the case with adults.

There is evidence that depressions may not be discrete, but rather may exist on a continuum throughout childhood and adolescence. That is, for young people, meeting exact requirements for duration and number of symptoms may have less importance than

ESSENTIAL FEATURES OF
PERSISTENT DEPRESSIVE DISORDER (DYSTHYMIA)

"Low-grade depression" is how these symptoms are often described, and they occur most of the time for 2 years (they are never absent longer than 2 months running). Some patients aren't even aware that they are depressed (though others can see it). They will acknowledge such symptoms as fatigue, poor concentration, poor self-image, and feeling hopeless. Sleep and appetite can be either increased or decreased. Patients may meet full requirements for major depressive episode, but the concept of mania is foreign to them.

The Fine Print

For children, mood may be irritable instead of depressed, and the time required is 1 year, not 2.

The D's: • Duration (more days than not, 2+ years) • Distress or disability (social, educational, occupational, or personal impairment) • Differential diagnosis (substance use and physical disorders; ordinary grief and sadness; adjustment to a long-standing stressor; bipolar disorders; major depressive disorder)

Coding Notes

Specify severity (Table 13.1).

Specify:

> **Early onset,** if it begins by age 20.
> **Late onset,** if it begins at age 21 or later.

Specify if:

> **With pure dysthymic syndrome.** Doesn't meet criteria for major depressive episode within preceding 2 years.
> **With persistent major depressive episode.** Does meet criteria, throughout preceding 2 years.
> **With intermittent major depressive episodes, with current episode.** Meets criteria now, but at times hasn't.
> **With intermittent major depressive episodes, without current episode.** Has met criteria, though doesn't currently.

Choose other specifiers from Table 13.2.

for adults. Such a finding would suggest the value of an Essential Features approach to diagnosis, rather than an absolute cutoff that depends on a critical number of depressive symptoms.

Once in place, an episode of MDD will last about 8 months in children who are referred for evaluation, with half or more experiencing recurrence within a few years. Childhood-onset depression is less likely to recur as later mood disorder than is depression of adolescent onset. There is a substantial risk (up to 40%) of developing later mania or hypomania, especially in a young patient with a history of psychosis, brief symptoms of hypomania, or a family history of bipolar disorders.

Merrill

"I didn't mean to hurt my little sister," was Merrill's chief complaint. Merrill was a second grader who was being held in a children's mental health unit on the basis that he was dangerous to himself or to other people.

There had been nothing remarkable about his gestation, delivery, or developmental milestones. In fact, according to his mother, he had been "a happy baby and a cheerful kid" until about halfway through kindergarten, when he was sent to live with his grandparents. Merrill's alcoholic father had deserted the family the year before, and his mother's new boyfriend earned his living selling crack cocaine. When police raided the residence, they found little in the refrigerator but drugs; Merrill's mother was jailed on a charge of child endangerment.

Merrill's mother said with a curl of her lip and a set of air quotes, "So to 'protect' the kids, the judge ordered them sent to live with my mother, and my stepfather molested Merrill. I tried to explain going in that he had molested me, too. But who was going to pay any attention to me?" After several months in jail, Merrill's mother was transferred to a mental facility for treatment of her MDD. A combination of Legal Aid and Prozac eventually won her release, but by that time her son was already showing symptoms.

Now Merrill never smiled; he always seemed either sad or angry. His sleep, appetite, and activity were about normal, but his teacher noted problems. A note sent home from first grade reported that "in class his attention wanders, and on the playground he doesn't join in games—he thinks he doesn't play well."

Despite his mother's return home, Merrill did not improve. In fact, for 2 months his behavior worsened. He would scream at other children and seemed to feel that they were making fun of him. His sleep decreased to about 5 hours a night; his appetite also fell off. Two weeks before his admission to the mental health unit, he began sticking pins into the skin of his hands. The day of admission, he tried to choke his 4-year-old sister. Then, isolated in his room, he made several superficial cuts on the side of his own neck with a pocketknife.

Merrill had received all of the usual childhood vaccinations and immunizations. He had no allergies, and his only previous hospitalization was for possible asthma when he was 3. He had received treatment with prednisone at that time and had had no respiratory problems since.

Now 32, Merrill's mother had been married and divorced three times. Merrill was the second youngest of her five children, whose ages ranged from 12 to 4 years. Between pregnancies, she had earned minimum wage as a school aide. Although her depression had responded to treatment with medication, the family was currently living on Social Security Disability Insurance.

Merrill was a rather thin child who was alert, made eye contact, and was reasonably cooperative. However, it took him an unusual amount of time to answer questions put to him, and he seemed less active than would be expected for an 8-year-old boy. Although his speech was slow and monotonous, his thoughts were linear and goal-directed. When asked about his mood, at first he said he felt "all right," but later admitted he had been feeling guilty because "I just keep doing bad things." He expressed remorse at having tried to harm his sister; he then admitted he wanted "to be dead," though he did not think he would try to cut himself again—"It hurt." He denied having anxiety, delusions, or hallucinations; his cognitive functioning was normal for his age. On the basis that he knew that he had been admitted to the hospital because of his recent behavior, his insight seemed good. The behavior itself, however, suggested strongly that Merrill's judgment had been deficient in recent weeks.

Evaluation of Merrill

The steps mentioned in this discussion are those outlined in the section "A Step-by-Step Approach to Diagnosing and Coding Mood Disorders," on page 235.

Step 1: What symptoms would qualify Merrill for a mood episode? Mood change was first noted by his mother when the two were reunited after her own incarceration. He seemed sad or angry (Criterion A1 for major depressive episode), but definitely different from his previous cheerful disposition (A). At first, his additional depressive symptoms seemed to include only loss of interest (A2: wandering attention in class) and poor self-image (he didn't think he played games well), so until the few weeks prior to his admission, he could not have qualified for any mood episode diagnosis.

Recently, however, Merrill had also lost sleep (A4) and appetite (A3), and he had expressed death wishes and suicidal behavior (A9); he even appeared to have psychomotor retardation (A5). These symptoms clearly interfered with his functioning at school and at home (B). Before concluding that Merrill qualified for a major depressive episode, his clinician would have to affirm that his symptoms had been present for most of every day, as DSM-5 requires for each of the symptoms we've mentioned. The clinician would also need to establish that there was no evidence of a general health problem (in children, look especially for trauma, multiple hospitalizations, or a chronic illness such as leukemia) that could account for his depressive symptoms (C). Absent such evidence, Merrill would fulfill the DSM-5 criteria and the Essential Features for major depressive episode (p. 236).

Step 2: Because Merrill had never had a manic or hypomanic episode, a diagnosis of a bipolar disorder would not be possible (though future episodes of mania or hypomania must be considered; initial depression in a patient with a bipolar disorder may be no different from one in a patient who will never have a manic episode). His major depressive episode would therefore be a part of MDD.

Step 3: With only one major depressive episode, his code and diagnosis so far would be F32.x major depressive disorder, single episode (Table 13.1).

Step 4: The severity code is determined from the guidelines provided for the current major depressive episode. Merrill's clinician regarded his depression as severe—not because he had so *many* symptoms, though there were more than the minimum, but because some of them (thoughts of death) were so serious. (Our advice: Regard DSM-5 criteria as guidelines, not shackles.) With no delusions or hallucinations, his code and diagnosis would now be F32.2 major depressive disorder, single episode, severe.

Step 5: None of the other episode specifiers would apply.

Step 6: Because this was Merrill's first episode of illness, neither would he have any course specifiers. This would end the evaluation of his MDD, and his diagnosis would read as follows:

F32.2	Major depressive disorder, single episode, severe
T74.22	Sexual abuse by grandfather
CGAS	50 (current)

Step 7: As an exercise, let's now suppose that even with treatment, Merrill had mild depressive symptoms for at least the next 6 or 8 months, more or less continuously. Let's say further that there were at least two of these symptoms, and that they persisted for at least a year (they would need to last 2 years for an adult). Then we would need to reevaluate him in the light of the criteria for persistent depressive disorder (dysthymia). If he didn't currently meet the full requirements for major depressive episode, we'd say that he had an early onset of persistent depressive disorder. The fact that during the past year he had had a major depressive episode would allow us to choose one of the longest specifiers in DSM-5:

F34.1	Persistent depressive disorder (dysthymia), early onset, with intermittent major depressive episodes, without current episode

A number of other conditions must be included in the differential diagnosis for depressive disorders. Considering the trauma Merrill had experienced, **adjustment disorder with depressed mood** would seem a possibility. Adjustment disorder (p. 311) is a diagnosis of last resort, to be used only if no other disorder can explain the symptoms. (Mood disorders are often misdiagnosed as adjustment disorder, especially in school-age children—a fact rendered regrettable because mood disorders are more treatable by far.) Patients with **anorexia nervosa** may look depressed and experience weight loss, but nowhere do we read that Merrill feared weight gain or had problems with his body image. Social impairment causes depression in some children who have **ADHD**; their hyperactivity may cause some to be viewed as having the mania of **bipolar I or II disorder**. Although Merrill had no phobias, compulsions, obsessions, or complaints of anxiety, in some children anxiety disorders (such as **separation anxiety disorder** or **generalized anxiety disorder**) may form part of the differential diagnosis. Of course, we'd consider **schizophrenia** whenever children or adolescents are so severely depressed or manic that they have psychotic symptoms. In those who present with somatic complaints, **somatic symptom disorder** must also be considered in the differential diagnosis of MDD.

Finally, let us consider disorders that may be comorbid with the mood disorders. These include **anxiety disorders** (found in about 40% of children with depression), **conduct disorder** (20% or more of depressed children), and **substance use disorders** (especially in adolescents). Also, be alert for ADHD and eating disorders, and for **specific learning disorders,** especially with impairment in reading.

The vignette of Corey (p. 286) presents another example of MDD.

F34.8 Disruptive Mood Dysregulation Disorder

For a generation or more, clinicians have been aware that chronic and severe irritability in children predicts emotional and interpersonal difficulties later in life. In recent years, some clinicians have sought to equate these behaviors with a form of bipolar disorder; as a result, such children have been treated with antipsychotic and mood-stabilizing medication. But many other clinicians see something else in the child who habitually flies off the handle at the slightest (or no) provocation: the antagonism of oppositional defiant disorder (ODD) or the impulsivity of ADHD. Or perhaps something new altogether?

That "something new" is now called disruptive mood dysregulation disorder (DMDD), a condition as controversial as its name is clumsy. Every few days, these children succumb to a burst of temper, during which they may threaten, yell, and even attack other people verbally, sometimes physically. These outbursts occur in a manner—and at times and places—that are not consistent with the child's developmental stage. And between eruptions, the child's mood is habitually angry or irritable.

This combination of problematic behaviors places children at risk for serious consequences at school, in their families, and with peers. Even patients with milder symptoms may find themselves excluded from traditional childhood experiences, such as party invitations and play dates. More severely affected children may be suspended from school and may even require constant supervision to prevent harm befalling them and others.

With the stakes so high, we'd like to be certain when we make this diagnosis. Unfortunately, there are a number of unresolved issues.

- Similar to other childhood disorders, DMDD is more common in boys than in girls—which of course places the diagnosis at odds with most mood disorders.

- Although DSM-5 criteria preclude the diagnosis prior to age 6, studies find that it is most common in preschool children, with only about a 1% prevalence after early childhood.

- The stability of the diagnosis is low; in one study, only one-fifth of the young participants retained the diagnosis at 2-year follow-up. (DMDD may evolve into unipolar depression or an anxiety disorder in adulthood, but not a bipolar disorder. It is classed with the depressive rather than the bipolar and related disorders in DSM-5.)

- A study by Margulies et al. (2012; see Appendix 1) found that the majority of inpatients ages 5–12 who were chronically irritable and explosive did not fulfill criteria for DMDD.

- In the Margulies et al. study, the diagnosis was almost threefold more likely when based on historical data than when based on observations in the hospital setting.

- In older children, DMDD must be discriminated from ordinary rebellion of adolescence, a transitional period where mood symptoms are common.

DMDD is strongly commingled with other mental disorders. For example, many children with this diagnosis could have received the diagnoses of ADHD or ODD when they were younger; perhaps as many as three-quarters of children diagnosed with DMDD will also meet criteria for ODD. In fact, some authors report that DMDD cannot be delimited from ODD and conduct disorder. Comorbidity has also been reported with other depressive disorders and ADHD.

Irritability predicts risk for mood and anxiety disorders in adults. Some studies have shown that even when irritable children don't have mental disorder as adults, they grow up to have difficulty getting along with others, to be downwardly mobile, and to be sporadically employed. They have a higher risk of being poor and uneducated, of engaging in illegal or risky activities, and suffering social isolation. Although it is not clear whether DMDD will help avert inappropriate diagnoses of bipolar disorders in children, it is obvious that children with such marked irritability are likely to have a rough time as they attempt to accommodate to adolescence and the adult world.

The relationship of DMDD to the spectrum of depressive disorders would seem to be tenuous, at best; except as something to rule out, the word *depressive* isn't even mentioned in the official DSM-5 criteria. In the event that it survives to another edition, might this diagnosis fit more comfortably in the chapter on disruptive, impulse-control, and conduct disorders, along with ODD? We predict that the diagnosis and categorization of children with severe temper outbursts will change substantially over the next few years. And we encourage readers to peruse new research for updates.

Kurt

"We get referrals from everywhere," the clinic intake worker said, "but this is the first one from a gym. A boxing instructor, no less. Miss Finch."

Kurt's parents had enrolled him at the gym because they thought he needed a safe outlet for his obvious energy and aggressiveness. Miss Finch had been welcoming and had taught him the basics of ring etiquette. But the next day, she'd called to say that he couldn't come back. The first time another kid had touched a glove to him in the ring, he'd exploded in a barrage of blows and invective. Miss Finch had had to drag Kurt away; the other kid's mother had complained. At home afterward, during the inevitable time out, he'd kicked a hole through his bedroom wall.

When Kurt was just a toddler, he was "prickly—you could hardly speak to him without causing him to cry or slam a door," his dad pointed out later. "Even when he was a baby. I was flying back home the day he was born, so I missed the delivery. But when I viewed the newborns in the nursery, they were all sleeping but one—a kid who'd screwed up his face with yelling so hard I thought he'd choke. 'Some dad's gonna have his hands full with that one,' the guy standing next to me said. Turned out, *that one* was Kurt!"

ESSENTIAL FEATURES OF
DISRUPTIVE MOOD DYSREGULATION DISORDER

For at least a year, several times a week, and on slight provocation, a child has severe tantrums—screaming or actually attacking someone (or something)—that are inappropriate for the patient's age and stage of development. Between outbursts, the child seems mostly grumpy or sad. The attacks and intervening moods occur across multiple settings (home, school, with friends). These patients have no manic episodes.

The Fine Print

The D's: • Duration and demographics (1+ years, and never symptom-free longer than 3 months running, starting before age 10; the diagnosis can only be made from ages 6 through 17) • Distress or disability (symptoms are present in all settings, severe in at least one—home, school, with other kids) • Differential diagnosis (substance use and physical disorders; trauma; major depressive disorder; bipolar disorders; ODD and ADHD; behavioral outbursts consistent with developmental age)

His first day in kindergarten, Kurt screamed at another child and overturned a heavy sandbox. Now, whether at school or in the neighborhood, other children wouldn't play with him because of his temper outbursts and generally sullen demeanor. "He's strong for his size," his mother said. "The other kids are afraid. Quite frankly, sometimes so am I."

When Kurt wasn't shouting, he was surly. "He seems always resentful, but of what, I haven't a clue," she continued. "Even at his own birthday party last month—family only, of course—he begrudged it that we gave his little sister a small present, so she'd feel included. Kurt got everything he'd asked for; she got a spangly barrette. Kurt belittled her and stalked out of the room—after he'd finished his cake."

Whenever his dad would try to talk to Kurt about his behavior, he'd blame his sister, the dog, or even the baby. "And whatever you ask, he'll *never* do it," he said. "He seems almost to delight in infuriating us."

Evaluation of Kurt

There are two main components to the diagnosis of DMDD, and Kurt abundantly fulfilled both: frequent, inappropriate outbursts of temper (Criteria C, B, and A) and in between outbursts, a mood that was mostly angry or irritable (D). According to his parents, Kurt had been this way since he was a very small child (E), and it affected every aspect of his life (F). His age, both current and at onset, was consistent with the requirements of diagnosis (G, H).

Then there are the exclusions that end this criteria set, the longest in DSM-5. There's no evidence in the vignette for a physical disorder or substance use (K), and his father's testimony would seem to rule out major depressive disorder (J) or a bipolar disorder (I).

Even when Kurt was a very young child, he was contrary and would easily have met criteria for ODD. But DSM-5 states that ODD and DMDD cannot be diagnosed at the same time, so we would have to put ODD aside for now, and only diagnose DMDD. (Also proscribed from comorbidity with this diagnosis are bipolar disorders and intermittent explosive disorder.) There are no specifiers on offer for Kurt's diagnosis:

F34.8	Disruptive mood dysregulation disorder
CGAS	55

N94.3 Premenstrual Dysphoric Disorder

To one degree or another, premenstrual symptoms affect 12% or more of women of reproductive age; half or more of adolescents experience some symptoms. The severe form, premenstrual dysphoric disorder (PMDD), affects nearly 2% of adult women. In adolescents, when these symptoms often begin, the prevalence of PMDD may be nearer 5%.

During their reproductive years, for perhaps a week out of each menstrual cycle, these young (and older) women will complain of fatigue and dysphoria (usually depression, anxiety, or anger). In addition, they will have physical symptoms that include breast sensitivity, weight gain, and abdominal swelling. Differentiation from major depressive episode and persistent depressive disorder (dysthymia) relies principally on timing and duration.

The consequences of PMDD can be serious—a (reproductive) lifetime of mood and other symptoms that may remit only with pregnancy and, ultimately, menopause. Patients may be completely unaware how seriously their negative moods affect their friends and families. Yet most will not be diagnosed or receive adequate treatment until they are in their 30s. Overall, this condition ranks high among mental disorders that are seriously underdiagnosed.

Aside from a genetic component, risk factors for PMDD include excessive weight, stress, and trauma (including a history of abuse). Anxiety disorders and other mood disorders, including bipolar conditions, can be comorbid. Adolescents and adults will probably differ little in their presenting symptoms, so we do not provide a vignette here. Interested readers can read about a patient with PMDD in *DSM-5 Made Easy* by James Morrison.

ESSENTIAL FEATURES OF **PREMENSTRUAL DYSPHORIC DISORDER**

For a few days before menstruating, a patient experiences marked mood swings, depression, anxiety, anger, or other expressions of dysphoria. She will also admit to typical symptoms of depression, including trouble with concentration, loss of interest, fatigue, feeling out of control, and changes in appetite or sleep. She may have physical symptoms such as sensitivity of breasts, muscle pain, weight gain, and a sensation of abdominal distention. Shortly after menstruation begins, she snaps back to normal.

The Fine Print

The D's: • Duration (for several days around menstrual periods, for most cycles during the past year) • Distress or disability (social, occupational, or personal impairment) • Differential diagnosis (substance use—including hormone replacement therapy—and physical disorders; major depressive disorder and persistent depressive disorder [dysthymia]; ordinary grief and sadness)

Coding Note

DSM-5 says that the diagnosis should only be stated as *provisional* until you've obtained prospective ratings of two menstrual cycles.

F32.8 Other Specified Depressive Disorder

F32.9 Unspecified Depressive Disorder

Use either other specified or unspecified depressive disorder when depressive symptoms are present, but not yet sufficient to warrant a more definitive depressive disorder diagnosis. (Use the other specified diagnosis when you wish to indicate the reason why a patient does not meet criteria for any other depressive disorder. For example, an adolescent who is currently depressed and too ill to give a complete history may not be able to state how long the symptoms have lasted.) These codes will be used infrequently; like most other specified or unspecified diagnoses, such a code should be changed to a more specific diagnosis once you obtain the additional relevant information. These patients must also not fulfill the criteria for adjustment disorder with depressed mood or adjustment disorder with mixed anxiety and depressed mood.

ASSESSING DEPRESSIVE DISORDERS

General Suggestions

Parents and teachers tend to be more accurate observers of young children's behavior, whereas the children themselves may provide more accurate information about emotions and associated somatic symptoms. Obviously, interviews with multiple informants will increase the likelihood of a complete and accurate clinical evaluation. A question about "three wishes" may yield statements indicating hopelessness or, in the case of a major depressive episode, even the wish for death.

Throughout the interview, don't be diverted from a possible depressive disorder diagnosis by the presence of somatic symptoms such as abdominal pain or headache. Young children tend to experience distressing feelings through somatic symptoms (headache, fatigue, abdominal pain), but they may also acknowledge feelings of sadness, hopelessness, and wishes to die. Most children respond to simple, concrete questions from a sympathetic, patient interviewer. Many children, lacking the vocabulary to understand what they experience, are relieved to have someone ask specifically how they feel. Classically, children and adolescents may experience irritability rather than sadness or frank depression. In general, irritability is found in MDD.

Although the criteria for depressive disorders are nearly identical for children and adults, we often forget that children and adolescents can have suicidal ideas and behaviors. Among young people ages 15–24, suicide is the third leading cause of death (after accidents and homicide). Even so, completed suicide is still a rare event; however, in a 12-month period, 16% of high school students seriously considered suicide, and 8% reported attempting it. When questioned closely, children as young as 6 who have MDD may admit to suicidal ideas. Very young children have little comprehension that life actually terminates at death, whereas older children generally understand the consequences of suicide. In any event, careful and repeated evaluation of suicidal potential is essential in any young person who has or has had a depressive disorder (or a major depressive episode in a bipolar disorder), along with evaluation of the potential for self-harm—which includes the presence of weaponry in the home.

Despite the fact that they may admit feeling sad, even older children may not realize that this is a change, let alone be able to pinpoint when these sad feelings began or how long they'd been present. Because a sense of time develops only in later childhood, it can be useful to relate timing to important events ("Did it start before your birthday [or Christmas, or in the first grade]?").

Cause of depression in children (as in adults) is undoubtedly multifactorial, so you will need to ask patient and parents about family history of mental disorders; prior experience with mood and other disorders (especially anxiety and substance use); trauma; interpersonal problems (peer interactions, romantic relationships for adolescents); and cognitive states (how do children view themselves or how they view their future?).

Developmental Factors

Young children may appear tearful and physically slowed down, and may talk less than is normal for them; the onset of depression can be even more insidious than in older children. In school-age children and adolescents, look for somatic symptoms such as headaches, low appetite, and abdominal pain. Sometimes failure to gain weight, or excessive sleepiness and inhibited overall activity level, may herald the diagnosis. Because language skills are not well developed in very young children, the observations of slumped posture, unwillingness to play, lethargy, sad face, slow speech, and monotonous tone of voice are extra important before age 5. Some young children (and even some adolescents) may not be able to identify what they feel as depressed mood; for them, irritability is an equivalent statement of mood for either major depressive episode or persistent depressive disorder.

Adolescents can describe symptoms more precisely than do younger children; they are also more likely to admit to guilt feelings, self-harm behaviors, and other symptoms characteristic of adult-style severe depression (psychomotor retardation, delusions, hopelessness). Of course, older children and adolescents alike may become so depressed that schoolwork and even friendships with classmates suffer. Adolescents may display their depressive illness in the form of problem behavior reminiscent of conduct disorder: promiscuity, petty crimes, and substance use.

BIPOLAR AND RELATED DISORDERS

The Diagnosis of Bipolar and Related Disorders in Young Patients

Were we discussing adults, this section would consider bipolar I, bipolar II, and cyclothymic disorders. Although these disorders can occur in children and adolescents, there's too little information about *how* they are manifested in young patients. Here's a brief summary of what we do know.

Like adults, most children with mood disorders have only depressions, but 1–3% of adolescents are found to have bipolar disorders. Even Emil Kraepelin, writing a century ago, mentioned that mania can occur before puberty; in fact, late adolescence is the most common time for onset of a bipolar disorder. Partly because mania is unusual in younger patients, and partly because of symptom overlap with ADHD, clinicians don't expect it and therefore often miss it. Irritability is often the main presenting mood; rapid cycling (more than four changes per year) and mixtures of mania and depression may be especially common in young patients. Of course, you can expect an abundance of the usual mania symptoms: labile mood, marked hyperactivity, reduced need for sleep, unrealistic plans for the future. Many patients have delusions, and some will hallucinate.

> How do you code a suicide attempt? Of course, it will be mentioned in the summary and in the body of your report, but this behavior is so important that it should be flagged, especially if it seems likely to be repeated. There is a Z-code number that can be assigned (Z91.5, personal history of self-harm). Use as many words as necessary to convey a complete, accurate message about a patient who shows suicidal behavior.

Sometimes even before clinical symptoms appear, children and adolescents with bipolar disorders may seem different from their peers. Toddlers may have mood or behavior problems, such as tantrums or trouble sleeping. Of course, these symptoms are also common during normal development, and the early onset of mood symptoms does not in itself predict a bipolar disorder.

Several features of depression may predict the eventual development of mania in children and adolescents:

- Rapid onset of depressive symptoms
- Psychomotor retardation during depression
- Mood-congruent psychotic depression
- Strong family history of mood disorders, especially bipolar disorders
- Manic symptoms that start in response to the use of an antidepressant medication, electroconvulsive therapy, or bright light therapy

Both children and adults with bipolar disorders spend more time being depressed than having mania or hypomania, and first episodes are typically depressed. By comparison with patients who have MDD, adolescents with bipolar disorders typically have mood disorders that are more severe and carry a prognosis for poorer overall functioning and greater comorbidity (especially anxiety disorders, oppositional defiant disorder, conduct disorder, and ADHD).

Cyclothymic disorder—which involves mood swings that do not meet criteria for any of the mood episodes—is infrequently diagnosed even in adults, and even more rarely in children. Nevertheless, we present its Essential Features below.

Tonya

When Tonya was 15, the police brought her to the hospital from her home. Her father had told them that she had threatened his life and was behaving bizarrely.

For several years, Tonya had been truant from school and had frequently run away from home. Intermittently, she had been remanded to a local alternative living center, where it was noted that her father drank heavily. A ninth-grade dropout, she had been expelled from a general equivalency diploma program several months previously for fighting.

Tonya's first encounter with mental health professionals had occurred 6 months earlier. Then, just after breaking up with her boyfriend, she discovered that she was 2 months pregnant. An impulsive overdose with her father's pain pills resulted in a rapid trip to a general hospital emergency room, where she was thought not to be acutely dangerous to herself and referred for psychotherapy. After the abortion, she appeared to have no symptoms of mood disorder.

ESSENTIAL FEATURES OF **CYCLOTHYMIC DISORDER**

The patient has had many ups and downs of mood that *don't* meet criteria for any of the mood episodes (major depressive, hypomanic, manic). Although symptoms occur most of the time, as much as a couple of months of level mood can go by.

The Fine Print

The D's: • Duration (2+ years; in children and adolescents, only 1 year is required) • Distress or disability (social, educational, occupational, or personal impairment) • Differential diagnosis (substance use and physical disorders; other bipolar disorders)

Coding Note

Specify if: **With anxious distress** (p. 240).

Her father had first noticed mood swings during the past 3 months. She had told him she'd felt low for about 2 days, followed by a high that lasted 8 or 9 hours. Because he assumed that she was "only high on crank," he didn't seek help for her. Besides, he added, to prevent him from forcing her to attend school, Tonya had once threatened to accuse him (falsely) of rape.

About 2 weeks before Tonya's current hospital admission, she awakened early one morning, her speech rapid and pressured. Throughout the day, she showed increasingly labile affect, moving from tears to laughter and back within a few minutes. Late that afternoon, her father finally called the police when she menaced him with a serrated steak knife. Although she insisted that he had raped her and three of her friends, the police officers responding to the complaint noted her obvious mental disturbance and transported her for evaluation.

Tonya had lived with her father for nearly all of the past 9 years (except for the 6 months when he was jailed for physically abusing her 11-year-old brother). Her mother, who was known to abuse drugs and who had been hospitalized several times for psychosis, had been out of the home since Tonya was in the first grade.

Tonya had been a happy, easy baby who was "always talking and on the go." Her developmental milestones occurred at the normal times. She did well through eighth grade and was valedictorian of her sixth-grade graduating class. It was when she began hanging out with known drug dealers in the neighborhood that she nearly flunked the first semester of ninth grade. At about this time, she also began fighting with other girls and became oppositional toward her teachers; finally, she had dropped out of school.

Upon admission, Tonya was disheveled and badly needed a shower. She seemed agitated and appeared to be in perpetual motion. Her speech was pressured, and she admitted that her thoughts were racing. Her mood was both angry and expansive, and she told several interviewers that she thought she had come to the hospital "to straighten you people out." During the admission process, she had difficulty focusing her attention and frequently muttered, "What was I saying? What was I saying?" She denied having visual hallucinations, but twice claimed that she could hear "heartbeats of the love of Jesus," which meant that she was the Second Coming. She repeatedly claimed that she was completely well, and that her father had all the problems; other than to reform the institution, she felt no need of hospitalization. She was alert and oriented, but would not cooperate further with cognitive assessment. Later testing revealed a Full Scale IQ of 125 and no cognitive deficits.

Although Tonya denied having disturbed sleep or appetite, both were noted to be markedly decreased from normal. She remained talkative and unable to focus on any task or to participate in milieu activities longer than a few seconds. Whenever these behavioral problems were pointed out to her, she would instantly become angry and defiant.

Her hospitalization stretched to 6 weeks. Tonya was eventually started on lithium; within a week her activity level decreased, and she was better able to focus on the topic at hand. Her affect became much less labile as well, and her mood appeared to stabilize. At discharge she was able to state, "Now I feel pretty good inside."

Evaluation of Tonya

Hyperactivity can be encountered in several other disorders. **ADHD,** perhaps the most prominent diagnosis in the differential list for juvenile bipolar disorders, typically starts at an earlier age than the usual manic episode, but it can be comorbid with bipolar I or II disorder. Tonya, however, had no history of problems with attention or hyperactivity prior to the eighth grade, and the symptoms of ADHD must be present before age 12. The **use of drugs** such as steroids or amphetamines (either prescribed or illicit) can produce psychotic symptoms that can also be confused with mania. Tonya's symptoms persisted after she was admitted to the hospital, markedly reducing the possibility that they were drug-related. (A drug screen might have helped reassure her caregivers, however).

Manic symptoms in adolescents are often accompanied by psychosis, which is too frequently misdiagnosed as **schizophrenia**. Although Tonya apparently had delusions at admission, her very considerable mood symptoms would weigh heavily against this diagnosis. DSM-5 makes an even stronger argument in the basic criteria for schizophrenia, which specify that the duration of any mood symptoms must be brief in relation to the duration of psychotic symptoms. Many patients in the throes of a manic episode may act out as though they had **conduct disorder** or, in more extreme cases, **antisocial personality disorder. Adjustment disorder with disturbance of conduct** is also sometimes suspected, probably due to the relative infrequency with which manias are encountered in this age group. However, adjustment disorders are near the bottom of the diagnostic hierarchy: we cannot diagnose one if the symptoms fulfill criteria for any other mental disorder.

Because Tonya's history accorded with none of the diagnoses mentioned above, we can proceed to evaluate how well her symptoms fit the mood disorders criteria. The steps mentioned here are those outlined in the "Step-by-Step" section (p. 235).

Step 1: During her recent episode, Tonya's mood seemed more angry than euphoric— not uncommon even for adults, but especially likely in children or adolescents. Earlier, she had been grandiose (Criterion B1 for manic episode); on admission, she admitted that her thoughts were racing (B4). For most of this time she talked a great deal (B3), seemed agitated (B6), was easily distracted (B5), and had a decreased need for sleep (B2) and a decreased appetite. Her physical health was good. Although there was some suspicion that she might have **abused drugs** earlier, she had no opportunity to do so during her hospitalization, during which her symptoms persisted (D). Although her symptoms had lasted far longer than the 1-week minimum for a manic episode, the fact that she had required hospitalization obviated the time requirement (A and C). She therefore easily met the criteria for a manic episode in both the Essential Features of Mood Episodes (p. 236) and DSM-5.

Step 2: It is now an easy step to the actual diagnosis (see the Essential Features of Mood Disorders Based on the Mood Episodes, p. 239). She had one building block, manic episode (Criterion A for bipolar I disorder). The abrupt onset and clear mood symptoms would rule out any psychotic disorder such as **schizophrenia** (Criterion B). The severity of her illness and the absence of *many* episodes would preclude the diagnosis of **cyclothymic disorder**; because she had a full-blown manic episode, she couldn't be diagnosed with **bipolar II disorder**.

Step 3: Tonya was now beginning to recover from a manic episode, and she had had no clear previous episodes. This would set her diagnosis as bipolar I disorder, most recent episode manic.

Step 4: Because her current manic episode included psychotic symptoms, Table 13.1 would direct us to code number F31.2—whatever we might think of the overall severity of her illness. (Obviously, she was pretty darned ill.)

Steps 5–6: No other episode or course specifiers (from the Essential Features of Mood Specifiers, p. 240) would apply.

In addition, the Z-code in the list below describes a feature of Tonya's environment that might complicate her subsequent treatment. Her full diagnosis would be as follows:

F31.2	Bipolar I disorder, current episode manic, with psychotic features
Z62.820	Parent–child relational problem
CGAS	45 (on admission)
CGAS	80 (at discharge)

F31.89 Other Specified Bipolar and Related Disorder

F31.9 Unspecified Bipolar and Related Disorder

A child or adolescent whose bipolar symptoms do not meet criteria for any better-defined bipolar disorder can be diagnosed with other specified or unspecified bipolar and related disorder (and should then be observed closely for symptom changes). As usual, the other specified diagnosis should be used if you wish to indicate the reason why criteria are not met for any other bipolar disorder.

ASSESSING BIPOLAR DISORDERS

General Suggestions

Of all the patients who are brought for evaluation and who can communicate adequately, those with mania may be the most difficult to interview. They typically believe that nothing is wrong, and they *know* that they have better things to do than speaking with a clinician. When a child or adolescent has mania, an added hardship may be the patient's aggressive activity level, which can pose a physical impediment to the therapeutic alliance. Fortunately, the compulsive talking of these patients serves as both a symptom and a vehicle for gathering information.

Most patients with mania feel hard-pressed to remain silent and will speak at length on just about any subject. Ask a question; then, by picking up on a word or phrase the patient has used, you can channel the subsequent barrage of speech toward the information you seek. Psychosis often accompanies juvenile mania—be sure to check for the presence of delusions and hallucinations. Remember that the diagnosis of a bipolar disorder is better made on the basis of longitudinal history than on an assessment of current symptoms. Also, rule out the use of substances that could induce mood symptoms.

Developmental Factors

Although juvenile mania strongly resembles that of adults, some differences have been noted. Children under the age of 8 may not appear to have discrete episodes, and regular cycling is uncommon before adolescence. Young patients' illnesses often begin insidiously and sometimes appear to be chronic. Children's moods are likely to be irritable rather than euphoric, and they are more likely than adults or adolescents to have psychotic features such as hallucinations. Young children are reported to have especially troubled premorbid personalities.

When mania occurs in young children, it may resemble ADHD or oppositional defiant disorder, in that the symptoms often include frequent fighting and swearing. Around puberty, children may experience mania as irritability or misbehavior that suggests conduct disorder or ADHD; sometimes they cycle continuously and rapidly. Another problem for diagnosticians is that ADHD is often comorbid with bipolar disorders. As a check against overdiagnosis of mania in prepubertal children, you should inquire about a family history of bipolar disorders.

OTHER MOOD DISORDERS

Depressive or Bipolar and Related Disorder Due to Another Medical Condition

Many medical conditions can cause depressive symptoms; some can cause manic symptoms as well. When you are evaluating a young patient with mood symptoms, it is always important to consider the possibility of medical problems.

Substance/Medication–Induced Depressive or Bipolar and Related Disorder

Substance use is a common and probably underrecognized cause of mood symptoms. It is essential to consider the possibility of substance use in young patients, especially those who suddenly present with mood symptoms but have no prior or family history of mood disorders. For symptoms, see the Essential Features of Substance Intoxication and Substance Withdrawal (pp. 403 and 404) and the Essential Features of Four Substance/Medication-Induced Mental Disorders (p. 405) in Chapter 24. Table 24.1 can help with wording and code numbers.

Nowhere does DSM-5 use age of onset as a criterion for mood disorders of children *or* adults. However, based on recent work, perhaps we should pay more attention to age, certainly when considering prognosis. Various indicators suggest that an early onset (during the early teen or even subteen years) of MDD carries with it a greater likelihood of adverse outcomes. These include comorbid illnesses (both physical and mental), repeated episodes of depression, future suicide attempts, the risk of loneliness (few long-standing friendships or never marrying), and symptoms that are generally more severe.

CHAPTER 14

Anxiety Disorders

QUICK GUIDE TO THE ANXIETY DISORDERS

The following conditions may be diagnosed in children and adolescents who present with prominent anxiety symptoms; comorbidity is the rule.

Primary Anxiety Disorders

Panic disorder. Patients with this disorder experience repeated panic attacks, together with worry about having additional attacks and other mental and behavioral changes related to them (p. 275).

Agoraphobia. Patients fear situations or places such as entering a store, where they might have trouble obtaining help if they became anxious (p. 275).

Specific phobia. These patients fear specific objects or situations. Examples include animals; storms; heights; blood; airplanes; being closed in; or any circumstance that may lead to vomiting, choking, or developing an illness (p. 270).

Social anxiety disorder. Patients imagine themselves embarrassed when they speak, write, or eat in public, or use a public urinal (p. 272).

Selective mutism. A child elects not to talk, except when alone or with select intimates such as family (p. 266).

Generalized anxiety disorder. Although they do not experience acute panic attacks, these patients feel tense or anxious much of the time (p. 279).

Separation anxiety disorder. A patient becomes anxious when separated from a parent or other attachment figure (p. 262)

Anxiety disorder due to another medical condition. Various anxiety symptoms can be caused by many medical conditions (p. 283).

Substance/medication-induced anxiety disorder. Various psychoactive substances produce anxiety symptoms that don't necessarily fulfill criteria for any of the above-mentioned disorders (p. 283).

Other specified, or unspecified, anxiety disorder. Use one of these categories for patients whose anxiety symptoms don't meet criteria for any of the diagnoses above (p. 283).

Other Causes of Anxiety and Related Symptoms

Anxiety symptoms can be found in patients with almost any other mental disorder. They are especially prevalent in major depressive episode in a mood disorder (where they may qualify for the specifier *with anxious distress*, p. 240); somatic symptom disorder (p. 328); and adjustment disorder with anxiety (p. 311). See also obsessive–compulsive disorder (p. 285) and the trauma- and stressor-related disorders (Chapter 7).

INTRODUCTION

In thinking about the anxiety disorders, keep the following points firmly in mind:

- The anxiety disorders are the most common of all mental health disorders, though how often they affect juveniles, especially young children, is not clear. For one thing, they have been studied in children and adolescents for a relatively short period of time. For another, young children often don't realize they are feeling anxiety—which they may express not by words but by behaviors such as clinging, crying, or freezing, and in physical symptoms such as stomachache, headache, fatigue, anorexia, or insomnia. Only recently have diagnostic criteria insisted that symptoms produce disability or distress; older studies that omit this criterion may exaggerate prevalence.

- That said, a major national survey reported that about 8% of adolescents (ages 13–18) had an anxiety disorder, with symptoms commonly emerging much earlier, often around age 6. Of these teens, only 18% received mental health care.

- The DSM-5 criteria are categorical—either you have a disorder or you haven't. (Shopworn analogy: There is no such thing as being a little bit pregnant.) However, many physical illnesses can be present in degrees, including diabetes, heart disease, and even cancer, and many mental health clinicians point out the value of dimensionality in diagnosis.

▨ The typical anxious child or adolescent can be diagnosed with more than one anxiety disorder. It is not yet clear whether this finding predicts multiple diagnoses (or *any* diagnosis) when this youngster grows up.

▨ Many anxious children and adolescents do not fully qualify for any well-defined DSM-5 anxiety disorder and must be diagnosed as having other specified, or unspecified, anxiety disorder.

▨ Until DSM-5, separation anxiety disorder was grouped with the disorders usually first diagnosed in infancy, childhood, or adolescence (which themselves have now been renamed neurodevelopmental disorders).

▨ Finally, remember that in many instances anxiety is a normal, even useful emotion that may change from one developmental stage to the next. It may take time to differentiate a child's normal, adaptive (to perceived threats) worries from anxiety that is a maladaptive expression of unrealistic fears or dysfunctional behaviors.

F93.0 SEPARATION ANXIETY DISORDER

The name encapsulates the symptoms—anxiety when a patient is separated from parents or other important caregivers. Separation anxiety disorder (SAD) often becomes most inhibiting in a school setting. However, other common sources of difficulty include reluctance to remain with babysitters or in day care, or, for older children and adolescents, fear of being alone at home. A precipitating event may be identified: a minor accident, illness, or operation; a move to a new house, classroom, or school; the loss of a pet, friend, or parent. Whereas trauma can cause the more serious posttraumatic stress disorder, don't forget that it can also precipitate the onset of SAD.

Any of these perceived threats can arouse anxiety in the patient, who characteristically first complains, then resists separating. Physical symptoms may serve as justification for remaining at home or clinging to or trailing after the parents. Ultimately, some patients refuse to be alone in a room, use the bathroom unaccompanied, or even sleep alone—despite creative "carrots and sticks" approaches tried by parents or extraordinary accommodations made by school authorities. This sequence usually progresses rapidly in younger children, but the process may be more insidious in adolescents.

SAD is sometimes confused with truancy, but the whereabouts of truants are usually unknown by parents or school authorities, whereas children or adolescents absent because of SAD are most likely to be found at home or with a parent. In any event, school avoidance is a highly visible, important aspect of childhood SAD. Indeed, it is often a classroom teacher or school psychologist who first suggests the correct diagnosis.

Because young children have difficulty talking about their anxious feelings, they commonly manifest SAD as somatic symptoms. Pediatricians who encounter children with headaches, recurrent abdominal pains, and muscle weakness are likely to treat these as physical disorders.

Children and adolescents are especially vulnerable to SAD at three stages: when they first begin kindergarten (5 years); when they shift to more complex peer social structures and learning environments (beginning of junior high, 11 years); and shortly after the onset of puberty (13–14 years). Perhaps 4% of grade school children have SAD; by junior high, the number falls to under 2%, so that SAD is the one anxiety disorder that reliably decreases in prevalence with advancing age. Girls with SAD outnumber boys in the general population; however, a boy with the condition is more likely to be referred for evaluation, causing the sex ratio in clinical populations to be approximately 1:1.

Genetic inheritance appears to be high on the list of causes for SAD. Children of parents with anxiety disorders and major depression are at special risk for developing SAD. It may also be especially prevalent in children who have serious medical physical illness—for example, those who are under treatment for cancer or cystic fibrosis, or who require dialysis for end-stage kidney disease. Occasionally, it is the parent who expresses anxiety about separation; if so, it is important to address this so that the parent can help the child develop resilience. Later in life, children with SAD may be at special risk for panic disorder and depressive disorders.

Eric

When he was 12 years old, Eric was referred for evaluation because he persistently feared losing his mother. When Eric was only 3, his father, a glazier working on a downtown office

ESSENTIAL FEATURES OF **SEPARATION ANXIETY DISORDER**

Because they fear what might happen to a parent or someone else important in their lives, these patients resist being alone. They imagine that a parent will die or become lost (or that *they* will), so that even the thought of separation can cause anxiety, nightmares, or perhaps vomiting spells or other physical complaints. They are therefore reluctant to attend school, go out to work, or to sleep away from home—perhaps even in their own beds.

The Fine Print

The D's: • Duration (6+ months in adults, though extreme symptoms—such as total school refusal—could justify diagnosis after a shorter duration; 4+ weeks in children and adolescents) • Distress or disability (social, educational, occupational, or personal impairment) • Differential diagnosis (mood disorders, generalized anxiety disorder, agoraphobia, posttraumatic stress disorder, panic disorder)

building, had died in a fall from a 12th-floor scaffolding. Eric's mother had gone back to work at a bank, and Eric seemed to accept day care relatively well. Yet as he was about to enter junior high, Eric's enthusiasm for school hit a snag. That summer, he had a number of dreams in which he could see his mother but could not reach her because they were separated by a wide ditch. "Maybe it was the Grand Canyon," he said. He lived just across the street from his elementary school, but the junior high was several miles from his home.

> *School phobia* is a term that was once used to describe the refusal of children to attend school. Of course, it was not usually school as such that a child feared, but the consequences of being away from home or parents. *School avoidance* (or *school refusal*) is a better term for a problem that can stem from a variety of causes, of which SAD is only the most frequent. Anxiety disorders, oppositional defiant disorder, mood disorders, substance use, academic impairment, intrafamilial discord, and being the victim of bullying or other trauma are among the other causes of school refusal. The important point is that school avoidance doesn't necessarily mean mental illness.

In the first week of seventh grade, Eric made several trips to the nurse's office. He repeatedly mentioned a worry that his mother's bank would be held up. He complained that he could not breathe, and twice his mother had to leave work and take him home. The second week he did not attend class at all because of abdominal pain. The pediatrician pronounced him physically healthy.

During his first mental health interview, Eric appeared verbal and cheerful. He denied symptoms of depression, anxiety, or panic attack. He acknowledged that his fears about his mother were probably exaggerated. "But I've only got one parent," he said. "You can't be too careful."

Evaluation of Eric

Whereas physical symptoms, persistent worry, troubled dreams, and fears about separation from a parent are common in very young children, they are developmentally unexpected in a boy age 12. Eric worried that his mother's bank would be held up (Criterion A2); he refused to go to school (A4); and he had trouble breathing and abdominal pain (A8). (At least three of the possible eight symptoms in Criterion A are required for diagnosis.) His symptoms had lasted longer than a month (B), and he was so distressed he couldn't attend class (C). Other possible diagnoses can be ruled out (D): He denied having **panic attacks,** and the circumstances of his symptoms were too limited for a diagnosis of **generalized anxiety disorder** (which is, however, often comorbid). Other conditions in which separation anxiety can be encountered include **psychotic disorders** and **posttraumatic stress disorder,** none of which could be supported by Eric's history. Although Eric had been bereaved, this had occurred long ago, and there was no evidence that he was still actively mourning his father. He denied symptoms of a **depressive disorder,** which co-occurs in up to half of these children. Eric's complete diagnosis would therefore be the following:

F93.0   Separation anxiety disorder
CGAS   70 (current)

ASSESSING SEPARATION ANXIETY DISORDER

General Suggestions

Very young children naturally go through a stage during which they object to separation from their parents, but this gradually diminishes between the ages of 3 and 5. Although such children may scream or have a tantrum as their parents get ready to leave, they calm down and carry on with their usual activities, once they are left in day care or with a babysitter. A child with SAD is less readily distracted, and such behavior will endure long past the age at which it is developmentally appropriate.

During history taking, look for symptoms (emotional or physical) that parallel the course of the school year—increasing when school is in session, waning on weekends or over the summer. Watch to evaluate the degree to which a young child clings to the parent in the waiting room. Does the resistance to parting increase as the time for separation draws nearer? Is the degree of distress so severe that you cannot interview the child alone? Ask the child, "What do you fear will happen?" The answer will probably involve scenes of disaster—a parent involved in a car crash, or the kidnapping or death of the child.

Carefully inquire about any family history of anxiety or mood disorder, and ask about comorbid conditions in the patient. ADHD is often found in young people with school refusal, as are mood and other anxiety disorders. You also want to know what the child does while staying home from school—is it something enjoyable that might be secondarily reinforcing the behavior? You also want to know how the parents react: Could their concern be adding to the child's insecurity?

Intense separation anxiety or other anxiety symptoms can occur in response to the experience or threat of trauma or abuse, and such a child may be too frightened to disclose the trauma. So ascertain whether a parent has been ill or injured, or whether family dissolution is imminent. If at all possible, meet (even briefly) alone with the child to inquire about traumatic experiences. Of course, if you suspect abuse, follow the child protective services' reporting laws in the jurisdiction where you work.

Developmental Factors

Young children with SAD may react to fears of parental separation by physically clinging to their parents or trailing them from room to room. They are more likely to report fear of harm to a parent, whereas older children and adolescents often describe physical symptoms or subjective feelings of distress. Older children may balk at leaving home to attend camp, sleep over with a friend, or even attend school. They may fear being home alone at an age when many teens begin babysitting younger children.

F94.0 SELECTIVE MUTISM

Children with selective mutism (SM) can speak fluently but remain silent except when alone or with a small group of intimates or family. The condition typically begins during preschool years, after normal speech has developed. Such a child, who speaks appropriately at home among family members but becomes relatively silent when confronted by strangers, may not attract clinical attention until starting school.

Most children with SM have normal hearing and intelligence. Those who come from immigrant families, who have a speech problem such as stuttering or delayed speaking, or whose primary language is other than that spoken in school are at special risk for SM. The usual pattern is that a child speaks fluently at home, but refuses to speak at school or when brought for evaluation. When these children do speak, sentence structure, vocabulary, and articulation are normal.

SM has traditionally been considered an uncommon disorder, but several recent surveys suggest that its prevalence in the general population is perhaps 0.5%, with girls somewhat more often affected than boys. There is frequently a family history of SM or social anxiety disorder; indeed, these often shy children may additionally meet criteria for social anxiety disorder. Although SM usually improves spontaneously after many weeks or months, the treatment process can be extremely frustrating for a therapist, whose young patient may remain completely silent during therapy sessions, even while gradually regaining normal speech when at school or with friends. In a small percentage, SM may persist into early adulthood. Some individuals develop other anxiety disorders, such as social anxiety disorder, in adulthood.

Kim

A tall, slender, tomboyish 7-year-old, Kim had stopped speaking with anyone but her mother, and then only when she was at home. The problem had begun abruptly 18 months earlier, when she was just finishing kindergarten. At about that time, her parents separated after 15 years of marriage, and her father left the family and moved to a distant city to live with a new girlfriend. Kim, her 9-year-old sister, and her mother were left behind.

Kim was born in New York City, where her grandparents had moved from Poland more than 60 years earlier. Her early growth and development were entirely normal; she had no

ESSENTIAL FEATURES OF **SELECTIVE MUTISM**

Despite speaking normally at other times, the patient regularly doesn't speak in certain situations where speech is expected, such as in class.

The Fine Print

The D's: • Duration (1+ months) • Distress or disability (social or educational impairment) • Differential diagnosis (unfamiliarity with the language to be used; a communication disorder such as stuttering; psychotic disorders; autism spectrum disorder; social anxiety disorder)

Coding Note

The first month of a child's first year in school is often fraught with anxiety; exclude behaviors that occur during this time.

history of stuttering or delayed speech. Whereas her previous functioning in school, both academically and with peers, had been good, her refusal to speak had now brought her to the brink of failure and had nearly severed her friendships. Instead of making her repeat the first grade, her teacher had recommended treatment.

Although Kim had stopped talking with her friends and was completely mute in class, she spoke normally at home with her mother and sister. In fact, her mother brought an audio recording of Kim's speech at home to the initial interview. On the recording, Kim talked at some length about a dance step she had seen on TV; twice she could be heard interrupting her sister. Although Kim refused to utter even one syllable with the examiner, she maintained good eye contact and promptly wrote out answers to questions. By this means, she denied any history of depression, hallucinations, or panic attacks.

Evaluation of Kim

Of course, Kim consistently failed to speak where she was expected to (Criterion A), and of course, it had interfered with her schooling (B) and lasted longer than a month (C). So the problem for Kim's clinician was to rule out any other possibilities, such as primary **disorders of language, learning,** or **hearing** that can produce the appearance of SM. None was apparent in Kim, who, as an American born to English-speaking parents, had no cause for discomfort with her native language (D). Once past these barriers, we have in SM a one-symptom disorder for which the symptom is completely self-evident.

However, several other conditions can present with mutism. **Severe intellectual disability** and **autism spectrum disorder** could be ruled out by Kim's history of normal development and progress through her first 5 years. The audio recording made clear that there was no evidence of another **communication disorder**. Although **social anxiety disorder** is often associated with SM, Kim indicated in writing that **anxiety** did not play a major role in her difficulties. Nowhere in these written communications or in her history was there evidence of **schizophrenia** or another **psychotic disorder**. Although children with severe **depression** may speak very little, that behavior tends to hold whether at home or away. So Criterion E is satisfied, and Kim's undisputed diagnosis would be this:

F94.0	Selective mutism
CGAS	51 (current)

ASSESSING SELECTIVE MUTISM

General Suggestions

There is something of a contradiction in the notion of interviewing anyone who won't speak. But of course, much that we seek to learn about any child comes from the history, and much else from observing nonverbal behavior. Learning that a child who utters nothing in the course of a half-hour session speaks fluently and at length at home strongly suggests SM. In the office, even such a child may be induced to communicate in whispers, in gestures, or by writing or drawing. Some creative clinicians have set up two phones in the exam room, and by that means been able to gain some interpersonal communication with children with SM—as long as they are not face to face with the children. (The use of telepsychiatry interviews may be a future tool to consider.)

Observing that a mute child appears *interested* in communicating may help sort out the differential diagnosis of one who has intellectual disability, just as warmth or responsiveness can help discriminate a child with selective mutism from one with autism spectrum disorder. Carefully note any apparent anxiety; some evidence suggests that selectively mute children may suffer from an extreme variety of social anxiety disorder. Such a child may also refuse to eat or write when with others. Angry children may try to control the environment by refusing to speak, but with patience in the interview and sincere regard for how angry that child feels, the resistance to speaking might diminish.

Developmental Factors

Because patients with SM speak normally at home, the behavior usually isn't noticed until they begin school. However, some normal children are reluctant to speak when they first begin school, so make the diagnosis only if the problem does not resolve spontaneously after a month in kindergarten or first grade.

PHOBIC DISORDERS

A *phobia* is a fear that is triggered by something. It produces clinically important anxiety symptoms, which can be panic attacks (they are cued) or more general symptoms of anxiety. Now let us consider the two main types of phobias, specific and social. (We consider agoraphobia separately below, together with panic attacks and panic disorder.) Specific phobia is a fear of situations (such as acrophobia—fear of heights) or objects (such as spiders or thunderstorms). A social phobia is a fear of some kinds of social or performance situations (such as speaking in public). In DSM-5, social phobia has been renamed social anxiety disorder, but the symptoms have remained essentially the same. We abbreviate it in this discussion as SOC, since separation anxiety disorder and several other disorders are commonly abbreviated SAD.

Specific phobia and SOC have many features in common that we can summarize:

- A defined condition triggers fear or anxiety.
- Whenever exposed to the trigger, the patient almost always experiences this feeling.
- Although adults usually have insight that their anxiety is excessive, children (and some adolescents) may not.
- Many adults with phobias first develop their symptoms during childhood or adolescence.
- A patient avoids the feared condition, or endures it with severe distress. (Children and adolescents may be less able than adults to avoid the stimulus.)
- The condition seriously affects the patient's life or causes marked distress. (Loss of blood pressure and fainting typically result from the blood–injection–injury type of specific phobia.)
- The symptoms must last for at least 6 months. In children, this requirement helps distinguish some transient fears—of strangers or the dark, for example—from developmentally normal behavior that can even have survival value.
- The symptoms aren't better explained by another anxiety disorder diagnosis. However, children and adolescents (and adults) with phobias usually have other major mental disorders as well, especially additional anxiety disorders.
- A final point applies only to SOC: People with medical or mental conditions that are disfiguring or cause unusual behavior may fear the scrutiny of other people. Therefore, we wouldn't diagnose SOC in, for example, a child or adolescent with trichotillomania if the only fear is that people might notice the hair pulling.

Although the symptoms of specific phobia and SOC may be somewhat different in juveniles (especially young children) than in adults, the criteria are fundamentally the same (see the Essential Features of each below).

Specific Phobia

Fears are nearly ubiquitous in children. In about 5% of children and 15% of teenagers, they cause a clinical level of distress, landing specific phobia among the most commonplace of the childhood mental disorders. Animal phobia typically begins at about the age of 7, fear of blood at 9, and fear of dental procedures at 12. Specific environmental phobias, such as claustrophobia, typically begin much later—about age 20. Fears of animals and environmental phenomena such as thunderstorms usually occur in females. DSM-5 notes that some children especially fear loud noises or costumed characters (such as Goofy and Ronald McDonald).

The following vignette describes one of Sigmund Freud's best-known patients. Our source is "Analysis of a Phobia in a Five-Year-Old Boy," in the *Standard Edition* of Freud's works (Vol. 10, pp. 5–149).

Little Hans

When Hans was not quite 5 years old, he developed a fear that "a horse would bite him in the street." That Freud associated this terror with Hans's fear of big penises and a desire to possess his mother sexually need not concern us here. In brief, here is the story.

Beginning in early January 1908, Hans would cry whenever he saw a horse. When taken to the park, he would grow "visibly frightened"; even when accompanied, he was reluctant to venture out of doors. He "always ran back into the house with every sign of fright if horses came along." This fear appeared to apply to any horse, whether it was being ridden or pulling a carriage or cart. When traffic was light and no horses were visible, however, Hans did not appear to be frightened. "How sensible!" he said. "God's done away with horses now." Other than when he was confronting a horse, he appeared to be a cheerful, healthy boy.

By May of that year, Hans's anxiety symptoms when he encountered a horse had largely disappeared. At follow-up 14 years later, he had remained asymptomatic, even during the divorce and remarriage of his parents.

Evaluation of Little Hans

How does this classic specific phobia stack up against DSM-5 criteria? The presence of horses (specific object) nearly always (Criterion B) triggered (cued) fearful crying and "every sign of fright" (A). Hans avoided proximity to horses whenever possible (C). There is no clear evidence that Hans ever realized his fears were disproportionate (D), but the presence of insight is not required for a diagnosis of specific phobia.

So far, so good—several of the criteria for specific phobia were met. But did his distress reach the level of clinical significance? To be sure, Hans cried when taken to the park, but that hardly constituted a clinically important event. He didn't attend school, and we read

ESSENTIAL FEATURES OF **SPECIFIC PHOBIA**

A specific situation or thing habitually causes such immediate, inordinate (and unreasonable) dread or anxiety that the patient avoids it or endures it with much anxiety.

The Fine Print

Children may express their fear by clinging or crying, raging or retreating, freezing or failing to speak.

The D's: • Duration (6+ months) • Distress or disability (social, educational, occupational, or personal impairment) • Differential diagnosis (substance use and physical disorders; agoraphobia; SOC; separation anxiety disorder; mood and psychotic disorders; anorexia nervosa; obsessive–compulsive disorder; posttraumatic stress disorder)

Coding Notes

Specify all types that apply with individual ICD-10 codes:

> **F40.218 Animal type** (spiders, snakes)
> **F40.228 Natural environment type** (thunderstorms, heights)
> **Blood–injection–injury type** (syringes, operations)
> > **F40.230 Blood**
> > **F40.231 Injections and transfusions**
> > **F40.232 Other medical care**
> > **F40.233 Injury**
> **F40.248 Situational type** (airplane travel, being closed in)
> **F40.298 Other type** (for instance, situations where the person could choke or vomit; for children, loud noises or people wearing costumes)

nothing of his interactions with friends. He didn't appear to be at odds with his family (with the possible exception of his father, whom he allegedly wanted to replace in his mother's affections). Fear of horses disrupted his activities only to the extent that he didn't go to the park much. He did feel distress, to the extent that clinical advice was sought. That would seem to fulfill the requirement of clinical significance (F).

However, the evidence suggests that Hans's fear of horses had dissipated in less than the minimum 6 months' duration DSM-5 requires for this diagnosis (E). Some might suggest that Freud's consultation had in some way shortened the duration of illness. It is as plausible, and perhaps more likely, that Hans never suffered from a "disorder" at all, but rather a simple childhood fear that vanished with later maturation. This conclusion is somewhat strengthened by the observation that Hans apparently had none of the conditions so often comorbid with phobic disorders.

Could Freud have mistaken Hans's condition for some other mental disorder (G)? His fear was not of being away from home in general, as would be expected with **agoraphobia**; nor were his spells of anxiety (we are not sure whether he ever had true panic attacks) uncued, as would be the case for **panic disorder**. We don't learn of other fears (robbers, kidnappers, train accidents) that could harm the family, as might be true in **separation anxiety disorder**.

Klein has noted that the diagnosis of specific phobia is among the least reliable for children, in part because the boundary between phobia and ordinary fears is imprecise. With the benefit of DSM-5 criteria, at the time of first evaluation Freud might have felt he needed more data or time before a definitive diagnosis could be made. Instead, if he could have reached for his DSM, he might have diagnosed something on the order of the following:

F41.9   Unspecified anxiety disorder
CGAS   60 (upon first evaluation)

F40.10 Social Anxiety Disorder

Youngsters who have SOC fear the scrutiny of others so greatly that they may have difficulty reciting in class, asking for a date, going to a party, performing before an audience, or even asking a teacher's help. The disorder typically begins in the preteen years and tends to become chronic. These children often grow up without friends and tend to develop depressive and substance use disorders; as adults, many do not marry. Note that this diagnosis cannot be given unless a child has developed sufficiently to have social relationships, and that the symptoms in children must occur with *peers*, not just with adults.

Children with SOC lack self-confidence and are excessively and age-inappropriately timid, perhaps to the point that they perform poorly in school or avoid playing with other children. One way DSM-5 tries to sort out clinically important distress from developmental phases is to require a duration of at least 6 months, which helps us disregard the transient social fears so common in many children. As many as 8% of adolescents (somewhat fewer for younger children) may have SOC, placing it among the most common mental disorders that affect young people.

Note the difference between SOC and agoraphobia: In both conditions, patients avoid certain social situations. However, in SOC the goal is to avoid embarrassing encounters, whereas in agoraphobia it is to avoid the anxiety symptoms themselves.

Some children with SOC are described as being extraordinarily shy; frequent comorbid conditions also include generalized anxiety disorder, specific phobia, and depressive disorders. Subsequent substance misuse and failure to complete schooling are often encountered in these children.

ESSENTIAL FEATURES OF **SOCIAL ANXIETY DISORDER**

Inordinate anxiety is attached to circumstances where others could closely observe a patient—public speaking or performing, eating or having a drink, writing, or perhaps just speaking with another person. Because these activities almost always provoke disproportionate fear of embarrassment or social rejection, the patient avoids these situations or endures them with much anxiety.

The Fine Print

In kids, symptoms must occur with peers, not just with adults.

The D's: • Duration (6+ months) • Distress or disability (social, educational, occupational, or personal impairment) • Differential diagnosis (substance use and physical disorders; mood and psychotic disorders; autism spectrum disorder; anorexia nervosa; obsessive–compulsive disorder; avoidant personality disorder; normal shyness; other anxiety disorders, especially agoraphobia)

Coding Notes

Specify if:

> **Performance only.** The patient fears public speaking or performing, but not other situations.

Rita

Twelve-year-old Rita was referred for evaluation after her Sunday school teacher reported to her parents: "Rita is a lovely little girl who seems to have a problem. She was to play a Wise Man in the Christmas pageant, but froze up completely when it came time to say her line." Although the Virgin Mary stage-whispered the line several times, Rita never could say it. The pageant finally went on without her verbal participation; afterward, she cried.

According to her mother, Rita had been a normal, happy infant and toddler. But although she made "about average" grades, she had never enjoyed school. When the other children went out to play at recess, she would stay in her seat, drawing or reading a storybook. In fourth grade, she complained that she hated to write on the chalkboard when the class did math. At first her teacher made her go up to the board anyway; eventually she was allowed to do most of her work at her seat.

The previous summer, Rita had attended camp for 2 weeks. She made nine whistle cords in the crafts tent, but no new friends. For 5 days after she returned, her lonely letters home continued to arrive.

At home, Rita played normally with her sister, who was almost 2 years younger than she. When her mother tried to start her in Brownies, she spent nearly all of every meeting she attended standing off to one side "looking completely miserable," though the Brownie leader repeatedly tried to engage her in singing and planning a field trip. Just after Christmas, her mother gave up the struggle, and she stopped attending.

Within a few therapy sessions, Rita formed a close, warm relationship with her clinician, to whom she confided a wish to be more like the other kids. But her self-consciousness continued to get in her way. "I can't stand to have everyone looking at me," she told the clinician. "It makes me feel like I'm burning up."

Evaluation of Rita

In addition to the 10 criteria DSM-5 enumerates for SOC, for kids there are two special notes. We've boiled all this down a bit for the Essential Features, but as usual, we'll go through everything right here.

For at least half a year (Criterion F), Rita feared not just social situations such as appearing in a play and playing with others at camp or Brownies (A); she also dreaded the embarrassment that they might entail (B). The situation must almost always cause anxiety (C), which in Rita's case seems likely from the history, though we'd need a diary to prove it. She responded principally by, whenever possible, withdrawing and avoiding these situations (D)—behavior that was out of proportion to any actual threat (E). Her distress and impaired social functioning were evident from her classroom and camp behavior (G).

Note that Rita's story demonstrates two features that differentiate children from adults. A child's response may be clinging, crying, freezing, withdrawing, or having tantrums (the note to Criterion C); and the note to Criterion A specifies that the anxiety must occur not solely when the child is in the company of adults, but with peers (Rita avoided camp activities and playground games).

Before making a definitive diagnosis, Rita's clinician would have to decide that her symptoms couldn't be explained better by **another medical condition** or by **substance use** or a **different mental disorder** (H). Because her symptoms persisted despite long familiarity (with the classroom situation, for example), we wouldn't try to explain her problem as due to a **temperamental variant**—a case of a timid child who warmed up slowly. The differential diagnosis also often includes **generalized anxiety disorder,** which frequently accompanies SOC, and **separation anxiety disorder**. Rita felt anxiety, but her distress was never expressed as actual panic attacks, ruling out a diagnosis of **panic disorder**. Her desire for social relationships differentiated her from children with **autism spectrum disorder** (I).

Rita's complete diagnosis is given below. In adults, **avoidant personality disorder** has been associated with SOC, and the two conditions show some overlap. Whereas no personality disorder diagnosis would be warranted now, her clinician should reevaluate Rita's personality characteristics when she is older.

F40.10   Social anxiety disorder
CGAS   55 (current)

PANIC ATTACKS, PANIC DISORDER, AND AGORAPHOBIA

As recently as a couple of generations ago, the ability of children and adolescents to develop repeated panic attacks was relatively ignored in the mental health literature. Now it is generally recognized that these symptoms can occur before puberty, even (rarely) in children as young as 5, and that the prevalence increases with age to the teen years. At some time during their lives, about 2% of adolescents have had enough symptoms to fulfill criteria for panic disorder; many more have had at least one isolated panic attack. Young girls and boys are about equally likely to be affected, though attacks are often more severe in girls. Females predominate among both adolescents and adults.

In children and adults alike, agoraphobia can develop in close association with panic disorder. For whatever reason (both hereditary and environmental factors are implicated), a patient begins to develop panic symptoms that eventually become full-blown panic attacks. The fear of recurrent symptoms spawns anxiety that persists between attacks. This anxiety can ultimately generalize to avoidance behavior that includes agoraphobia—the fear of being away from home, especially where escape might be difficult or help not available when needed. Classically, this was in the *agora*, the Greek marketplace—but it can occur in theaters, shopping malls, or many other places away from home. Although the two conditions are not always linked, this order of onset often occurs. The prevalence of agoraphobia in adolescents is around 2%.

Further evidence of the continuum between juvenile and adult anxiety disorders is the fact that many adults who report panic attacks first had symptoms prior to their middle teens—some as young as 10. Although the exact symptoms may differ, it seems clear that the overall syndromes of panic attack and agoraphobia are the same for children, adolescents, and adults (though adolescents may be somewhat less likely to worry about having future episodes). The Essential Features are presented below.

Hank

Hank knew exactly when his trouble began. It had been the previous year, in his seventh-grade prealgebra class. He had aced the first two questions and was just organizing his answer to a brief essay question about factoring when his test paper started swimming before his eyes.

"Like, it shimmered, you know? Like heat waves coming off a hot pavement."

"Besides the swimming, did you notice anything else?" asked the interviewer.

Hank shook his head. "No. In a few minutes it went away, and I finished the exam. But

ESSENTIAL FEATURES OF **PANIC ATTACK** AND **PANIC DISORDER**

A panic attack is a fear (sometimes stark terror) that begins suddenly and is accompanied by a variety of classic "fight-or-flight" symptoms—plus a few others: chest pain, chills, heat sensations, choking, shortness of breath, rapid or irregular heartbeat, numbness or tingling, sweating, nausea, dizziness, and trembling. As a result, these people may feel unreal, as if they are losing control, or dying.

In panic disorder, the patient fears future panic attacks that are not anticipated or tries to avert them by taking (ineffective) action such as abandoning an exercise program or avoiding places where attacks have occurred.

The Fine Print (for Panic Disorder)

The D's: • Duration (1+ months) • Distress or disability (social, educational, occupational, or personal impairment) • Differential diagnosis (substance use and physical disorders; other anxiety disorders; mood and psychotic disorders; obsessive–compulsive disorder; posttraumatic stress disorder; actual danger)

Special note: Panic attack (see the first paragraph of these Essential Features) is not a codable disorder and can occur in conditions other than panic disorder (which is coded F41.0). Thus panic attack may serve as a specifier to posttraumatic stress disorder, other anxiety disorders, and other mental disorders, including eating, mood, psychotic, personality, and substance use. It is even found in medical conditions affecting the heart, lung, and gastrointestinal tract.

a few days later I was writing an essay during English class. My hand shook so much and my fingers felt so weak that I couldn't hold the pencil. The teacher sent me to the nurse's office. I thought I was going to faint on the way."

"Did you feel anything else during that episode?"

"I could feel my heart beating, really hard. That scared me—I guessed I was having a heart attack. The nurse said I was hypoventilating and made me breathe into a paper bag."

"Hy*per*ventilating," said the interviewer. "Did the bag breathing help?"

"Yeah, hyperventilating. It got better after a while."

Hank sat slumped a little in his chair, his forehead resting lightly on the fingers of his hand. He had begun having attacks outside of class, too, he said. They were mostly the same—a tight chest, constricted breathing, palpitations, and the fear that he was terribly ill. Although examinations always seemed to cause an attack, more and more they would spring up any time, even when he wasn't at school. "It'll happen within seconds, right out of the blue."

From Hank's parents, the interviewer had already obtained quite a lot of information. Because he was bright and articulate, his grades at first hadn't suffered much. His parents were both professional people who didn't delve too deeply into their son's inner feelings—or perhaps he had chosen not to reveal them. In any event, until he began cutting school, they'd noticed nothing wrong. "First he didn't want to take the school bus," his father said, "said it always made him jumpy. Then he just didn't ever *leave* home. Said he'd get by on home study. It's been that way ever since."

Hank's birth had been a full-term, normal delivery; he was the second of two planned and well-loved children. He and his sister had both done well throughout their private school education. Neither had had prior emotional difficulties, though Hank had "seemed somewhat nervous" for most of the winter and spring when he was 5. He had clung to his mother the first few days she tried to leave him at kindergarten, but was soon distracted by the playthings in the classroom. Neither of his parents had noticed any recent problems with eating or sleeping. He had no unsavory friends, and as far as they were aware, he had never used drugs or alcohol.

Hank had been silent for some time. "So you started staying home?" the interviewer prompted.

"Yeah. I kept thinking I'd have another attack at school. Pretty soon, I couldn't stand going anywhere by myself—you know, without Mom or Dad."

Hank was pleasant to talk to, even funny as he described some of his problems. He made good eye contact with the examiner, smiled appropriately, and spoke clearly in well-

ESSENTIAL FEATURES OF **AGORAPHOBIA**

These patients almost invariably experience inordinate anxiety or dread when they have to be alone or away from home. Potentially, there's an abundance of opportunities: riding a bus (or other mass transit), shopping, attending a theatrical entertainment. For some, the triggers may be as ordinary as walking through an open space (flea market, playground), being part of a crowd, or standing in a queue. When you dig down, these people are afraid that escape would be impossible or that help (in the event of panic) would be unavailable. So they avoid such situations or confront them only with a trusted friend—or, if all else fails, endure them with lots of suffering.

The Fine Print

The D's: • Duration (6+ months) • Distress or disability (social, educational, occupational, or personal impairment) • Differential diagnosis (substance use and physical disorders; other anxiety disorders; mood and psychotic disorders; obsessive–compulsive disorder; posttraumatic stress disorder; separation anxiety disorder)

constructed sentences. He had never had delusions or hallucinations, and denied ever using drugs. He readily admitted that he had a problem and said that he wished he could go back to school. "I can learn algebra at home. But, heck, I'm missing sex ed."

Evaluation of Hank

Spoiler alert: Hank's symptoms require the diagnosis of two anxiety disorders, which we'll take one step at a time.

First, how do his episodes of anxiety fit the criteria for panic disorder? His episodes were recurrent and unexpected, occurred suddenly, lasted a few minutes, and then were gone. Some of Hank's panic attacks were triggered (cued) by a test situation or by going to the store, but others had no apparent precipitant (Criterion A). The symptoms he experienced included shakiness (A3), pounding heart (A1), shortness of breath (A4), "tight chest" (A6), and feeling faint (A8). The diagnosis requires only four of these symptoms.

For longer than a month (B), Hank worried that he would have more attacks (B1) and stayed home from school to try to avoid them (B2). His parents' report about the absence of any diagnosed **medical conditions** (such as hyperthyroidism) that could cause panic attacks was considered accurate (C). Although it seemed evident that Hank did not use alcohol or drugs, the clinician wisely verified this by questioning both Hank and his parents directly—and separately (also C). Of course, caregivers must be alert to the possibility that some actual threat or danger could be causing any patient's panic symptoms.

No other anxiety or mental disorder would seem to explain Hank's symptoms better (D). His panic attacks weren't limited to social situations (such as speaking in public or, in older patients, asking for a date), as in **social anxiety disorder,** or to limited situations such as being confronted with a spider, as in **specific phobia.** Although there had been hints of separation anxiety when he was very young, the duration was brief. Hank's fears also differed from those of **separation anxiety disorder,** in that the focus of his anxiety was having another panic attack, not the physical separation from his parents.

After Hank's panic disorder was well established, he developed the fear of being away from home alone (Criterion A5 for agoraphobia)—so that was where he stayed, unless accompanied by a parent. He had also stopped using the school bus (A1); anxiety in two types of situations is required for the diagnosis of agoraphobia. He feared he'd have another attack at school (B); being on the school bus always made him jumpy (C). He avoided school and the bus (D), despite the fact that there wasn't any actual danger (E). From Hank's own statements, we infer that the symptoms were persistent (F), and he was certainly impaired for attending school (G). These symptoms weren't any better explained by another anxiety diagnosis than was the panic disorder (I)—which, you'll notice, itself isn't mentioned as a rule-out in this criterion. And so, at last (!) we can say that he fulfills the criteria for agoraphobia.

Many patients, even children, will have more than one anxiety disorder. **Generalized**

anxiety disorder is often comorbid, but Hank's worries were circumscribed rather than being about a number of different problems. In addition to one or more other anxiety disorders, Hank's clinician should look carefully for evidence of a mood disorder—especially **major depressive disorder** or a **bipolar disorder,** which commonly co-occur in patients who have panic attacks; the anxiety disorder often starts first. Based on our current information, Hank seemed to be bearing his difficulties without this sort of complication: His affect was generally good, even humorous, and there was no evidence of problems with appetite or sleep. He would need to be evaluated later for symptoms of **avoidant personality disorder,** which is also sometimes comorbid in patients with agoraphobia. Always inquire about trauma, because posttraumatic stress disorder can include panic attacks.

The criteria for agoraphobia explicitly encourage us to make two diagnoses when appropriate, and that's what we will do for Hank:

F41.0	Panic disorder
F40.00	Agoraphobia
CGAS	60 (current)

F41.1 GENERALIZED ANXIETY DISORDER

Children who have generalized anxiety disorder (GAD) worry about a variety of situations or events. Their worry is something they cannot control—worry that is out of all proportion to the objective seriousness of the situation. They may feel anxiety when anticipating situations in which their behavior or performance will be assessed by others.

As applied to children and adolescents, DSM-III-R called this behavior overanxious disorder of childhood (OAD). However, researchers realized that OAD is similar to, and probably on a continuum with, adult GAD; therefore, the two diagnoses were combined. Even as of this writing, much of our information on childhood GAD comes from studies of OAD. Children typically worry about "kid things"—grades, tests, being bullied, athletic ability—but they may also experience more adult concerns, such as worries over natural disasters or the family's fiscal health. Some studies have found that nonreferred children also worry about many issues, only not as intensely as children diagnosed with GAD.

A large minority of children will at one time or another have enough symptoms to meet the old DSM-III-R criteria for GAD (or OAD). But in DSM-5, symptoms must be important enough clinically to cause distress or impair functioning; then the lifetime prevalence of GAD in general adolescent populations falls to about 2%. These figures are still substantial, and GAD probably accounts for about one-third of child referrals to an anxiety disorder clinic. As with other anxiety disorders, girls are probably somewhat more likely to be affected. At this writing, the prognosis is still unclear; a 2009 report notes that no specific outcome has been demonstrated, and even cites evidence that GAD in children and adults may actually represent different conditions. Quite frankly, the research on GAD in children has been so mixed with older reports of OAD that we can only await further studies to clarify outcome.

Gerald

Gerald's parents said that he'd always been a "worrywart," and everything about Gerald seemed to confirm their opinion. Last year, he told the interviewer, he had worried that he was too short to play basketball; he had grown quite a bit in the fifth grade, but he worried that he still couldn't shoot well. He was also afraid that he wasn't very popular: He'd been elected class vice-president, but not president. His dad had told him that vice-president was a responsible position, but Gerald wasn't having any of that. "He's always trying to reassure me," said Gerald. "Besides, I think he and Mom are getting a divorce. They fight an awful lot." Recently, he had decided not to join the Boy Scouts—he knew he could never learn to tie knots. "When he isn't worrying," his dad said, "he's asleep."

Gerald was the second of three brothers. The other two had always seemed pretty normal, rough-and-tumble kids, according to their parents, both of whom worked as clerks at a Department of Veterans Affairs medical center. Gerald's physical health was excellent, but he was "the most cautious kid in six counties," his dad said. When all three boys got skateboards for Christmas one year, Gerald put his in the closet after a couple of trial rides. He never touched it again.

Although Gerald had always been a good student, his fifth-grade teacher had lately remarked that his mind seemed elsewhere. "Something seems to be troubling him," she had said at the fall parent–teacher conference. "Some days he's just cranky with everyone; other days he gets up and wanders around the room. He wasn't like that last year at all."

ESSENTIAL FEATURES OF **GENERALIZED ANXIETY DISORDER**

Hard-to-control, excessive worrying about a variety of issues—health, family problems, money, school, work—results in physical and mental complaints: muscle tension, restlessness, being easily tired and irritable, experiencing poor concentration, and trouble with insomnia.

The Fine Print

Only one physical or mental complaint is required for a GAD diagnosis in children.

The D's: • Duration (on most days for 6+ months) • Distress or disability (social, educational, occupational, or personal impairment) • Differential diagnosis (substance use and physical disorders, mood and other anxiety disorders, OCD, PTSD, realistic worry)

Gerald denied that he was depressed or on drugs. "But," he said, "I know I worry too much—everyone says so. I can't help it. I've tried closing the door in my mind on these problems, but it keeps popping open again." Although he denied having any of the somatic symptoms typical of a panic attack, he did admit to feeling "wired" whenever he thought about his problems. Then moving around would sometimes help him feel better.

Evaluation of Gerald

Gerald's worries were numerous and always present (Criterion A). They included his physical abilities, his schoolwork, his popularity, and even the integrity of his own family. That's the point of GAD: A patient finds plenty to worry about. Even though Gerald struggled for control (B), it cost him considerable distress (D), and the vignette implies that his schoolwork was about to suffer. Gerald's anxiety symptoms included inattention (C3), restlessness (C1), and irritability (C4). DSM-5 requires only one of these symptoms for children and adolescents, three or more for adults. Neither drug use nor medical illness could account for Gerald's symptoms (E).

The criteria for GAD include the usual laundry list of anxiety disorders that must be ruled out as a focus of anxiety: **panic disorder** (Gerald had had no panic attacks), **social anxiety disorder** (his fears were multiple and varied), **obsessive–compulsive disorder** (his worries only concerned everyday problems, not contamination, and we don't read that they were intrusive), **separation anxiety disorder** (his anxiety was not limited to concerns about separation from parents), and **posttraumatic stress disorder** (we don't know of any traumatic event). Other disorders that must be ruled out include **anorexia nervosa** (anxiety about being fat), anxiety as a symptom of **ADHD,** and **somatic symptom disorder** (anxiety about physical complaints). Of course, some of these same disorders may be comorbid with GAD. In summary, the vignette provides no evidence that another diagnosis might explain Gerald's symptoms better than GAD (F). His diagnosis would be as follows:

F41.1   Generalized anxiety disorder
CGAS   70 (current)

ASSESSING DISORDERS INVOLVING PANIC, AGORAPHOBIA, OTHER PHOBIAS, AND GENERALIZED ANXIETY

General Suggestions

Young children will not understand the term anxiety, so you will need to ask, "Are there things that frighten or worry you?" The responses will be quite varied, ranging from darkness to germs to snakes to strangers to visits to the dentist. Depending on the history the parents give, it may be necessary to run through a list of other possibilities: animals, bee stings, being lost or teased, burglars, death, inability to breathe, making errors, and poor grades. Not all of these will constitute phobias—some young patients will worry about competence in school or sports, the future, and various physical complaints, whether real or imagined. What does the patient fear as dire outcomes for self, for family members, for close friends, or for pets? Be sure to ask whether the child is afraid of water (in one study, 98% of children with phobias listed water).

Behavioral traits that suggest an anxiety disorder include avoidance, clinging, crying, and school refusal. Some children may become restless or have difficulty concentrating. Even a long latency before speaking can suggest an extremely cautious child who may ultimately develop an anxiety disorder. Children tend to express anxiety by physical symptoms, of which the most common are stomachaches or recurrent abdominal pain, fatigue, disrupted sleep, headaches, and diffuse limb/muscle aches ("growing pains").

Children and adolescents with panic disorder probably won't spontaneously mention their panic symptoms; you will have to ask. They are most likely to report tremors, palpitations, dizziness or faintness, trouble breathing, sweating, and fear of losing control or dying.

Developmental Factors

Young children often respond timidly to new situations. Indeed, caution is normal in children of any age and may have self-protective value. Youngsters with phobias will show even more reluctance than other children to interact in new situations, perhaps hugging the wall at a birthday party or demanding that a parent remain with them the entire time. As the criteria for various disorders specify, fear or anxiety in young children may be conveyed by crying, clinging, or temper outbursts rather than the more classic anxiety responses. And they may not understand what it means to *avoid*, well, anything; you may have to depend on information from their parents.

A patient's age will to some extent determine the content of a phobia: Younger children will be afraid of the dark or animals, whereas older children or adolescents may fear nuclear disaster or other societal calamities. Panic attacks are unusual before puberty, but are increasingly encountered after adolescence. Adolescents will typically report agoraphobia or fears relating to sex or failure. Although adults will usually have insight into the irrationality of the fear, young children often don't recognize that their fears are unreasonable.

An 8-year-old child should be able to answer questions about anxiety symptoms. Older children and adolescents can keep diaries to record the nature, timing, precipitation, and duration of their anxieties. They can also usually express the imagined consequences if exposed to the object of fear. For example, ask, "What do you think will happen if a dog runs into the room?" Those who develop phobias in adolescence may experience a decline in functioning, just as adults do. However, you may have to compare a young child's actual school progress with what's expected, based on testing or teacher estimates.

OTHER ANXIETY DISORDERS

F06.4 Anxiety Disorder Due to Another Medical Condition

Many medical conditions can cause symptoms of anxiety. Usually these will be similar to the symptoms of panic disorder or generalized anxiety disorder. In general, anxiety symptoms in a young patient will not be caused by a medical disorder, but it is most important to identify those that are.

Substance/Medication–Induced Anxiety Disorder

Many substances can produce anxiety symptoms. These may occur during either intoxication (or heavy use, in the case of caffeine) or withdrawal, and they may take the form of panic, generalized anxiety, or phobias. As always in young patients, it is important to consider the possibility of substance use when symptoms develop suddenly and when no history of such symptoms exists. For symptoms, see the Essential Features of Substance Intoxication and Substance Withdrawal (pp. 403 and 404) and the Essential Features of Four Substance/Medication-Induced Mental Disorders (p. 405) in Chapter 24. Table 24.1 can help with wording and code numbers.

F41.8 Other Specified Anxiety Disorder

F41.9 Unspecified Anxiety Disorder

Many adult patients who feel distressed have anxiety symptoms that don't qualify for a specific DSM-5 diagnosis. Although the data are still lacking, we have no reason to believe that this finding will be different for children and adolescents. You can use the other specified or unspecified category for those patients whose symptoms are too few, too confusing, or too poorly described to permit a more precise diagnosis. (Use the other specified diagnosis when you wish to indicate the particular reason why criteria for another anxiety disorder are not met.) Before assigning a child or adolescent to either of these categories, be sure to consider adjustment disorder with anxiety or with mixed anxiety and depressed mood.

CHAPTER 15

Obsessive–Compulsive

and Related Disorders

QUICK GUIDE TO THE OBSESSIVE–COMPULSIVE AND RELATED DISORDERS

Obsessive–compulsive disorder. These patients are bothered by repeated thoughts or behaviors that appear senseless, even to them (p. 285).

Body dysmorphic disorder. Physically normal patients persistently believe that parts of their bodies are misshapen or ugly (p. 291).

Trichotillomania. Pulling hair from various parts of the body is often accompanied by feelings of "tension and release" (p. 289).

Excoriation disorder. Patients so persistently pick at their skin that they traumatize it (p. 291).

Hoarding disorder. An individual accumulates so many objects (perhaps of no value) that they interfere with life and living. Although hoarding begins when the patient is young, it doesn't usually come to clinical attention until much later (p. 291).

Obsessive–compulsive and related disorder due to another medical condition. Occasionally, obsessions and compulsions can be caused by another physical illness (p. 294).

Substance/medication-induced obsessive–compulsive and related disorder. Rarely, use of a substance can lead to obsessive–compulsive symptoms that don't fulfill criteria for any of the above-mentioned disorders (p. 294).

Other specified, or unspecified, obsessive–compulsive and related disorder. Use one of these categories for disorders with prominent obsessional or compulsive symptoms that do not fit neatly into any of the groups above (p. 294).

INTRODUCTION

In this chapter, we consider disorders involving thoughts and behaviors that are often intrusive, repetitive, and time-consuming. (The DSM-5 chapter on these disorders is new to the DSMs.) Obsessive–compulsive disorder (OCD) is the best known of these, but there are others—skin picking, hoarding, checking for body defects. Initially, at least, some of these behaviors carry with them a whiff of pleasure, such as the relief of tension a teenager might feel when tweaking out a strand of hair, or the fun some people get from collecting before it has morphed into the burden of hoarding.

The features that bind together this group of conditions include youthful onset, similar comorbidity, family history of OCD, response to the same kinds of treatment, and perhaps dysfunction in the frontostriatal brain circuitry (caudate hyperactivity).

F42 OBSESSIVE–COMPULSIVE DISORDER

For generations, we mental health clinicians have known of OCD. What we have not recognized is that, far from being rare in young people (as was once thought), OCD is actually relatively common, occurring in up to 2% of all children and teenagers. OCD begins earlier in boys, who, as younger children, outnumber girls with the disorder by perhaps 2:1; at puberty, the ratio drifts toward parity. Mean age of onset is about 10 years, earlier in boys than girls. Although the outlook is good relative to adult-onset OCD, in about 40% of children the disorder persists into the adult years. Fully half the adults with OCD first become symptomatic as children.

Until recently, we have failed to appreciate just how often this debilitating condition begins in early childhood. Part of the explanation is that children may keep secret their obsessive thinking and compulsive behavior. They may control repetitive rituals relatively well in public settings (such as school), only letting down their guard at home. Even parents are sometimes surprised to learn the extent of their children's disability. With parents' ignorance and children's reluctance to ask for help, many youngsters with OCD remain undiagnosed and untreated for months or years.

Like adults, children and adolescents experience compulsions more frequently than obsessions. Young children often don't have obsessional thinking that accompanies their compulsions—just "an urge to do it." The content of children's obsessions most often concerns dirt and contamination, sex (including the possibility of homosexuality), and religious and other moral concerns. These naturally lead to compulsions of cleaning, checking (to ensure that a behavior has truly been accomplished), and repetition. Adolescents are especially prone to religious or sexual obsessions; concerns about cleaning are rare. However, the content of these thoughts and behaviors tends to change with time, so that today's symptoms may be forgotten tomorrow—supplanted by other obsessional ideas and compulsive behaviors. Major depression is often comorbid, as are anxiety and tic disorders; the presence of a comorbid condition predicts a worse prognosis.

Like most other mental conditions, OCD appears to stem from a variety of causes. Foremost among them is heredity, with rates ranging around 50%. However, many patients have no known family history at all. Some cases appear to involve an immune response to infectious disease (pediatric acute-onset neuropsychiatric syndrome, or PANS, associated with streptococcal infections), which has also been implicated in tic disorders (see sidebar, p. 215).

Although OCD is sometimes episodic, it more commonly runs a chronic course. Follow-up studies of varying length find that although most patients continue to have symptoms, the disorder may remit in some 40% or more by the time they are adults. Early onset, severe symptoms, long duration, comorbidity, and a first-degree relative with OCD all predict persistence of symptoms into adulthood.

Corey

When he was 15, Corey tried to buy a gun. He was tall and had been shaving for a couple of years, and he might have succeeded if he hadn't written his actual telephone number on the form for the 5-day waiting period. The clerk thought he looked depressed, and called Corey's mother after he left the shop.

"That's how I ended up here instead of the morgue," Corey told his clinician the day after he was admitted to a locked mental health unit. "Anything seemed better than feeling rotten all the time."

Information from a number of sources supported a diagnosis of a mood disorder. Several teachers had noticed that Corey's concentration had been impaired for a month or more; his grades had plummeted. His mother had worried that he wasn't eating; his father had observed that he'd seemed to lose interest in the basement color photo-processing lab they had worked on all winter. Corey himself complained of several weeks' sleeplessness and chronic fatigue; he said he felt guilty that he had let his father down about the lab ("I knew he enjoyed it"). His family doctor had said he was physically healthy.

After a diagnosis of major depressive disorder and 10 days' treatment with an antidepressant, Corey improved enough that his name came up in a discharge-planning conference. "What about the compulsions?" asked the evening nurse, who had doubled back that morning to fill in.

"What compulsions?" everyone else wanted to know.

The nurse hadn't known about them either, until Corey's roommate had finally spilled the beans during group therapy. It took Corey 3 hours to get ready for bed. Everything had to be done in a certain order—teeth first, 10 strokes per tooth from roots to crown, beginning with the left upper molars. If he lost count, or if he thought he did, he started over. Toothbrushing alone sometimes occupied 45 minutes.

ESSENTIAL FEATURES OF **OBSESSIVE–COMPULSIVE DISORDER**

The patient has distressing obsessions or compulsions (or both!) that occupy so much time they interfere with accustomed routines.

The Fine Print

Obsessions are recurring, unwanted ideas that intrude into awareness; the patient usually tries to suppress, ignore, or neutralize them.

Compulsions are repeated physical (sometimes mental) behaviors that follow rules (or are a response to obsessions) in an attempt to alleviate distress; the patient tries to resist them. The behaviors are unreasonable, meaning that they don't have any realistic chance of helping the obsessional distress.

The D's: • Distress or disability (typically, the obsessions and/or compulsions occupy an hour a day or more or cause social, educational, occupational, or personal impairment) • Differential diagnosis (substance use and physical disorders; "normal" superstitions and rituals that don't actually cause distress or disability; depressive and psychotic disorders; anxiety and impulse-control disorders, Tourette's and other tic disorders; obsessive–compulsive personality disorder)

Coding Notes

Specify degree of insight:

> **With good or fair insight.** The patient realizes that these thoughts and behaviors are definitely (or probably) not true.
> **With poor insight.** The patient thinks that the OCD concerns are probably true.
> **With absent insight/delusional beliefs.** The patient strongly believes that the OCD concerns are true.

Specify if:

> **Tic-related.** The patient has a lifetime history of a chronic tic disorder.

"If I don't get it right, I feel awful. I squirm." Corey admitted that he didn't know what would happen if he didn't "get it right," but he worried that it could be pretty terrible. "It even sounds dumb to me. Like, rationally, what could possibly happen? But being rational doesn't seem to have much to do with it."

After Corey finally finished brushing his teeth, he would shower—scrubbing away with his washcloth for 100 strokes per body part at a time, until the hot water ran out. He mentally divided his towel into four segments: the first for his face and neck, the second for his arms and legs, the third for his upper body, and the fourth for "everything that's left over." There had been a few times 6 or 8 months ago, not long after his rituals began to get out of hand, when he became confused about which part of the towel he had used and commenced the whole showering process again. But cold showers and soggy towelings had taught him to pay close attention to the details of his drying process. Other rituals would follow—how many steps to take, which objects to touch (or untouch if he got it wrong), how to arrange his slippers, how to take off his bathrobe—as he physically got, or tried to get, into bed.

Although Corey's bedtime rituals had begun only about a year ago, even as a small child he had had a variety of fears and obsessional thoughts. "Mainly, I'd count things. You know—how many steps it took to get from one block to the next; how many breaths; how many ceiling tiles, or holes in ceiling tiles, in the classroom. There's nearly 10,000 in my room here."

From the time Corey was 5, his mother noted, he had been afraid of a possible terrorist attack. When he would open his eyes in the morning, the light streaming through his window would sometimes be so bright that he would start counting seconds as he waited for the blast that seemed certain to come. She added that the family history was negative for mental disorders—except for her husband's brother, who had developed a facial tic when he was a teenager. It had lasted until he committed suicide when he was 31.

Evaluation of Corey

Corey's current OCD symptoms were largely limited to compulsions; obsessions by themselves would also qualify him for this diagnosis. He felt that he had to repeat these behaviors (primarily his bedtime rituals, although his earlier behavior of counting was also still present—Criterion A1). He carried out these behaviors according to strict rules (number of strokes, arranging his slippers, touching), and he felt that if he didn't follow the rules, something awful would happen (A2). It didn't matter that he couldn't define the consequence; this simply underscored the fact that there could be no realistic relationship between the behaviors and the consequences they were intended to avert. The symptoms were important, in that they both caused him distress and wasted a lot of time (B). The family doctor found no evidence of **substance use** or a **medical condition**; the latter would be important to rule out, since obsessive–compulsive behavior has been reported in Lyme disease and streptococcal infections (C). Although as a younger child he might not have had insight into the excessive or unreasonable nature of his symptoms, he did now. The specifier *with good insight* therefore applies.

There is no evidence to support a different mental disorder, such as an **anxiety disorder** or a **different condition related to OCD**, as the source of his symptoms (D). Corey had not reported **panic attacks**, and his fears were of some vague retribution that could occur, not of those typical of the more **specific phobia** or **social anxiety disorder**. Patients with

generalized anxiety disorder also worry a lot, but about a variety of situations that seem realistic (see, for example, the history of Gerald given earlier). Obsessive–compulsive symptoms are often encountered in patients with tic disorders including **Tourette's disorder,** which should have been considered (and quickly rejected) in Corey's case.

Depressions like Corey's are frequently encountered in OCD and are often the reason patients come for evaluation. Corey had more than enough symptoms to diagnose major depressive disorder (see p. 239): For at least 2 weeks (Criterion A for MDD) he had had depressed mood (A1), poor concentration (A8), decreased appetite (A3), loss of interest (A2), insomnia (A4), fatigue (A6), and a suicide plan (A9). They caused him much distress and interfered with school (B); we've already ruled out substances and other illnesses as possible causes (C). Because he was not psychotic and had no history of prior mood disorder, he would be diagnosed as having major depressive disorder, single episode, severe (see Table 13.1).

Because it more urgently required attention, we list Corey's major depressive disorder first:

F32.2	Major depressive disorder, single episode, severe
F42	Obsessive–compulsive disorder, with good insight
CGAS	45 (on admission)
CGAS	70 (on discharge)

F63.3 TRICHOTILLOMANIA

A "passion for hair pulling" (the literal meaning of the word *trichotillomania*) was first described over 100 years ago. Today it is found in at least 1 in 200 persons in the adult population (the actual rate could be several times greater), though it usually begins before puberty. The prevalence in childhood has yet to be accurately defined. Girls and boys are both affected, though the ratio in adults is perhaps 10:1. Despite their discomfort, patients seldom complain about or even mention their symptoms, so relatively few mental health professionals—fewer still who specialize in children and adolescents—have ever encountered a case.

Trichotillomania (see the Essential Features, p. 290) is simply defined. DSM-5 no longer requires a rising sense of tension that is relieved when the patient pulls out a strand of hair. Indeed, a substantial number of patients describe the behavior as occurring "automatically" at times when they are thinking about other matters. However, some individuals still report experiencing the tension-and-release phenomenon.

The head is most often involved, though the affected hair can be growing on any part of the body—face, brows, lashes, extremities, and (in adolescents and adults) underarms and pubic area. Chewing or mouthing of the hair often occurs; about 10% of patients swallow it. However, development of a bezoar (such as Eve's in the case vignette) is unusual. Hair pulling is much more common in children than in adults, suggesting that the usual outcome is spontaneous resolution.

Eve

When Eve was 13, she developed acute abdominal pain that gradually worsened over 4 weeks. Her family doctor could make no diagnosis, but one evening the cramping became so severe that her parents rushed her to the urgent care department of their community hospital. An X-ray revealed something blocking her small intestine. It required surgery to remove the object—a bezoar, or hairball, nearly 2 inches in diameter.

That discovery prompted the doctor to look closely at Eve's scalp. "In several patches of scalp the size of a half-dollar, I saw a pattern of thinning of hair, with the characteristic intermingling of long and short hairs growing back in a pattern typical of chronic hair pulling," read the report that accompanied Eve to the mental health counselor. "This conclusion was subsequently confirmed by a dermatologist."

When questioned about her habit, Eve readily admitted that she had been pulling out her hair, a strand or two at a time, for many months. Though she didn't seem to understand why it happened, she acknowledged that many times a day she would feel increasingly "wired." After several minutes of rising tension, she would twirl a single hair around her ring finger, then gently tug until the strand came away at the root. If no one was watching, she would then roll the strand over and over in her mouth until it was as compact as her tongue could make it. As she swallowed, the sense of tension would evaporate. Although the hair pulling produced no sense of pain, she noted that her scalp seemed to itch where her hair was growing back.

Eve was a slender girl whose figure had barely begun to develop. She wore her blond hair tucked under a knit cap, which she resisted removing. Once the cap was off, it was easy to see why she preferred to wear it. Downy, new, short hairs sprouted in the patches where hair was either missing or thinned.

The initial interview revealed no information to suggest another diagnosis. Eve denied

ESSENTIAL FEATURES OF **TRICHOTILLOMANIA**

Repeated pulling out of the patient's own hair results in bald patches and attempts to control the behavior.

The Fine Print

The D's: • Duration ("recurrent") • Distress or disability (social, educational, occupational, or personal impairment) • Differential diagnosis (substance use and physical disorders; mood and psychotic disorders; body dysmorphic disorder; OCD; ordinary grooming)

having any other mental or physical problems (among other issues, her mother had reported no evidence of hallucinations, delusions, depression, obsessions, or compulsions). As she slouched in her chair, she grumbled, "I just wish I could stop. I hate wearing that hat, and the kids all call me 'Baldy.' But if I don't do it, I just feel grody."

Evaluation of Eve

The facts of Eve's hair pulling speak for themselves: It was recurrent (Criterion A) and it caused distress (C). We'll have to infer from her statement about wishing to stop that she had repeatedly attempted to do so (B). Eve's hair pulling had lasted several months, though there is no absolute time requirement for diagnosis. Children often do not report the tension-and-release phenomenon (which DSM-5 no longer requires for adults, either). Eve, however, spontaneously noted that her unpleasant sensation of feeling "wired" (or "grody") abated once she had completed her ritual.

In an evaluation of patchy hair loss, **other medical conditions** (especially **dermatological disorders**) must be considered (D). Eve had no evidence of such a problem, or of another mental disorder (such as a **psychosis**, **OCD**, or **factitious disorder**) that could explain her symptoms better (E). Her entire diagnosis would be as follows:

F63.3	Trichotillomania
CGAS	70

F45.22 BODY DYSMORPHIC DISORDER

L98.1 EXCORIATION (SKIN–PICKING) DISORDER

F42 HOARDING DISORDER

Some studies suggest that even people without body dysmorphic disorder (BDD) can become distressed upon prolonged gazing into a mirror. But when dissatisfaction with an aspect of personal appearance becomes so intense that a person begins to engage in repetitive behaviors (see the Essential Features of BDD, p. 292), a diagnosis of BDD may be warranted. Early onset of BDD is more gradual, more severe, and carries with it greater comorbidity, including attempts at suicide.

People with excoriation disorder pick or dig at their skin, sometimes to the point that it causes physical damage (pitting, scarring)—in addition to the psychological trauma of shame and embarrassment.

Although hoarding disorder tends to begin young, two features protect children and adolescents from the full extent of the problem: (1) Kids don't have full control over their environments ("Clean your room, Billy"). (2) It takes years to accumulate a mountain of stuff, pushing the age of total involvement well into young adulthood or beyond.

Each of these conditions typically begins during the teen years, though clinical attention may not be sought until many years later. Each disorder has a prevalence of perhaps 2% in the general adult population; BDD and excoriation disorder are distributed more or less equally between males and females, whereas hoarding disorder may be more typical of males.

All three disorders tend to be familial. For BDD and excoriation disorder, OCD in a first-degree relative is a risk factor, and major depressive disorder may be comorbid. Hoarding disorder has been found in 16% of children with learning disabilities.

Clinicians who care for children and adolescents are not often presented with these conditions, so we have provided no vignettes here. Interested readers can find more about these disorders in *DSM-5 Made Easy* by James Morrison.

ESSENTIAL FEATURES OF **BODY DYSMORPHIC DISORDER**

In response to a miniscule, sometimes invisible physical flaw, the patient repeatedly checks in a mirror, asks for reassurance, or picks at patches of skin—or makes mental comparisons with other people.

The Fine Print

The D's: • Distress or disability (social, educational, occupational, or personal impairment) • Differential diagnosis (substance use and physical disorders; mood and psychotic disorders; anorexia nervosa or other eating disorders; OCD; illness anxiety disorder; ordinary dissatisfaction with personal appearance)

Coding Notes

Specify if:

> **Muscle dysmorphia form.** These people believe that their bodies are too small or lack adequate musculature.

Specify degree of insight:

> **With good or fair insight.** The patient realizes that these thoughts and behaviors are definitely (or probably) not true.
> **With poor insight.** The patient thinks that the BDD concerns are probably true.
> **With absent insight/delusional beliefs.** The patient strongly believes that the BDD concerns are true.

ESSENTIAL FEATURES OF **EXCORIATION DISORDER**

The patient repeatedly tries to stop recurrent digging, scratching, or picking at skin that has caused lesions.

The Fine Print

The D's: • Duration ("recurrent") • Distress or disability (social, educational, occupational, or personal impairment) • Differential diagnosis (substance use and physical disorders; psychotic disorders; OCD; body dysmorphic disorder; stereotypic movement disorder)

ESSENTIAL FEATURES OF **HOARDING DISORDER**

These patients are in the grip of something powerful: the overwhelming urge to accumulate stuff. They experience trouble—indeed, distress—when trying to discard their possessions, even those that appear to have little value (sentimental or otherwise). As a result, things pile up, cluttering up living areas to render them unusable.

The Fine Print

The D's: • Duration (not stated, other than "persistent") • Distress or disability (social, educational, occupational, or personal impairment) • Differential diagnosis (substance use and physical disorders; mood and psychotic disorders; major neurocognitive disorder [dementia]; OCD; normal collecting)

Coding Notes

Specify if:

> **With excessive acquisition.** If symptoms are accompanied by excessive collecting, buying, or stealing of items that are not needed or for which there is no space available.

Specify degree of insight:

> **With good or fair insight.** The patient realizes that these thoughts and behaviors cause problems.
> **With poor insight.** The patient mostly believes that hoarding isn't a problem.
> **With absent insight/delusional beliefs.** The patient strongly believes that hoarding isn't a problem.

F06.8 OBSESSIVE–COMPULSIVE AND RELATED DISORDER DUE TO ANOTHER MEDICAL CONDITION

SUBSTANCE/MEDICATION-INDUCED OBSESSIVE–COMPULSIVE AND RELATED DISORDER

F42 OTHER SPECIFIED OBSESSIVE–COMPULSIVE AND RELATED DISORDER

F42 UNSPECIFIED OBSESSIVE–COMPULSIVE AND RELATED DISORDER

Quite frankly, these diagnoses are pretty darned uncommon, even in adults. Occasionally, you might need to use a diagnosis of other specified or unspecified obsessive–compulsive and related disorder, but the other two are so infrequently encountered that their chief value is the reminder that we should *always* be alert to the possibility of an "organic" causation of a mental disorder. In any patient. Always.

ASSESSING OBSESSIVE–COMPULSIVE AND RELATED DISORDERS

General Suggestions

Due to shame or embarrassment, neither children nor adolescents are likely to mention obsessions and compulsions, or their related behaviors, spontaneously. You will probably have to ask young patients a question like this: "Have you ever felt you had to do something, or had certain habits, that might seem senseless to you but that you felt you just had to keep on doing?" Be prepared to give some examples, such as dressing or bathing or bedtime routines that must be done a certain number of times, rituals that involve repeatedly checking the stove or oven to be sure it is off, or looking repeatedly into a mirror. A cap may be worn indoors to conceal a bald spot. (Because skin picking so often involves the face, it may be more obvious.)

Be sure to query family members about their own behaviors: Because the demands of OCD are insatiable, siblings and parents, in trying to help an affected child or adolescent cope, sometimes become enmeshed in carrying out the very behaviors they would like to discourage. Brace yourself for quite a few false positives; many children have the odd obsession or compulsion without meeting criteria for diagnosis.

Obsessions often center on themes of contamination (germs, dirt), danger (to self or others), the drive for symmetry, and morality (scrupulosity). Compulsions include washing for cleanliness, carefully drawing numbers or letters until they are perfect, and ordering things into appropriate groupings. Rituals can be quite elaborate, and are much more likely to be reported by parents than to be observed during an office visit. Symptoms tend to change over time, so that in the course of a year or two a young patient may sequentially develop counting, washing, and ordering rituals.

Developmental Factors

OCD and related symptoms also tend to change with increasing age. Preoccupation with counting and symmetry is especially prevalent in grade school children; concerns about cleanliness become more prominent during adolescence. It is important not to diagnose OCD in children who are merely experiencing typical developmental rituals, such as games with stringent rules ("Step on a crack and break your mother's back") and hobbies that require careful attention to detail (collecting stamps, match covers, and the like).

CHAPTER 16

Trauma- and
Stressor-Related Disorders

Ever since the publication of DSM-III in 1980, the diagnostic manuals have famously maintained an "atheoretical" approach. That is, causes are not stated for the disorders described. However, in this DSM-5 chapter (new to the DSMs), the cause is explicitly stated, and it is presumed to be something traumatic or stressful in the patient's history.

QUICK GUIDE
TO THE TRAUMA- AND STRESSOR-RELATED DISORDERS

Primary Trauma- and Stressor-Related Disorders

Reactive attachment disorder. There is evidence of pathogenic care in a child who habitually doesn't seek comfort from parents or surrogates (p. 297).

Disinhibited social engagement disorder. There is evidence of pathogenic care in a child who fails to show normal reticence in the company of strangers (p. 297).

Posttraumatic stress disorder. An individual with this disorder repeatedly relives a severely traumatic event, such as a natural disaster (p. 303).

Acute stress disorder. This condition is much like posttraumatic stress disorder, except that it begins during or immediately after a highly stressful event and lasts a month or less (p. 303).

Adjustment disorder. Following a stressor, an individual develops symptoms that disappear once the cause of stress has subsided (p. 311).

Other specified, or unspecified, trauma- and stressor-related disorder. Patients whose stress or trauma appears related to other presentations may be classified in one of these categories (p. 316).

Other Disorders That Can Result from Trauma or Stress

Problems related to abuse or neglect. A large number of codes can apply to the sort of difficulty that arises from neglect or from physical or sexual abuse of children or adolescents (or adults) (p. 441).

Separation anxiety disorder. The patient becomes anxious when separated from parent or home (p. 262).

F94.1 REACTIVE ATTACHMENT DISORDER

F94.2 DISINHIBITED SOCIAL ENGAGEMENT DISORDER

Reactive attachment disorder (RAD) and disinhibited social engagement disorder (DSED) are probably quite rare, but extremely serious, disorders of early childhood. Underlying them is the fact that for adequate growth and development, a child needs consistent social stimulation and affective feedback from the relationship with a parent or some other familiar, sensitive caregiver. This attachment relationship serves to mediate the balance between security and exploration, and it may be different for a mother, a father, and for others. When the relationship is faulty—care is inconsistent or the parent is neglectful of physical or emotional needs or is abusive—a disorder of attachment can develop. DSM-5 has transformed the two subtypes of the old reactive attachment disorder of infancy or early childhood into two separate disorders, RAD and DSED.

Lacking a preferred attachment to anyone, infants and toddlers with RAD withdraw from social contacts; if they interact at all, they tend to be shy or distant. Such a child may display indifference to the departure of the parent or other primary caregiver. As you can see, RAD can look a bit like a depressive disorder.

In contrast, DSED is characterized by overly familiar social relationships. The infant or toddler does not exhibit age-appropriate wariness of strangers, but approaches all with equanimity and apparent lack of fear. Children with Williams syndrome, caused by a deletion of about 26 genes from chromosome 7, have behaviors similar to DSED (as well as physical abnormalities). It is in part to exclude children with known medical causes for the behavior that the criteria continue to require evidence of parental neglect or absenteeism.

In both RAD and DSED, the child must be old enough (9 months) to form attachments, and (as noted above) both disorders appear to be almost vanishingly rare, confined almost exclusively to high-risk populations. And even in children who have suffered abuse or who have been institutionalized, the prevalence of RAD is only 10%; the prevalence of DSED is about twice that. Once they have been placed into families where they can receive secure nurturing, children with RAD are quite likely to become securely attached, whereas children with DSED may be more likely to retain symptoms.

The DSM-5 diagnoses of RAD and DSED are unusual in two ways. Aside from a couple of sleep–wake disorders, they are the only conditions that were created from the division of a DSM-IV category. (The *International Classification of Diseases* took this step in its 10th revision back in 1992.) And, of all the conditions that can originate in childhood, these are the only two that appear not to apply at all to adults.

ESSENTIAL FEATURES OF **REACTIVE ATTACHMENT DISORDER** AND **DISINHIBITED SOCIAL ENGAGEMENT DISORDER**

	Reactive attachment disorder	Disinhibited social engagement disorder
Apparent cause	Adverse child care (abuse, neglect; caregivers insufficient or changed too frequently). Presumption of causality stems from evidence such as a temporal relationship of the inadequate care to the disturbed behavior.	
Symptoms	A child withdraws emotionally (neither seeks nor responds to soothing from an adult). Such children will habitually show little emotional or social response; far from having positive affect, they may experience periods of unprovoked irritability or sadness.	A child becomes unreserved in interactions with strange adults. Such children, rather than showing typical first-acquaintance shyness, will show little hesitation to leave with a strange adult; they don't "check in" with familiar caregivers; and they readily become excessively familiar. In so doing, they may cross normal cultural and social boundaries.
Demographics	Begins before age 5; child has developmental age of at least 9 months.	
Differential diagnosis	Autism spectrum disorder, intellectual disability, ADHD	
Specify if:	Persistent (symptoms present longer than 1 year)	
Specify if:	Severe (all symptoms present at a high level of intensity)	

Shawna

Almost since she could walk, Shawna had been overly friendly. When she was 3, a social services caseworker referred her to the mental health clinic. Neither the caseworker nor her mother could stop her from running up to any stranger while shopping, or, later, from striking up a conversation with strangers of either sex. Once she had accompanied a newfound friend to his home for cookies. Fortunately, she had been returned to the yard of her home unharmed; however, despite a memorable spanking, she remained "willing to go off with anyone."

Shawna's mother was trying to rear two daughters alone while completing her own high school education and working evenings in a variety store. The children were watched by a series of neighbor girls, one of whom had dropped out of school in the ninth grade; another might have smoked pot while on duty.

Shawna's behaviors had seemed to worsen after her sister was born. The previous summer, the two girls had lived with their maternal grandmother. The grandmother had reported a gradual reduction in Shawna's impetuous behavior after their second month together, but it recurred once the girls returned to their mother.

When she first met the interviewer, Shawna immediately ran up to him, arms outstretched, squealing with delight and calling, "Daddy! Daddy!" During the interview, she paid her mother hardly any attention. At first she clung to the interviewer's leg, repeatedly requesting to be picked up, asking for a shoe ride, and engaging in other familiarities. As she became increasingly provocative and difficult to manage, her mother offered to "whack your butt," but she neither followed up on the threat nor made other attempts to manage Shawna's behavior. The interviewer finally suggested a walk outside to continue the interview. Away from the presence of her mother, Shawna confidently took his hand and trotted along, chattering about the dolls she had discovered in the playroom. Throughout that portion of the session, Shawna focused well on the topics at hand and used age-appropriate verbal and nonverbal communications.

Evaluation of Shawna

Instead of showing a child's usual reluctance to engage with strange adults, Shawna readily approached them (Criterion A1 for DSED) and, without fear, would talk with anyone (A2). She had even gone off with a brand-new acquaintance for cookies (A4). During the interview, she ignored her mother rather than checking back with her, as would be consistent with typical behavior for her age (A3). Although it would be unusual to diagnose **ADHD** at this age, it must be considered in any impulsive child. However, Shawna appeared to focus her attention when sufficiently engaged and showed evidence of self-control in situations other than at home (for example, when she was staying with her grandmother—

Criterion B). Similarly, she did not show the negative behavior that would be expected in **oppositional defiant disorder**, or the violation of rights or rules found in **conduct disorder**. Although formal testing was not attempted at this interview, her overall intellectual functioning appeared about normal for her age, so **intellectual disability** seemed unlikely. There was nothing about her communication or socialization that would suggest **autism spectrum disorder**.

Rather, Shawna's too-ready acceptance of a strange male interviewer suggested a disturbance of social relatedness that is typical for DSED. Pathogenic care was evidenced by repeated changes of babysitters and her mother's prolonged absences from the home (C2). Some of her developmentally inappropriate behavior remitted once she experienced a more stable environment (staying with her grandmother), suggesting a causal relationship between care and behavior (D). Of course, she was developmentally older than 9 months (E).

Her history of nondiscriminating sociability went back at least a year, which would justify the specifier of *persistent*. However, in our clinical judgment, her symptoms were not of sufficient intensity to justify the added specifier of *severe*; that judgment is further reflected in Shawna's CGAS.

F94.1	Disinhibited social engagement disorder, persistent
CGAS	70 (current)

Randall

When Randall was 4, he experienced his first kiss.

"For sure, he never got one from his birth mother," remarked Bernice, his foster mom; she had made good use of the information she'd received from child protective services. "She was 16, and much more interested in boys and doing drugs. And *her* mother was a God-fearing woman who didn't at all approve of any kid born without benefit of clergy—kept Randall at arm's length, she did."

Then Grandma died, and next in line was an aunt who had three school-age kids and plenty of commitments on her time, without wasting any of it on affection. Randall's cousins were all boys who weren't much focused on a baby, either.

Randall spent his time in a playpen, learning to talk from the TV. By all accounts, he wasn't mistreated. "He just wasn't treated at all," Bernice remarked. She didn't think he'd even been out of the house, except to run around by himself in the fenced yard. "He had more or less toilet-trained himself, so he didn't even get that kind of attention." Room at the table was limited, so he was given his meals apart from the rest of the family.

So, when Bernice's kiss arrived, "It just sat there on his face. He didn't react at all, just accepted it, no emotion involved. The way he does with most things." Bernice had had several foster kids and knew the drill, but he had ignored the plush rabbit she had tucked into his arms. He ate the gelatin dessert she made, but didn't show any real enthusiasm for it, either.

"The first week he was with us, he fell on the sidewalk and scraped up his face. He snuffled and just turned away, his nose dripping blood. He let me take care of it, but he didn't cry. In fact, I don't think he reacted at all. Again."

Randall seemed smart enough. Right away, he knew where the bathroom was and which was his bedroom—and he stayed out of everyone else's. He also quickly picked up how to operate the rather complicated home theater system. "And that's where he wanted to spend his time, watching TV. His behavior isn't all that strange—he doesn't focus on twirling objects, and he doesn't say weird things. He just doesn't interact much at all."

"He doesn't really acknowledge the presence of others in the room," Bernice finished up. "He never smiles. When he's with Mort and me, he just looks glum. Like he hasn't a friend in the world. And from what I understand, I guess that's just about right."

The division of RAD and DSED into separate disorders in DSM-5 has provoked concern that this forced dichotomy may be simplistic. Some children may appear inhibited at an early age, but then become disinhibited later. Another worry is that the DSM-5 criteria require children to be seriously affected before either diagnosis can be made. Yet, as is true for other diagnoses in the manual, precursor or "high-risk" disturbances may foreshadow a later, full-blown disorder that early intervention could forestall.

Because the literature on attachment behaviors is complex, some writers suggest that criteria other than those of DSM-5 may better identify this group of children; others have even suggested that a name change could help promote understanding and differentiation from insecure attachment. It has also been noted that other DSM-5 diagnoses, especially major depressive disorder and avoidant/restrictive food intake disorder, may be equally appropriate for a small child who fails to thrive. Finally, why is it that the same set of circumstances (neglect) can produce two such widely different outcomes? Clearly, we are by no means finished with changes to the definition of these two conditions.

Evaluation of Randall

This is going to read a lot like the evaluation of Shawna. The requirements for DSED and RAD are, after all, structured with high similarity.

The pieces of the RAD diagnosis are all there. First, there was the required minimal seeking of comfort from adults (Criterion A1) plus limited (OK, in Randall's case, zero) response to any comfort that was offered (A2); both are required. His persistent emotional and social pathology was shown by his lack of an emotional response to other people (B1) and, as nearly as Bernice could tell, complete lack of positive affect (B2). Indeed, his predominant affect, when he showed any at all, was sadness (B3). Two of these B criteria are needed to qualify.

What could be the cause? We would blame his patently pathological early childhood care—the lack of affection and stimulation shown by a paucity of affection and only the TV for company (C1)—which, from its temporal relationship, we would assume had caused the behavior (D). Bernice's testimony did not include behavioral peculiarities suggestive of autism, but his clinician would want to briefly review the Modified Checklist for Autism in Toddlers—Revised (M-CHAT-R; see Appendix 1 for details) to help rule out **autism spectrum disorder** (E). Obviously, he met the demographic requirements—onset before age 5 (F) and a developmental age of at least 9 months (G).

Because his disturbed attachment behaviors had lasted throughout his short life, he should receive the specifier of *persistent*. We don't think anyone will quarrel with our judgment as to the severity specifier.

Although pathological care is implicit in the description of RAD, we've elected to use the code for child neglect, too. RAD can be related to neglect, abuse, or inconsistent caregiving; we'd like to codify Randall's specific history.

| F94.1 | Reactive attachment disorder, persistent, severe |
| Z69.010 | Encounter for mental health services for victim of child neglect by parent |

ASSESSING REACTIVE ATTACHMENT AND DISINHIBITED SOCIAL ENGAGEMENT DISORDERS

General Suggestions

In evaluating an infant or toddler with RAD or DSED, it is of course necessary to establish the nature of the child's interactions with the parent. Abnormal attachment interactions are likely to intensify during stress, such as in new situations, when a young child often feels insecure and turns to the parent for comfort. If the parent leaves the room, the child's sense of insecurity may be reawakened. The clinical evaluation affords many opportunities to observe the response to stress, the recovery of security, and the exploration of the new setting. A careful and detailed history of such experiences during the child's development, and observations of comfort and exploration during the evaluation, constitute the basic elements of an attachment assessment.

These two disorders call for working carefully yet effectively with both the patient and the parent. You may need to redirect a disinhibited patient you have just peeled off your leg, taking care neither to encourage the behavior nor to reject the child; a relaxed, friendly, nonintrusive attitude permits an inhibited child time to become comfortable with the interview situation and with you. Dealing with the parent may necessitate even greater caution, to preempt resistance and reduce the suspicion and hostility that may be the natural lot of parents whose behavior qualifies for this disorder. Of course, a friendly, open attitude is likely to carry you far. But certain interviewing techniques may help set the informant at ease:

- Begin with other topics. Although we generally discourage spending much time in small talk, there is value in a few moments of nonthreatening information gathering to demonstrate your compassion and establish rapport.

- To relieve embarrassment, suggest an excuse for unfavorable information—for example, "Working two jobs makes every minute with your child doubly precious."

- Emphasize the positive: "Shawna's doing very well in a number of areas."

- Consider the value of multiple sessions to obtain the greatest information about patient's and caregiver's behaviors.

Developmental Factors

By definition, RAD (though not DSED) must begin before a child's fifth birthday. At this writing, there are still no data that would suggest greater prevalence of either subtype at any particular age.

F43.10 POSTTRAUMATIC STRESS DISORDER (AND F43.0 ACUTE STRESS DISORDER)

The cause of posttraumatic stress disorder (PTSD) is an emotion—fear, helplessness, horror—evoked by an overwhelming event. For children and adolescents, those events are pretty much the same as for adults: accidents or severe illness; physical or sexual abuse; violence (especially prevalent wherever drugs are readily available); and the disruption caused by war or by environmental catastrophes (fires, earthquakes, or tornadoes). Even incidents that are only "near-misses," such as leaving the shelter of a tree moments before it was struck by lightning, can qualify as a precipitant.

Of course, it takes more than a traumatic event to create PTSD. Otherwise, how can we explain the fact that the same stressor may produce symptoms in one individual but not in another? Several factors may be involved:

- Duration and severity of the stress for the individual and the duration of the evoked terror

- How rapidly rescue occurs

- The emotional stability of the child or adolescent, and the preexistence of other disorders

- Reactions shown by parents and extended family members
- The community's social network
- Gender, with girls somewhat more likely than boys to become symptomatic

Some estimates place the occurrence of PTSD among American children and teenagers as high as 1 million per year. And the incidence may be increasing, especially among those who live in stress-ridden inner cities. One study found that 40% of inner-city teenagers had experienced at least one traumatic event by the age of 18. Of these, as many as 25% develop PTSD. In other studies, half or more of children involved in traffic accidents or who sustained other forms of physical trauma developed symptoms of PTSD. Although juvenile PTSD may be among the most underrecognized of mental health disorders, there is also some evidence that young patients can recover quickly—perhaps two-thirds do so within the first 18 months of developing symptoms. However, some remain symptomatic well into adulthood.

The requirements for PTSD and its sibling, acute stress disorder (ASD), keep changing. Now, in DSM-5, there is even a special set of criteria for children age 6 and under. Below, we've listed the Essential Features of PTSD (and ASD) for adults and adolescents, and then provided a table that compares the PTSD requirements for young children and for ASD. But right here, to provide an outline for these somewhat complicated disorders (the official DSM-5 PTSD criteria require 3½ pages, by far the most pages in the book), we'll outline in plain language what you need to know.

Of course, there must first be a precipitating traumatic event that the person experiences personally or sees (not just on TV), or learns has occurred to a friend or relative, or is repeatedly exposed to—someone (obviously an adult) who has to collect body parts, for example.

After the trauma, the patient must experience symptoms in four domains (see the Essential Features for a fuller explanation):

1. Dreams or other intrusion symptoms
2. Avoidance of memories or other reminders
3. Negative moods or thoughts associated with the trauma
4. Changes in arousal

These requirements also hold for young children, though the form they take may differ from that in adults, and the total number of symptoms required is fewer than for adults.

In ASD, symptoms develop soon after the trauma and persist for a month or less. There must be a total of 9 or more symptoms out of a possible 14 that are drawn from all of the four groups mentioned above. Any patient with ASD whose symptoms last longer than 1 month will have to be rediagnosed as having PTSD.

ESSENTIAL FEATURES OF
POSTTRAUMATIC STRESS DISORDER (AND ACUTE STRESS DISORDER)

Something truly awful has happened. One patient has been gravely injured or perhaps sexually abused; another has been closely involved in the death or injury of someone else. As a result, for many weeks or months these patients:

- Repeatedly relive their event, perhaps in nightmares or upsetting dreams, perhaps in intrusive mental images or dissociative flashbacks; a young child may reenact it in play. Some people respond to reminders of the event with physiological sensations (racing heart, shortness of breath) or emotional distress.
- Take steps to avoid the horror: refusing to watch films or television or to read accounts of the event, or pushing thoughts or memories out of consciousness.
- Turn downbeat in their thinking: with persistently negative moods, they express gloomy thoughts ("I'm useless," "The world's a mess," "I can't believe anyone"). They lose interest in important activities and feel detached from other people. Some experience amnesia for aspects of the trauma; others become numb, feeling unable to love or experience joy.
- Experience symptoms of hyperarousal: irritability, excessive vigilance, trouble concentrating, insomnia, or an intensified startle response.

The Fine Print

A person can become eligible for a PTSD or ASD diagnosis even if the only exposure was hearing that a close friend or relative was traumatized (violent or accidental), or through repeated exposure to the aftermath, as happens to police, firefighters, or other emergency workers who respond initially.

For PTSD in young children, the second and third bullet points in the list above are combined. For ASD, the symptom requirements differ slightly. See Table 16.1.

The D's: • Duration (1 month or more after exposure for PTSD, 3 days to 1 month for ASD) • Distress or disability (social, educational, occupational, or personal impairment) • Differential diagnosis (substance use and physical disorders (especially traumatic brain injury); mood and anxiety disorders; normal reactions to stressful events)

Coding Notes

Specify if:

With delayed expression. Symptoms sufficient for diagnosis didn't accumulate until at least 6 months after the event.

With dissociative symptoms:
   Depersonalization. This indicates feelings of detachment, as though dreaming, from the patient's own mind or body.
   Derealization. To the patient, the surroundings seem distant, distorted, dreamlike, or unreal.

In Table 16.1, we've outlined and compared the key features of the two versions of PTSD and of ASD.

Monica

When Monica was 5, she nearly died in an earthquake. With her best friend, Erin, she had been riding in a car driven by Erin's mother. Coming home from an after-school party for a classmate's birthday, they were just ready to leave the expressway when the car began to pitch from side to side. Monica, buckled into the right side of the rear seat, glanced at her friend just as a piece of the overpass fell onto the left half of the car. That was the last she ever saw of either Erin or her mother.

It was nearly 2 days before rescuers could get to the car. They found Monica physically unhurt, though hungry and cold. When a metalworker finally cut through the side of the car with an acetylene torch and brought her out, the television reporters took to calling her the "miracle girl."

After a physical checkup at the hospital, Monica went home with her father. Of course, she had been reunited with both her parents, but her mother was too distraught to care for her; besides, it was Monica's week to live with her father. Since the parents' trial separation had begun, she and her sister, Caroline, had spent that summer and fall shuttling between their parents. Through heavy sedation, her mother agreed that Monica should return to afternoon kindergarten as soon as possible. "We both thought she should get back on the horse," her father explained.

The following Monday she was back in class, but right away her teacher noticed that something was wrong. Monica had always loved the rhythm band, but now she would leave the circle and roam aimlessly. She couldn't even be enticed by her favorite instrument, the triangle. At times she would put her forearm across her eyes. "It looked just like she was trying to shut out the light," her teacher told the clinician. "I tried to talk to her about it, but she'd wander off. It seemed as if we just didn't have her with us any more."

Her father had also noticed the change, but he kept thinking, "She'll come out of it." Besides, he said, he only saw her for a week at a time, and he and his wife didn't talk much about anything, even the children. He knew that Monica had begun wetting the bed once again, after nearly 2 years of being dry at night, and that now she nearly always cried when-

TABLE 16.1. Comparison of PTSD in Preschool Children, PTSD in Older Children/Adolescents/Adults, and Acute Stress Disorder

Young child (≤6 years) PTSD	Adult/adolescent/older child PTSD	Acute stress disorder
Trauma		
Direct experience	Direct experience	Direct experience
Witnessing (not just TV)	Witnessing	Witnessing
Learning of	Learning of	Learning of
	Repeated exposure (not just TV)	Repeated exposure (not just TV)
Intrusion symptoms (1/5[a])	*Intrusion symptoms (1/5)*	*All symptoms (9/14)*
• Memories	• Memories	• Memories
• Dreams	• Dreams	• Dreams
• Dissociative reactions	• Dissociative reactions	• Dissociative reactions
• Psychological distress	• Psychological distress	• Psychological distress *or* physiological reactions
• Physiological reactions	• Physiological reactions	
Avoidance/negative emotions (1/6)	*Avoidance (1/2)*	
• Avoids memories	• Avoids memories	• Avoids memories
• Avoids external reminders	• Avoids external reminders	• Avoids external reminders
	Negative emotions (2/7)	
		• Altered sense of reality (self or surroundings)
	• Amnesia	• Amnesia
	• Negative beliefs	
	• Distortion → self-blame	
• Negative emotional state	• Negative emotional state	
• Decreased interest	• Decreased interest	
• Detached from others	• Detached from others	
• No positive emotions	• No positive emotions	• No positive emotions
Physiological (2/5)	*Physiological (2/6)*	
• Irritability, anger	• Irritability, anger	• Irritability, anger
	• Reckless, self-destructive	
• Hypervigilance	• Hypervigilance	• Hypervigilance
• Startle	• Startle	• Startle
• Poor concentration	• Poor concentration	• Poor concentration
• Sleep disturbance	• Sleep disturbance	• Sleep disturbance
Duration		
>1 month	>1 month	3 days–1 month

[a]Fractions indicate the number of symptoms required from the number possible in the following list.

ever she had to go anywhere in the car. But it was 9-year-old Caroline who finally tipped him off to the extent of Monica's deterioration. Monica had trouble falling asleep, and nearly every night she awakened screaming about some dream she'd had—"monsters, or something," Caroline explained. Several times she had been observed playing "earthquake" with a set of blocks that she repeatedly tumbled onto her dolls.

Caroline had tried to talk to their mother, who was still somewhat in shock herself. "She just shakes her head when I try to tell her about Monica," Caroline said. "She cries a lot."

During his time with the children, 3 weeks after the earthquake, their father took Monica for an evaluation. He reported that she had been born after a full-term, normal pregnancy and that as far as he could remember, her developmental milestones had been normal. "No use asking their mother. She insists that both girls are perfect, have never been sick a day in their lives. Not even a cold." But he was pretty sure that Monica had had no previous health problems or allergies. The only family history of mental disorder he knew of was in some of his wife's relatives—her father had had a serious problem with alcohol, and her older brother had shot and killed himself when he was quite young. The reasons had never been determined.

Monica would only enter the playroom accompanied by her father. She was a serious-looking, dark-haired child who, with his urging, spent several minutes surveying the contents of the room before carefully seating herself on the edge of a wooden chair and adjusting her dress so it fell well below her knees. Throughout the interview, she never made a single spontaneous comment, though she would respond to questions from the interviewer. On two occasions, she replied "I don't know" or "I don't remember" to questions about what happened in the car the day of the earthquake. Toward the end of the session, the interviewer placed the doll house squarely in front of Monica and began to play with it. Monica showed her first spark of enthusiasm when she took the little girl doll and stuffed it into the pink plastic toilet. "We don't need her any more," she explained. "She died."

Evaluation of Monica

Monica's event was traumatic by anyone's standards. Not only did it threaten her own life (Criterion A1), but in her presence it took the lives of Erin and her mother (A2); only one of these two A criteria is required. We can surmise Monica's emotional reaction, but showing fear, horror, or some other direct response to the trauma is no longer necessary to fulfill the diagnostic requirement about the event itself. In the next paragraphs we will discuss Monica's symptoms in light of the DSM-5 requirements for young children. Had she been only a couple of years older, we'd have to use a slightly different set of criteria (see Table 16.1).

Visual flashbacks are uncommon in children, but Monica relived the event in three ways (only one is required): through distressing dreams about monsters (children may not be able to relate dream content to their trauma, B2); by playing "earthquake" (traumatic play) with her dolls (B3); and by crying whenever she had to take a car ride, an external event that seemed to symbolize her traumatic event (B4). She showed avoidance and numbing through refusal to talk (C2), the aversion to car rides (C1), and reduced interest in her schoolwork (C4). (The patently obvious play with the "dead" doll might be read as a reaction to intrusive images—B1—but we'll resist interpreting beyond the data.) Her sleep problems (D5) and poor concentration (D4) suggested hyperarousal. Her symptoms caused serious distress and impaired school functioning (F). There was no evidence of physical injury or substance use (G). At the time of her interview, Monica had been symptomatic for just over 5 weeks (E), so her diagnosis would be PTSD.

If she had been evaluated several weeks earlier, might she have been diagnosed as having ASD? The stressors required are the same as for PTSD, but the time frame is compressed to 30 days or less. Many of the same symptoms must be present, but there is no requirement for representation from each of the categories mentioned in PTSD. Instead, there must be at least nine symptoms in total—more than double the requirement for PTSD in a young child). Based on current information, Monica had eight of these symptoms. Had we seen her a couple of weeks earlier, we'd have claimed clinician's privilege, thrown caution to the winds, and diagnosed her anyway with ASD.

Prominent among the symptoms found associated with PTSD are depression and anxiety, the categories that usually form the backbone of the differential diagnosis. Monica had too few depressive symptoms to warrant an independent diagnosis of **major depressive disorder** (though future clinicians would need to watch for suicide attempts), and no symptoms of any other **anxiety disorder** (especially **phobias**). In some patients, reduced attention span and hyperactivity can be confused with **ADHD**; in others, reluctance to talk about the event could be construed as **oppositional behavior**. For Monica, we can safely discard these interpretations. We would diagnose an **adjustment disorder** only if the stressor were milder (not life-threatening) and if the specific PTSD symptoms—and other specific diagnoses—were absent.

Because comorbidity is the rule with juvenile PTSD, clinicians must also ask about symptoms related to the **misuse of substances,** as well as the additional symptoms that might allow an additional diagnosis of **reactive attachment disorder, disinhibited social engagement disorder,** or **separation anxiety disorder.** Preexisting **learning disorders** may be exacerbated. Other possible comorbid disorders include **panic disorder, generalized anxiety disorder**, and **non-rapid eye movement sleep arousal disorder (sleep terror** or **sleepwalking type).** None of these was evident in Monica's case.

Note that the criteria for PTSD allow the stressor to be one that has been vicariously experienced. Could Monica's mother, whose inability to provide emotional support may have contributed to Monica's symptoms, have been suffering from a degree of PTSD herself?

Monica didn't have prominent dissociative symptoms, and there was certainly no delay between the trauma and the onset of her symptoms, so no specifiers would be given. Her full diagnosis would be as follows:

F43.10   Posttraumatic stress disorder
CGAS   50 (current)

ASSESSING POSTTRAUMATIC STRESS DISORDER
(AND ACUTE STRESS DISORDER)

General Suggestions

Of all the DSM-5 diagnoses, PTSD (as well as ASD) presents some of the greatest challenges to interviewers. One impediment lies in the diagnostic criteria, which are more
numerous and more complicated than those for most other commonly diagnosed
mental disorders. And then the nature of the trauma is sometimes so extreme that
children and adults alike do often try to forget either the actual incidents or the feelings they experienced at the time.

Allow a cooperative child or adolescent to report the entire event spontaneously. When no specific event is obvious, you may have to mention a number of possible stressors (such as natural disasters or physical or sexual trauma) to prompt recall.
Drawing or dramatizing trauma can facilitate communication and data gathering in
a younger child. Of course, history obtained from parents or other informants will
guide your emphasis.

Beware of inducing false memories in suggestible individuals; some authorities
recommend audio-recording or even video-recording interview sessions, to preserve
the exact feeling-tone of questions and answers, and thereby to counter possible
legal challenges. We point out that some data-gathering methods are extremely controversial and will be rejected by many child mental health professionals.

The abuse of trust that accompanies sexual or physical abuse may cause some
children or adolescents to have difficulty expressing their feelings, even to the most
sympathetic of interviewers. Accurate information may be especially difficult to obtain
in cases of suspected parental abuse. Whenever possible in such a case, interview each
informant separately and alone.

The length of time since the trauma occurred may affect the symptom picture
you observe. Immediately after the incident, there may be acute anguish and the
appearance of shock—the patient moves slowly, as if dazed. Later, there may be gradual withdrawal that, accompanied by other symptoms, can be mistaken for depression. It is easy to diagnose a mood disorder and ignore the PTSD.

Developmental Factors

Young children are especially likely to develop PTSD symptoms. They may talk less
than before, complain of physical symptoms (headache or abdominal pains), or repeti-

tively act out their anxieties. Such play may specifically reenact the causative trauma: For example, a 6-year-old who had fallen out of a boat repeatedly "drowned" a GI Joe doll in the bathtub as he worked through his reactions. Others may regress to muteness, bedwetting, thumb sucking, or immature speech.

Older children develop anxiety or depressive symptoms; they, too, may regress to an earlier developmental stage (crying when frustrated, "forgetting" what they have already learned well, doing chores to the standards of a younger child). Adolescents may engage in dangerous counterphobic play that may come to light only as historical material. Whereas adults may relive the traumatic incident in flashbacks or dreams, most children have only the latter, the content of which may take the form of monsters or other frightening images.

ADJUSTMENT DISORDER

With some studies reporting that a third of children and adolescents admitted to an inpatient treatment facility have a diagnosis of adjustment disorder (AD), it is a prevalent diagnosis—especially among patients who have serious medical illnesses. Indeed, it is too popular, according to some writers who believe that clinicians often use it because it lacks the pejorative baggage of, say, conduct disorder or even a bipolar disorder. A conservative estimate is that 4% of children develop mental symptoms as the result of some commonplace environmental stressor.

Stressors commonly associated with AD include divorce, illness of a parent, beginning or changing to a new school, rejection by peers, and severe personal illness (such as Type I diabetes). The diagnosis is made about as often in boys as in girls, and seems to occur more often among children whose parents are experiencing marital problems. Bullying and victim status have also been associated with emotional difficulties during adolescence.

Whereas some writers have included bereavement as a stressor, DSM-5 specifically rules out uncomplicated bereavement (though a grief reaction that is especially intense or lasts an exceptionally long time, beyond what would be considered normal for that person's age or culture, could be considered a precipitant for AD). AD with depressed mood is by far the most common subtype diagnosis made in adults, but for adolescents, AD with disturbance of conduct may be more common yet.

More than half of patients with AD have comorbid disorders. The presence of a comorbid diagnosis does not appear to affect the rate of recovery from the AD; indeed, by definition, once the stressor abates, recovery *always* occurs. Subsequently, many children with AD will be found to have another, better-defined illness. Although critics point out that the criteria for AD are among the flimsiest in DSM-5, the requirement that symptoms last no longer than 6 months after the stressor resolves may be too restrictive. Some studies report that symptoms last an average of 7 months.

ESSENTIAL FEATURES OF **ADJUSTMENT DISORDER**

A stressor causes someone to develop depression, anxiety, or behavioral symptoms—but the response exceeds what you'd expect for most people in similar circumstances. After the stressor has ended, the symptoms may drag on, but not longer than 6 more months.

The Fine Print

The D's: • Duration (starts within 3 months of stressor onset, stops within 6 months of stressor end) • Distress or disability (social, educational, occupational, or personal impairment) • Differential diagnosis (just about everything you can name: substance use and physical disorders; mood and anxiety disorders; other trauma- and stressor-related disorders; somatic symptom and related disorders; psychotic disorders; conduct and other behavior disorders; milder reactions to life's stresses; uncomplicated bereavement)

Coding Notes

Specify:

> **F43.21 With depressed mood.** The patient is mainly tearful, sad.
>
> **F43.22 With anxiety.** The patient is mainly nervous, tense, or fears separation).
>
> **F43.23 With mixed anxiety and depressed mood.** Symptoms combine the preceding.
>
> **F43.24 With disturbance of conduct.** The patient behaves inappropriately or inadvisedly, perhaps violating societal rules, norms, or the rights of others.
>
> **F43.25 With mixed disturbance of emotions and conduct.** The clinical picture combines emotional and conduct symptoms.
>
> **F43.20 Unspecified.** Use for other maladaptive stress-related reactions, such as physical complaints, social withdrawal, or work/academic inhibition.

Specify if:

> **Acute.** The condition has lasted less than 6 months.
>
> **Persistent (or chronic).** 6+ months duration of symptoms, though still not lasting more than 6 months after the stressor has ended.

Kerrilynn

Just 1 week after her 12th birthday, Kerrilynn learned that she was seriously ill. For several weeks her parents had ignored her complaints that she felt tired and warm, but when her joints began to ache, they finally took her to the pediatrician. After a routine blood test, her doctor consulted with a hematologist, who did a bone marrow smear that left her with a painful right hip. The two doctors spoke with her parents, and then all four of them told Kerrilynn that she had acute lymphocytic leukemia. "What's that?" she asked.

She later admitted to an interviewer that it had frightened her. "I didn't think I'd die," she said, "but I knew it had to be something pretty bad—everyone was so kind." She spent several weeks receiving transfusions and starting chemotherapy, which made her sick. She cried when her hair fell out.

According to her father, she kept it together pretty well until she returned to school, some 6 weeks after she was diagnosed. Some of her classmates taunted her and called her "Baldy." On the playground, one boy pulled off her wig and for several minutes played keep-away with it. A teacher overheard the class bully explain to her that within a few weeks, she'd be "pushing up daisies."

Although Kerrilynn physically responded well to treatment, she soon became moody and sullen. She stopped attending her Girl Scout meetings and refused even to talk to friends on the telephone. Several evenings, her mother found her crying in her room, but she refused to talk about her feelings. She repeatedly picked fights with her older sister, whom she said she hated. A month of plummeting grades led to a conference with her school counselor, who reported to her parents that she had two wishes—to be dead and to go to Disneyland. The following day she ran away from home and was gone for nearly 6 hours. A policeman found her in the back seat of an abandoned Buick, attempting to have intercourse with a badly frightened 13-year-old boy. "I'm going to die anyway, so I wanted to see what it was like," she told the nurse that evening when she was admitted to the psychiatric ward of a children's hospital.

Kerrilynn and her sister were both wanted children born to middle-class parents. Her developmental milestones had occurred at the expected times. Other than her current illness, there had been no previous operations or major illnesses. She'd experienced menarche at the age of 11, but her periods had stopped shortly before she was diagnosed with leukemia. She had no environmental or medication allergies, and she emphatically denied any substance misuse. The family history was completely negative for any mental health disorder.

Kerrilynn denied having problems with sleep or appetite, or any somatic symptoms such as heart palpitations or chest pain. She had had no phobias, obsessional ideas, sense of impending doom, or flashbacks or other evidence of reliving incidents from her recent past. She was very interested in learning what delusions and hallucinations were, and finally laughed and said that she wasn't *that* sick.

For the first several days of her 2-week psychiatric hospitalization, Kerrilynn spent most of her spare time reading stories about horses. The hospital's classroom teacher noted that she was bright, focused her attention well, and quickly caught up with her class in areas where she had fallen behind during the previous 3 months.

Evaluation of Kerrilynn

As in most evaluations, the first step in evaluating Kerrilynn would be to determine whether she had the symptoms necessary for the diagnosis. In the case of AD, this might seem almost unnecessary, inasmuch as hardly any symptoms are actually required. However, Kerrilynn's presenting symptoms were important for two reasons: to determine subtype diagnosis, and—far more pressing—to rule out better-defined DSM-5 conditions.

Her initial symptoms suggested a mood disorder: low mood, crying, irritability, and expressing a wish to die (Criterion A; because the alternative was Disneyland, that wish did not seem firmly held, however). By themselves, these would be insufficient to diagnose a major depressive episode, and Kerrilynn did not have vegetative or other symptoms to flesh out the diagnosis of **major depressive disorder**. Of course, the duration had been far too brief for **persistent depressive disorder (dysthymia)**.

She had no symptoms that would suggest **panic disorder**, and she denied anything resembling **obsessive–compulsive disorder** or a **phobic** or **social anxiety disorder**. Could her disturbance be a form of **posttraumatic stress disorder**? Being told that she had a life-threatening illness was certainly an awful experience, but there was no evidence that it in some way repeatedly intruded upon her consciousness. She had had no **psychotic symptoms** and denied the **use of substances** such as alcohol. Once she was admitted to the psychiatric ward, it was clear that she had no evidence of a **cognitive disorder**.

However, could Kerrilynn's one or two rather alarming behavioral problems indicate **conduct disorder**? For one thing, the time course was wrong: At most, she had been having problems with fighting for only a month or two (hardly what we would call persistent). Her sexual acting out might qualify if she had *forced* the boy, but his participation appeared to have been voluntary, if futile. The running away was brief and occurred only once. Her symptoms of defiance were too brief and too few for **oppositional defiant disorder**. Although we can't completely exclude a developing **personality disorder**, symptoms would have to be enduring for any such diagnosis; and **antisocial personality disorder** cannot be diagnosed at all prior to the age of 18. **Uncomplicated bereavement** is ruled out by the absence of recent deaths in her family (D).

Therefore, we can conclude that no other mental diagnosis could reasonably explain Kerrilynn's symptoms (C). They *did* occur within 3 months of two serious stressors (again, A): first, being told that she had a life-threatening illness, and then the rejection by peers. Considering her academic and social impairment (B), the diagnosis of AD seems to fit like a glove, though we would need the passage of time to be sure that the symptoms really disappeared once the stressors abated (E).

Kerrilynn presented with a combination of depressive and behavioral symptoms that dictate the subtype and code number we assign. *With mixed disturbance of emotions and conduct* isn't commonly used, but of the six possibilities, it best fits her symptoms. A duration of less than 6 months justifies the specifier *acute*. Although the DSM-5 criteria do not specifically require using the term *provisional* for AD that has not yet resolved, they should; her clinician did, awaiting the resolution of symptoms within 6 months of resolution of the stressors. The bullying and taunting she sustained from her schoolmates fits into the Z-code for social exclusion or rejection, though in listing it, we'll use language specific to Kerrilynn's situation. Her diagnosis would therefore be as follows:

F43.25	Adjustment disorder, acute, with mixed disturbance of emotions and conduct (provisional)
C91.01	Acute lymphocytic leukemia, in remission
Z69.4	Social exclusion or rejection (rejection by peers)
CGAS	55 (on admission to psychiatric ward)
CGAS	81 (on discharge)

ASSESSING ADJUSTMENT DISORDER

General Suggestions

Even in the face of severe stressors such as life-threatening illness or organ transplantation, the first task is to rule out all other DSM-5 diagnoses. This usually translates into a careful search for the symptoms of major depressive disorder, generalized anxiety disorder, and conduct disorder. The second task is to search for stressors, which tend to be everyday problems of nearly any type or severity. If you don't already know, ask the patient about problems in school (grades, peer relations) or at home (parental divorce, parental or personal illness, one parent imprisoned or away for an extended period on military duty). Younger children may poorly verbalize answers, which can be sought in play. Always, however, when a child or adolescent has been exposed to more unusual stressors (physical or sexual abuse, natural disasters), look first for symptoms of posttraumatic stress disorder.

As long as symptoms persist, the diagnosis demands frequent reevaluation to be sure that another, potentially more serious diagnosis has not supervened. Many patients with AD have coexisting mental diagnoses, such as enuresis and ADHD.

Developmental Factors

Depressive symptoms by themselves are much less likely with AD in young children, who will have behavioral symptoms more than half the time. Instead of complaining of feeling tired, sleepy, or not having sufficient energy, children may withdraw or, in contrast, become fidgety, inattentive, and irritable.

AD is probably best regarded as a diagnosis of "almost last resort," to be made only after all other possible, more specific DSM-5 categories have been eliminated. The absolute last resort would be some form (see the Introduction to this book, p. 8) of the powerful other specified or unspecified mental disorder, which has several advantages:

- It recognizes that a child or adolescent is ill, without forcing a diagnosis before all the data are in.
- Therefore, it decreases the likelihood of an inaccurate diagnosis, especially one that might be pejorative.
- By preventing closure, it encourages ongoing thought about complicated or confusing patients.

F43.8 OTHER SPECIFIED TRAUMA– OR STRESSOR–RELATED DISORDER

F43.9 UNSPECIFIED TRAUMA– OR STRESSOR–RELATED DISORDER

Use the other specified or unspecified category for a patient for whom there is an evident stressor or trauma, but who does not meet the criteria for any of the diagnoses described above. The other specified category should be used when you wish to specify the reason why the other criteria are not fulfilled (DSM-5 gives several examples).

CHAPTER 17

Dissociative Disorders

QUICK GUIDE TO THE DISSOCIATIVE DISORDERS

Primary Dissociative Disorders

Dissociative amnesia. A patient cannot remember important information that is usually of a personal nature and related to stress (p. 319).

Dissociative identity disorder. Additional identities or personalities intermittently seize control of the patient's behavior.

Depersonalization/derealization disorder. A patient has episodes of detachment, as if observing the patient's own behavior from outside. Some patients feel that the world is unreal or odd. In either case, there is no actual memory loss.

Other specified, or unspecified, dissociative disorder. Patients who have symptoms suggestive of any of the disorders above, but who do not meet criteria for any one of them, may be placed in one of these categories.

Other Disorders Involving Dissociation

Memory loss and other dissociative symptoms can also occur in posttraumatic stress disorder and acute stress disorder (p. 303), substance intoxication and withdrawal (p. 402), conversion disorder (p. 324), somatic symptom disorder (p. 328), panic disorder (p. 275), the sleepwalking type of non-rapid eye movement sleep arousal disorder (p. 371), borderline personality disorder (p. 432), and cognitive disorders (Chapter 25). They may also be reported in malingering (p. 443).

INTRODUCTION

The term *dissociation* originated 400 years ago, but only during the 20th century has it been applied to thought. It occurs when one group of normal mental processes is cut off from the rest; we define it as a loss of the normal relationships between the different groups of mental processes, so that at least one group—consciousness, identity, memory, or perception—appears to function independently. The phenomenon of dissociation is found in a variety of mental illnesses other than psychosis, including somatic symptom disorder as well as posttraumatic and acute stress disorders. When dissociative symptoms are encountered in the course of other mental diagnoses, a separate diagnosis of a dissociative disorder is not ordinarily given.

In fact, authorities still vigorously argue about the DSM dissociative disorders: Do they deserve their own category, or should they be folded into other chapters? Dissociative identity disorder (DID), famous in its DSM-III-R incarnation as multiple personality disorder, is especially controversial: Many clinicians feel that this condition is sometimes induced in susceptible patients by (largely North American) therapists who are particularly interested in these strange phenomena. A 2011 survey found only 244 childhood cases of DID, nearly two-thirds of which had been reported from just four U. S. research groups.

In two of the dissociative disorders, patients experience memory loss that is *not* caused by physiological or structural disorders of the brain. The third, depersonalization/derealization disorder (DDD), comprises episodes of detachment in which individuals feel as though they are detached observers of their own behavior or as if their surroundings are unreal.

Amnesia experienced in the dissociative disorders can take several forms:

- In *selective amnesia*, certain events are not recalled.

- In the most common form, *localized amnesia*, all the events of a particular time period are gone.

- Patients with the rare *generalized* form of amnesia forget pretty much everything, including personal identity and the ability to perform skills they once had mastered; these are the patients who wander into police stations or health care facilities and sometimes attract publicity as attempts are made to identify them.

Theoretically, a child or adolescent can have any of the dissociative disorders, but none has been extensively reported in young patients. DID and DDD may begin in childhood but are usually not diagnosed until maturity. For this reason, and because of the controversy surrounding the status of the dissociative disorders in general, we have chosen to limit our discussion. We focus here on dissociative amnesia (DA), which DSM-5 notes can present in any age group from young children upward. Even so, it isn't common in youngsters.

F44.0 DISSOCIATIVE AMNESIA

The most frequent cause of amnesia is a medical condition, such as the use of substances, a blow to the head, or the effects of a brain operation. However, in patients with DA, no such medical condition can account for the inability to remember certain important events that have occurred in one or multiple episodes over a period of time. This loss of memory is sufficiently serious to cause distress or to interfere with functioning in some important way. Its Essential Features are given below.

DA usually begins suddenly, and the time lost to the amnesia can be brief or extended—a matter of hours or days to several months. The cause most frequently given is emotional stress or trauma, such as the sense of betrayal a child might feel at being forced into a sexual relationship with a trusted adult. Some of these incidents have come to light in spectacular fashion when an adult, an adolescent, or an older child finally recalls the event and accuses a parent or other adult. In many of these cases, the accused adult has successfully challenged the allegation as induced factitiously by an overzealous therapist. Organizations are now devoted to supporting victims of this so-called *false-memory syndrome*, although sorting out victims from perpetrators has sometimes occupied courtrooms for months.

Whenever a patient with DA engages in apparently purposeful travel from home or in wandering in a bewildered fashion, the specifier *with dissociative fugue* can apply (and the code number changes). These episodes can occur following a severe stress, and they are seldom if ever reported in children.

ESSENTIAL FEATURES OF **DISSOCIATIVE AMNESIA**

Far beyond common forgetfulness, there is a loss of recall for important personal (usually traumatic or distressing) information.

The Fine Print

The D's: • Distress or disability (social, educational, occupational, or personal impairment) • Differential diagnosis (substance use and physical disorders; major neurocognitive disorder (dementia); posttraumatic stress disorder; dissociative identity disorder; somatic symptom disorder; ordinary forgetfulness)

Coding Note

If relevant, specify:

F44.1 With dissociative fugue

Rosalind

In her junior year of high school, Rosalind tipped the scales at nearly 300 pounds. Despite 3 years of faithfully attending Weight Watchers, she had recently gained another 35 pounds. This had prompted the referral for psychotherapy.

Rosalind proved an excellent candidate for therapy: She was intelligent, clear in her thinking, and unafraid to disagree with an authority figure. Although she didn't lose an ounce, within a couple of months she made real progress in understanding her problems. "It really spooked me," she said during one session. "I had just been watching TV when an image occurred to me and I shut off the sound with the remote. I could see myself in bed with my father, back when I was about 6. He was lying on top of me, with his pants down, and I had a lot of pain between my legs." Over the next few weeks, Rosalind reported more such memories. She was now sure that her father had had intercourse with her repeatedly over a 3-year period.

At this point, her therapist got her permission to interview others in her family. The additional information was shocking, even to a clinician with decades of experience working with mental patients. Her brother Bert (older by 7 years) confirmed not only that he had had suspicions about their father's involvement with Rosalind, but that in fact he had been involved at the same time in an incestuous affair with their mother. Both relationships had lasted until their father was jailed on unrelated charges; he later died in a knife fight in the prison yard. Before long, their mother found a boyfriend and lost interest in Bert.

At no time since the age of 10 had Rosalind experienced any sense of lapses in time; nor had she ever "awakened" to find that she had wandered from home. Other than a lifetime of obesity, her history was unremarkable. Her overall physical and mental health were both good, and she denied any use of drugs or alcohol. A physical exam revealed no neurological cause for concern.

Evaluation of Rosalind

Rosalind's lack of memory for a prolonged period of incest easily fulfills Criterion A for DA. The absence of alternative personalities during any of these periods would rule out **dissociative identity disorder**. Of course, the repeated sexual attacks by her father would qualify as severely traumatic incidents; nevertheless, **posttraumatic stress disorder** and **acute stress disorder** would be eliminated from consideration, in part because she did not reexperience the incidents in flashbacks or dreams. And her intact cognitive abilities would rule out any **cognitive disorders** as a possible cause of memory loss (D). She denied **substance use** and other **medical problems** such as head trauma or seizures (C), and she did not complain of physical problems, as would be the case in **somatic symptom disorder**. There was no evidence at all to suggest **factitious disorder**. The fact that her brother corroborated the memories she developed while in therapy militates strongly against a false-memory syndrome explanation for her story (which, we should note, is not a disorder recognized by DSM-5).

In fact, the only serious problem remains with the DSM-5 (and Essential Features) requirement for distress/disability (B) at her episode of localized amnesia. We could postulate that Rosalind's obesity was a consequence of her childhood trauma (hence related to her amnesia), and that this was a serious consequence. We could, but we'd be going somewhat beyond the data. Indeed, there were many issues in Rosalind's story that troubled her, perhaps least among them the amnesia. The text of DSM-5 does not discuss this issue at all; we feel that it may be an example of boilerplate terminology that has not been well thought through in context. In any event, the other aspects of her amnesia story are persuasive enough that we're going to assert clinicians' privilege and make the diagnosis anyway. There were no episodes of travel from home or confused wandering, so the specifier would not apply.

F44.0	Dissociative amnesia
E66.9	Morbid obesity due to excess calories
GAF	80 (current)

ASSESSING DISSOCIATIVE DISORDERS

General Suggestions

Assessing memory and other dissociation-related mental functions in anyone can be a challenge, but doing so in a child can be especially difficult. Due to inattention or brain immaturity, young children normally have memory gaps. And children are acutely aware of the desires of adults, so it is all too easy for an interested, sympathetic clinician to inadvertently influence the direction of a child's narrative. Whenever you are attempting to assess apparent amnesia or other dissociative symptoms in a child or teenager, you need to be doubly careful to enter into the project with no agenda or expectation beyond learning the truth.

Besides maintaining an open mind, you should adopt a casual approach, ask open-ended questions, and try to minimize the opportunity for distortion. Avoid penetrating glances and repeated questions about sensitive areas. Material that seems significant and needs exploration in depth may be more safely assessed across multiple interviews. When the possibility of sexual or physical abuse exists, consult with the child protective services agency in your community to determine whether the interview should be conducted by someone trained in forensics. Depending on the laws in your community, you could also consider obtaining permission to audio-record or video-record interviews, thereby documenting that you have not asked leading questions or otherwise unduly influenced a patient's answers. Finally, watch for behaviors that may be associated with dissociative disorders in children or adolescents. These include excessive daydreaming, forgetting names of familiar people, losing track of time, having vivid imaginary playmates, and frequently talking to oneself.

Developmental Factors

Younger children may become preoccupied with an activity that can make them appear oblivious and unresponsive to their surroundings. During imaginative play, children may imbue dolls or toys with personalities and other qualities that help them form a reciprocal relationship. Of course, this statement holds for any diagnosis; it is the basis for using play materials and fantasy in evaluations with a young child.

The symptoms of dissociating adolescents closely resemble those of adults.

Even experienced mental health professionals express considerable confusion about how to proceed with questions regarding alleged sexual or physical abuse in children or adolescents. Sexual exploitation and other forms of child abuse are crimes. This fact is sometimes overlooked in the quest for diagnostic information or approaches to treatment. If we fail to understand the legal consequences of a decision to begin a line of questioning about possible abuse, not only do we risk the emotional health of our patients; we may compromise the outcome of a critical investigation or subsequent trial. We recommend in the strongest terms that professionals who work with such children become familiar with the laws in their jurisdiction that concern the reporting and investigating of abuse.

CHAPTER 18

Somatic Symptom

and Related Disorders

QUICK GUIDE TO THE SOMATIC SYMPTOM AND RELATED DISORDERS

Primary Somatic Symptom and Related Disorders

Somatic symptom disorder. A young patient (usually an adolescent) has unexplained symptoms that cause excessive worry or investment of time in activities related to health care. It is found more commonly in females (p. 328).

With predominant pain (specifier for somatic symptom disorder). Either the pain in question has no apparent physical or physiological basis, or it far exceeds expectations suggested by a patient's objective physical condition (p. 332).

Conversion disorder (functional neurological symptom disorder). These patients complain of altered voluntary motor or sensory functions that have no identifiable physiological or anatomical cause (p. 324).

Illness anxiety disorder. A physically healthy patient has the unfounded fear of a serious, often life-threatening illness such as cancer or heart disease.

Psychological factors affecting other medical conditions. A patient's mental or emotional issues influence the course or care of a medical disorder (p. 334).

Factitious disorder. In order to gain attention, an individual either consciously fabricates personal symptoms (factitious disorder imposed on self) or causes someone else, often a child, to have symptoms (factitious disorder imposed on another) (p. 338).

Other specified, or unspecified, somatic symptom and related disorder. These are catch-all categories for unexplained somatic symptoms that fail to meet criteria for *any* of the better-defined DSM-5 disorders listed above (p. 336).

Other Causes of Somatic Complaints

Pain with no apparent physical cause is characteristic of some patients with a major depressive episode (p. 239). Patients who use substances may complain of pain or other physical symptoms that result from the effects of substance intoxication or withdrawal (p. 402), or such complaints may represent efforts to obtain the substance of choice. Finally, in malingering, people devise symptoms for material gain (obtaining money or drugs, avoiding work or punishment). Malingering is only infrequently diagnosed in adolescents and *never* in young children (p. 443).

INTRODUCTION

Although somatic symptom and related disorders often have their roots in childhood and adolescence, they have been little studied in juveniles, especially young children. Indeed, most of these disorders apply poorly to children, partly because the older (DSM-III and DSM-IV) criteria were not written with them in mind. For example, somatic symptom disorder (SSD) is frequently encountered in adult mental health populations, but its very low apparent frequency in children may have been influenced by DSM-III and DSM-IV criteria for somatization disorder, which emphasized behaviors that can only be expected after puberty. DSM-5 has so liberalized the criteria for what it now calls SSD that this argument no longer applies; however, other arguments do apply, and we make them in a sidebar below (p. 331).

CONVERSION DISORDER (FUNCTIONAL NEUROLOGICAL SYMPTOM DISORDER)

A *conversion symptom* occurs when there is (1) a change in how the body functions (2) in the absence of any apparent physical or physiological malfunction. For years, a third requirement was stated—namely, that it occur under the influence of an emotional conflict. In DSM-5, that requirement has been deleted from the criteria for conversion disorder (CD), though many would argue that it is still important to note.

Many conversion symptoms (so called because they supposedly transform emotional distress into physical manifestations) suggest the presence of neurological deficits where none exist. DSM-5 calls these *functional neurological symptoms*; indeed, they are sometimes called *pseudoneurological symptoms*. Examples include a patient who complains of total deafness but flinches when a paper bag is burst nearby, or one who claims the inability to speak, yet can whisper.

Conversion symptoms include both motor and sensory deficits. Although the list of possible symptoms is long, only a few have been much reported in young children. They include fatigue, muscle stiffness and pains, abdominal distress, and pseudoseizures. (Patients may also complain of headache, painful menses, and other bodily pains. When *only* pain symptoms occur, however, these are given a DSM-5 diagnosis of SSD with predominant pain.)

Older children and adolescents may report classical pseudoneurological symptoms, such as numbness or tingling of extremities (paresthesias), partial paralysis, and trouble walking. Other conversion symptoms can include blindness, double vision, deafness, inability to speak (aphonia), difficulty urinating, difficulty swallowing (which may be reported as the sensation of lump in the throat—*globus hystericus* in a much older literature), loss of consciousness, amnesia, and hallucinations.

Though it can begin as early as 4 years and incidence increases with age, CD is rarely diagnosed in young children; childhood prevalence estimates place it at about 2–4 per 100,000. In a study of childhood psychogenic movement disorders, only 2 of 15 child or adolescent patients had had onset prior to the age of 10. In both adults and children, females outnumber males by perhaps 3:1.

In an apparent paradox, low prevalence rates may result from the seeming ubiquity of conversion-type symptoms in children. For example, think of the child who complains of feeling nauseated prior to a dreaded arithmetic test. This is *not* malingering; the child truly feels ill. Most often, because the stress underlying such a complaint is patently obvious and education must be pursued, the child is sent trudging off to school anyway. Only in extraordinary circumstances do such complaints cause enough distress to require clinical attention or interfere with functioning; hence the rarity in children of a diagnosis for behavior that is common.

Under what circumstances is CD likely to be diagnosed? In adults, it may be found among those who are economically deprived, poorly educated, and medically unsophisticated. Similar factors might well obtain in children and adolescents. CD may also be fostered in families where illness is used as a form of communication or as metaphor. In a large minority of cases, conversion symptoms develop in those who earlier have experienced genuine somatic disease and now may unconsciously use it for some sort of gain. Common antecedents include the stresses of bullying, parental separation, and death of a friend or relative, and other stressful events.

Diane

When Diane was only 4, she was started on valproic acid for petit mal epilepsy, which had been diagnosed via EEG. A therapeutic dose was achieved within a few weeks, and her staring spells abruptly stopped. For the next 10 years, Diane took her medicine religiously twice a day. Only once or twice, as she neared adolescence, did she ever look at the videos her parents had made of her during one of her spells.

ESSENTIAL FEATURES OF **CONVERSION DISORDER**

The patient's symptom or symptoms—altered sensory or voluntary motor functioning—seem clinically inconsistent with any known medical illness.

The Fine Print

A "normal" exam or a bizarre test result is not enough to affirm the diagnosis; there must be positive supportive evidence. Such evidence would include a change in findings from positive to negative when a different test is used (or the patient is distracted), or impossible findings such as tunnel vision.

The D's: • Distress or disability (social, educational, occupational, or personal impairment) • Differential diagnosis (substance use and physical disorders; mood or anxiety disorders; body dysmorphic disorder; dissociative disorders)

Coding Notes

Specify if:

> **Acute episode.** Symptoms have lasted under 6 months.
> **Persistent.** Symptoms have lasted 6+ months.

Specify: **{With} {Without} psychological stressor**

Specify type of symptom:

> **F44.4 With weakness or paralysis; with abnormal movement** (tremor, dystonia, abnormal gait); **with swallowing symptoms;** *or* **with speech symptom**
> **F44.5 With attacks or seizures**
> **F44.6 With anesthesia or sensory loss**
> **F44.6 With special sensory symptom** (hallucinations or other disturbance of vision, hearing, smell)
> **F44.7 With mixed symptoms**

Diane had a sister, Deirdre, who was 3 years older. Deirdre was a honey blonde, senior class president, and student coordinator of the school science fair. Diane had stringy, carrot-red hair and little scholastic aptitude. Her freshman year was the first time the two sisters had ever attended the same school together. On the evening of the homecoming dance, to which Deirdre had been invited by several boys (and Diane by no one), Diane experienced the first in a series of staring episodes that continued throughout that year.

Her valproic acid level was reassessed and found to be clinically acceptable; nonetheless, the dose was gradually raised, almost to the point of toxicity, but without effect. Next she was tried on a series of other anticonvulsants, then on combinations of these medications. Several times she improved temporarily, only to relapse into staring episodes, which now were occurring as often as four or five times a day. To her evident distress, she was almost completely unable to participate in extracurricular activities.

Near the end of her freshman year, Diane was admitted to a neurology unit for inpatient observation with continuously monitored EEG. On none of the seven recorded episodes of staring did her EEG show the 3-cycles-per-second, spike-and-wave pattern of discharges that had been present years earlier. During each episode she was unresponsive when nursing staff or family members spoke to her, but twice the neurology resident aborted the episode by tickling the bottom of her foot. When a therapist later observed that her pseudoseizures probably served to remove her from competition with her older sister, Diane remarked, "Deirdre's beautiful and smart, and I'm nothing!"

Evaluation of Diane

Ruling out **general medical** or **neurological disease** (Criterion C) is a cardinal task for any clinician evaluating a patient for CD—or any other mental disorder, for that matter. Diane's case was confounded by the fact that, as is often true of young people who have genuine epileptic seizures or pseudoseizures, she had both. However, even had no physical cause been found, this would not have been sufficient for a CD diagnosis: Many apparent conversion symptoms later turn out to be caused by physical disease or a different medical or mental disorder.

The fact that Diane's seizures (Criterion A) could be aborted by a noxious stimulus (tickling) suggested that they were indeed conversion symptoms. Some writers recommend bringing on an episode through suggestion, but we worry about this procedure's ethical implications (trust) and consequences for outcome (reinforcement of symptomatology we'd rather eliminate). In any event, the lack of EEG abnormality provides the clinical evidence required for a definitive diagnosis (B).

Identification of a probable psychological stressor is no longer required for diagnosis (DSM-IV included it), but it is something to watch for, partly because it can provide grist for subsequent therapy. No evidence suggests that Diane was consciously feigning her seizures (in fact, she seemed upset when she couldn't engage in after-school activities), as would be the case in **malingering**. Diane's distress and disability vis-à-vis after-school activities were obvious (D).

Diane would also need to be carefully investigated for other somatic symptoms to rule out **somatization disorder**, which is by far the better-defined (in DSM-IV), more common diagnosis. Somatic symptoms can also occur in patients who have **major depressive disorder** or **posttraumatic stress disorder**. The case vignette provides no evidence concerning any abnormal character traits, but we would want to watch Diane carefully for the emergence of a **personality disorder**. Note that the principal symptom type determines the exact code number:

F44.5   Conversion disorder with seizures, acute episode, with psychological stressor

G403.09   Petit mal epilepsy, well controlled

CGAS   70 (on admission)

F45.1 SOMATIC SYMPTOM DISORDER

SSD is the latest iteration of *hysteria*, a mental diagnosis that dates to the time of the ancient Egyptians and Greeks. It has more recently been called *Briquet syndrome*, for the French physician who in the 19th century first described the typical presentation of multiple physical and mental symptoms. DSM-IV called it *somatization disorder*, which we discuss in the accompanying sidebar (p. 331). Because SSD has been so recently defined, most of what we can say about it must be drawn from studies of its diagnostic predecessors.

The somatic symptoms in question often last for many years, perhaps a lifetime of waxing and waning as first one, then another symptom appears. They can lead to a variety of undesirable sequels: loss of time from work or school, unnecessary surgical procedures, prescription of harmful medications. At its worst, the disorder can alienate patients from their families; suicides have been reported.

According to DSM-5 criteria, SSD must last at least 6 months. There is no mandated minimum age for onset; typically it begins by the age of 30, but in nearly every case the onset is far earlier—sometimes as young as 4 or 5. As defined by DSM-5, SSD may affect as many as 5–7% of adult women, though with the more restrictive criteria of DSM-IV somatization disorder, the prevalence in the adult population is probably closer to 1%. It is rare in men; its prevalence in adolescents is unknown. Like somatization disorder, SSD probably runs in families, transmitted both through genes and the environment.

Somatization disorder has accounted for as many as 8% of mental health clinic visits by women; the DSM-5 criteria for SSD may render it more prevalent yet. Nonetheless, clinicians often overlook it, perhaps because comorbid mental disorders are more obvious, or perhaps because of the complicated DSM-IV criteria. However, we consider it well worth putting time into its detection: A valid diagnosis can down the road save endless hours of contradictory tests, fruitless treatment, and heartbreaking complications.

Wilma

Wilma was only 17 when she was hospitalized for suicidal ideas, but she agreed with her mom that she'd been sickly and hypochondriacal most of her life. By the time she was 16,

ESSENTIAL FEATURES OF **SOMATIC SYMPTOM DISORDER**

Concern about one or more somatic symptoms leads the patient to express a high level of health anxiety by investing excessive time in health care or being excessively worried about the seriousness of symptoms.

The Fine Print

The D's: • Duration (6+ months) • Differential diagnosis (DSM-5 does not state one, but we would cite substance use and physical disorders; psychotic, mood, or anxiety disorders; trauma- or stressor-related disorders; dissociative disorders)

Coding Notes

Specify:

> **With predominant pain.** For patients who complain mainly of pain (see p. 332).
> **Persistent.** If the course is marked by serious symptoms, lots of impairment, and a duration greater than 6 months.

Consider the following behaviors related to seriousness of the patient's symptoms: excessive thoughts, persistent high anxiety, excessive time/energy expended. Now rate severity:

> **Mild.** One of these behaviors.
> **Moderate.** 2+.
> **Severe.** 2+ plus multiple somatic complaints (or one very severe complaint).

she had had two laparotomies for abdominal pain, retention of urine that required catheterization, headaches for which she had consulted a neurologist, and menstrual periods so heavy and painful that she had to remain home from school several days each month. (The only physical finding had been a cervical polyp, which her gynecologist said could not have caused the trouble.)

Wheezing and chest pain—her family physician had pronounced them "no big deal"— were accompanied by severe anxiety attacks. When she was only 14, an ophthalmologist could find no physical cause for a prolonged episode of visual blurring ("For days, I thought I must have a brain tumor"). Recently she had also been evaluated for vomiting spells, which she thought might be related to severe food intolerance (for several years, the very thought of coconut, celery, and peanut butter had nauseated her); again, however, no pathology had been found. Frequent, dramatic mood swings and numerous claimed suicide attempts had led to a diagnosis of bipolar I disorder. For several months she had taken lithium until she became "allergic" to it.

The second of four siblings, Wilma called her family life "a disaster." Her mother had a long-standing drinking problem; her father gambled; a cousin had died accidentally from an overdose of heroin.

In the hospital, Wilma was at first tearful and distraught. Within a few hours, however, she became interested in a college freshman who had been admitted to deal with his cocaine use. In the evening they were seen giggling together in a corner of the dayroom; later that night, they eloped from the hospital.

Evaluation of Wilma

Wilma easily fulfilled the DSM-5 requirements for SSD. She had had not one but numerous somatic symptoms that were distressing and interrupted her life (Criterion A). Although the exact behavior varied depending on the symptom (and only one of these behaviors is required for diagnosis), she had had persistent, disproportionate concern (B1) and high anxiety (B2), and had overall devoted far too much time and energy to her symptoms (B3). These behaviors had existed for years, far beyond the minimum 6 months required (C).

The criteria for DSM-IV somatization disorder (see the sidebar) are far more demanding, yet Wilma fulfilled them, too: *pain*, in head and abdomen and with menstruation and urination; *gastrointestinal*, food intolerance and vomiting spells; *sexual and genitourinary*, excessively heavy menses; and *pseudoneurological*, urinary retention. There is no evidence that over the years she had intentionally faked her symptoms, which might warrant a diagnosis of **malingering**, or that she was consciously striving for deception, as in **factitious disorder imposed on self**.

In addition, like so many other patients with a lot of somatic symptoms, Wilma had been treated for severe **mood disorder**. Should she also receive a mood disorder diagnosis? To some degree, this is a matter of judgment. Although she might at one time have met strict criteria for a major depressive episode, the added diagnosis of a mood disorder could encourage a subsequent clinician to use inappropriate somatic treatment when behavioral management might be more effective. In any patient who tends to somaticize, it is vital to ask about other disorders and behaviors that often co-occur: **substance-related disorders** and **personality disorders** (especially **histrionic personality disorder**, though **borderline** and **antisocial personality disorders** are also sometimes diagnosed).

Wilma's condition had lasted far longer than the minimum of 6 months and was replete with many symptoms and much disability and distress. We would therefore add the specifiers to the full diagnosis:

F45.1	Somatic symptom disorder, severe, persistent
GAF	65 (on admission)

The most significant issue with DSM-5 SSD is that the criteria have been so very much simplified from the requirements for somatization disorder—the term for the DSM-IV disorder it replaces—that many, many more people will qualify for the diagnosis.

DSM-5 Made Easy by James Morrison includes a more complete discussion of the 60-year march through various names and criteria sets. Each of these required counting up a certain number of physical symptoms to a minimum required for diagnosis; follow-up studies demonstrated that such an approach resulted in a highly reliable method of ascertainment. The DSM-5 approach was published without data and without substantial testing—indeed, with only the hope that it can discriminate a valid disease entity.

We worry that it will not succeed. And because young patients especially should not be unnecessarily lumbered with a diagnosis that could serve to obscure other, more treatable conditions, we recommend use instead of the older criteria set for somatization disorder. To that end, we have reprinted them (from *DSM-IV Made Easy*, also by James Morrison) below. Note that in each of the four symptom categories below, the specific symptoms are listed in approximate descending order of frequency.

Somatization Disorder Criteria

- Starting before age 30, the patient has had many physical complaints occurring over several years.
- The patient has sought treatment for these symptoms, or they have materially impaired social, work, or personal functioning.
- The patient has at some time experienced a total of at least eight symptoms from the following list, distributed as noted. These symptoms need not be concurrent.
    - Pain symptoms (four or more) related to different sites, such as head, abdomen, back, joints, extremities, chest, or rectum, or related to body functions, such as menstruation, sexual intercourse, or urination.
    - Gastrointestinal symptoms (two or more, excluding pain), such as nausea, bloating, vomiting not during pregnancy, diarrhea, or intolerance of several foods.
    - Sexual symptoms (at least one, excluding pain), including indifference to sex, difficulties with erection or ejaculation, irregular menses, excessive menstrual bleeding, or vomiting throughout all nine months of pregnancy.
    - Pseudoneurological symptoms (at least one), including poor balance or coordination, weak or paralyzed muscles, lump in throat or trouble swallowing, loss of voice, retention of urine, hallucinations, numbness to touch or pain, double vision, blindness, deafness, seizures, amnesia or other dissociative symptoms, or loss of consciousness other than with fainting. None of these is limited to pain. *(continued)*

> ■ For each of the symptoms above, one of these conditions must be met:
>   ✓ Physical or laboratory investigation determines that the symptom cannot be fully explained by a general medical condition* or by the use of substances including medications, *or*
>   ✓ If the patient does have a general medical condition, the impairment or complaints exceed what would generally be expected, based on history, laboratory findings, or physical examination.
> ■ The patient doesn't consciously feign the symptoms for material gain (as in malingering) or in order to occupy the sick role (as in factitious disorder).
>
> *Here is one area at least where we can agree with the DSM-5 approach: The weight of evidence collected to date suggests that requiring a lack of medical explanation for the symptoms in question is not helpful to the diagnosis, and that the full weight of all somatic symptoms (medically explained or not) is the best predictor of health outcome.

WITH PREDOMINANT PAIN (SPECIFIER FOR SOMATIC SYMPTOM DISORDER)

We usually think of pain in terms of its cause. Most of the time, for most humans, the etiology is something that can be seen, felt, or deduced from medical tests—an infected thumb, a sore throat, a twisted loop of bowel. Such pain is not a mental disorder. But a substantial number of individuals react to pain more strongly than seems warranted by its nature. That is, they generally conform to the requirements of DSM-5 SSD by reacting more strongly or at greater length to pain than do most people. When that is the case, the specifier *with predominant pain* can be used. (In this discussion, we abbreviate SSD with this specifier as SSDPP.)

Unlike the DSM-IV criteria for pain disorder (as a disorder in its own right), SSDPP does not require clinicians to judge that a psychological factor has created, worsened, or maintained the pain. However, clinicians and parents will continue to look for evidence that a given pain symptom does not spring from a defined organic state. Although none of the following factors is definitive, they can suggest psychological causation:

■ Pain begins after psychological trauma.

■ Stressful events increase the pain.

■ Disability is worse than seems reasonable for the cause.

■ There is evidence of secondary gain (such as avoiding school or punishment).

Headache and abdominal pain lead the list of pain sites for children. For example, in one study, 22% of children interviewed over 4 years reported recurrent abdominal pain; girls outnumber boys by about 2.5:1. However, the number of children for whom this finding is clinically important is undoubtedly much lower.

The experience of pain is subjective, so its measurement relies on the threshold of the sufferer and the judgment of the person who evaluates it. This is a difficult enough task for an adult patient; it approaches the Herculean for a young child, who has fewer experiences that can serve as reference points of severity. Response to a placebo is often positive, regardless of whether the patient suffers from organic pain or something else.

The origins of SSDPP are still not known. Children, adolescents, and adults alike may use pain and other physical symptoms to communicate emotional distress or a need for comfort; certainly a family pattern of illness behavior can influence a child's or adolescent's response to pain. Although the roots of SSDPP may ultimately be found in a young patient's genetic predisposition, factors specific to the patient's own social circumstances—school problems or lack of social support from the parents, for example—may also play a role.

Jordan

On a Saturday afternoon in early October, during the second period of his team's soccer match against another third-grade class, Jordan gradually became aware that his stomach was hurting him. At the time, he was tending goal—his favorite position—and he didn't tell anyone until after the match, but that evening his parents took him to the urgent care department at their HMO. After X-rays and lab tests proved entirely normal, he was sent home. He soon recovered, but intermittently during the following weeks, he experienced abdominal pain.

Now it was nearly Christmas, and Jordan had spent nearly 10 days (off and on) at home, complaining of cramping pain. Several more visits to the doctor and a variety of increasingly complicated laboratory and radiological tests revealed no pathology. In desperation, the pediatrician referred them to the HMO's mental health department.

According to the social worker who interviewed them, Jordan's was a "Dick and Jane" sort of family on the surface. They lived in a quiet suburb, owned a dog and a cat, and appeared to have had no serious social or financial problems. His dad's job entailed reasonable hours, good pay, and no travel out of town. Jordan's mother hadn't taught school since just before Jordan and his twin sister, Sarah, were born. Now she stayed home to care for them and their 3-year-old sister. A dour woman who looked older than her 38 years, she complained during the interview of her own ill health. Over the years she had evidently consulted a variety of physicians and other clinicians, but the social worker knew of no definitive diagnosis that had ever been made.

Jordan was a good student who liked school, and his grades had not yet suffered. He had cried when he was told that he couldn't finish the soccer season with his team, but his mood had otherwise remained good throughout the fall. He always fussed when his pain kept him home from school, and he carefully followed the regimen his doctor advised.

Evaluation of Jordan

In most respects, Jordan's history would seem to qualify him for a diagnosis of SSDPP. His recurrent abdominal pain had led to numerous episodes of treatment and had caused him to miss a number of days of school (Criterion A). A great deal of effort had been expended to try to pinpoint the cause (B3), though in truth it was not clear how much of this effort had been at Jordan's and how much at his parents' instigation. No **medical disorder** often associated with recurrent abdominal pain (such as abdominal migraine, ulcerative colitis, Crohn's disease, or fructose malabsorption) had been identified. However, ruling out organic illness is not a requirement for SSDPP; indeed, DSM-5 states explicitly that the diagnosis can be made in the presence of another medical condition.

Always described as cheerful, Jordan did not appear to have another mental condition, such as **major depressive disorder**. There was no evidence of a desire to be sick or intent to deceive, which would suggest **factitious disorder** or **malingering**, respectively; indeed, he enjoyed school and objected to remaining at home when stricken. Nothing even hinted at an incipient **personality disorder**.

Here's a stumper: The overall duration of Jordan's abdominal complaints had been just shy of 3 months. Criterion C for SSD states only that a symptom (or series of symptoms) should be "persistent (typically more than 6 months)." But it does not clearly state an operational time period and does not elaborate on the criterion in the text. We, however, would be loath to apply such a diagnosis to a child who is monosymptomatic and has such a relatively brief history. As a result, we would have to give Jordan some diagnosis that would help us (and all future clinicians) maintain an open mind about the etiology of Jordan's pain.

R10.4	Abdominal pain, unknown etiology
CGAS	70 (current)

If we were more confident that he did have a disorder involving somatization, we might opt for this:

F45.8	Other specified somatic symptom disorder (somatic symptom disorder with brief duration)

At this point in his medical saga, however, even that would be a stretch.

F54 PSYCHOLOGICAL FACTORS AFFECTING OTHER MEDICAL CONDITIONS

DSM-IV suggested six sorts of psychological factors that can affect the treatment of a medical disorder. Though clinicians treating children and adolescents may not often employ these designations, they are occasionally useful. DSM-5 doesn't list these specific categories, but they provide a useful way to remind us of issues that can affect the course of treatment. If more than one psychological factor is present, choose the most prominent one.

- *Mental disorder.* Peter's obsessive–compulsive disorder causes him to doubt that he has taken his insulin; at age 16, he's already had several episodes of low blood sugar due to overdose.

- *Psychological symptoms* (insufficient for another DSM-5 diagnosis). With few other mental symptoms, Scooter's fearfulness causes him to run away instead of accepting the chemotherapy the pediatrician recommended for his leukemia.

- *Personality traits or coping style.* Tracey has fought with authority figures since early adolescence; now she refuses to wear the splint she needs to protect her broken arm.

- *Maladaptive health behaviors.* Jason knows that smoking causes his asthma to flare up, but he desperately wants acceptance with the popular kids at school.

ESSENTIAL FEATURES OF **PSYCHOLOGICAL FACTORS AFFECTING OTHER MEDICAL CONDITIONS**

A physical symptom or illness is affected by a psychological or behavioral factor that precipitates, worsens, interferes with, or extends the patient's need for treatment.

The Fine Print

The D: • Differential diagnosis (other mental disorders, such as panic disorder, mood disorders, somatic symptom and related disorders, posttraumatic stress disorder)

Coding Notes

Specify current severity:

Mild. The factor increases medical risk
Moderate. The factor aggravates the underlying medical condition
Severe. The factor causes an emergency room visit or hospitalization.
Extreme. The factor results in severe, life-threatening risk.

First, code the name of the relevant medical condition.

▨ *Stress-related physiological response.* April's family needs her to get a college scholarship; twice now, when scheduled to sit for the SAT, she's gotten a migraine.

▨ *Other or unspecified psychological factors.* Terry has a fear of needles. Her parents mistrust vaccinations, so they didn't push her to start her HPV series.

F45.8 OTHER SPECIFIED SOMATIC SYMPTOM AND RELATED DISORDER

Examples of conditions that might be assigned the other specified diagnosis include *pseudocyesis* (false pregnancy), transient hypochondriacal states, total environmental allergy syndrome, and unexplained physical symptoms lasting less than 6 months. However, it is doubtful whether the first three of these would ever apply to young patients. The case of Jordan (described above in regard to SSDPP) illustrates the application of the other specified diagnosis to a child.

F45.9 UNSPECIFIED SOMATIC SYMPTOM AND RELATED DISORDER

The unspecified category should be reserved for patients who do not meet criteria for any of the disorders described in this DSM-5 chapter, but who nonetheless seem to have a somatic symptom and related disorder.

ASSESSING SOMATIC SYMPTOM DISORDERS

General Suggestions

A clinical interview is not usually the appropriate venue for validating physical complaints. Volumes could be (indeed, have been) written describing tests for discriminating conversion symptoms from physically or neurologically based pathology. (For example, patients with genuine blindness comply when asked to sign their names, whereas patients with pseudoblindness may just scribble; any conversion symptom may decrease when a patient is being distracted. DSM-5 describes several other examples.) Although many mental health practitioners don't routinely perform such tests, they can look for a complicated medical history (multiple hospitalizations and many trials of medication) and for patterns of behavior and personality characteristics that distinguish patients with a tendency to somaticize.

The affective tone used to describe the physical complaints can provide useful information in a teenager who giggles or otherwise appears unconcerned when describing serious symptoms. This characteristic is called *la belle indifférence*, which means "lofty indifference." (Rather than responding with indifference, most young patients with mental or physical illness are frightened by their symptoms.)

The following features include some of the characteristics typical of histrionic personality disorder, which often accompanies somatic symptoms.

- A presentation that may be either overly dramatic or, paradoxically, blasé
- A seductive manner toward the examiner
- Constant attention seeking
- Excessive emphasis on the patient's own physical attractiveness
- Vagueness when recounting historical data
- An apparent need for frequent praise or reinforcement

On the other hand, remember that although the following factors can *suggest* that a patient is somaticizing, they are *not* diagnostic:

- A patient's anxiety or somatic symptom is increased by stress (stress or conflict can worsen physical symptoms, too).
- The symptoms seem too intense for real illness (individuals vary tremendously in their reactions to pain or dysfunction).
- The patient seems sensitive or dramatic (many people with histrionic or other personality disorders are physically healthy).
- The presenting symptom seems bizarre (physical illness and other major mental disorders can begin with highly unusual symptoms).

Because somatic symptom disorders are strongly correlated with childhood abuse, it is especially important to consider the possibility of sexual or physical abuse in young patients with these diagnoses. Also remember that a person's culture can modify how symptoms are expressed.

Above all, when you are assessing any of these disorders, be alert for the possibility of physical disease; missing one can be dangerous for the patient and at best embarrassing for you, the clinician. DSM-5 states that SSD can be diagnosed in the face of genuine physical pathology; however, we don't want to risk shrugging off remediable disease states on the basis of a presumed emotional origin.

Developmental Factors

It is developmentally normal for a young child to react temporarily to a minor injury by complaining of pain, limping, or even howling. In the usual course of events, a few minutes of diminishing parental attention to the injury will be repaid when the child, too, shifts attention elsewhere. When children do develop conversion symptoms, they tend to have numbness or tingling of extremities (paresthesias), paralyses, pseudoseizures, and trouble walking.

Among young children, boys and girls are about equally likely to develop conversion symptoms; after puberty, girls are more likely to be affected. Other studies find that fatigue, back pain, and blurred vision can be experienced by children of any age. Adolescent concern with normal body parts and functioning is developmentally appropriate, and should be considered pathological only when it endures and causes clinically important distress or impairs functioning.

The way children react to pain changes as they mature. Very young children may request hugging or other maneuvers as a distraction from severe, recurrent pain. Older children are often better able to understand and rationalize the need for painful medical procedures. Tolerance to pain also increases as a child grows; an 8-year-old can shrug off an injury that would make a toddler scream. The physical complaints most frequently reported by prepubertal children are recurrent abdominal pain and headache, with abdominal pain occurring at an earlier age. Older children and adolescents will complain of extremity pain, muscle aches, and neurological symptoms.

The major precursor to the DSMs, the Washington University criteria for mental disorders (popularly referred to as the "Feighner criteria" after the first author of a seminal paper), included mood symptoms in the criteria for somatization disorder. These symptoms were dropped in DSM-III, allowing clinicians to make multiple diagnoses—for example, somatization disorder plus major depressive disorder. An unintended consequence was that the change allowed clinicians to forget that mood and anxiety symptoms—even psychotic behavior—often accompany and are even intrinsic to somatization disorder.

F68.10 FACTITIOUS DISORDER

Patients with factitious disorder (FD) feign symptoms, but not for financial or other gain, which is the case in malingering. Rather, they do it for some other motive—perhaps to obtain sympathy or attention for themselves. Some publications call this "occupying the sick role." FD has borne a variety of other names—most prominently *Münchausen syndrome*, after the storied 18th-century Baron von Münchausen, who wandered Europe concocting tall tales about his adventures.

When the same person both causes and bears the symptoms, DSM-5 calls the disorder FD imposed on self (FDIS). It is thought to begin early in life, and it is occasionally (though not often) diagnosed in older children and adolescents. But there is another such situation that more typically involves children: Rather than personally feigning illness, the perpetrator attempts to induce or falsify symptoms in someone else. DSM-5 calls this factitious disorder imposed on another (FDIA) and, for the first time ever, includes it as a part of the official manual. (DSM-IV said it needed more study and called it FD by proxy.) FD had its own chapter in DSM-IV, but DSM-5 groups it with the somatic symptom and related disorders.

In about three-quarters of the cases, the mother of a child is the instigator responsible for the behavior, but occasionally it will be a father, grandparent, babysitter, or other primary caregiver. Only rarely does the perpetrator have psychosis; usually there is a personality disorder, substance use disorder, or some other mental condition. Many perpetrators have a background in health care, and some have had a personal history of abuse or FD. Often they work hard to appear as excellent caregivers for a child.

In children under age 16, being the victim of FDIA is uncommon, occurring at the rate of about 1 per 200,000 per year; for those a year old or younger, the rate increases perhaps fivefold. (Older children must, of course, collude to some degree in the deception.) Boys and girls are about equally affected, and are usually 4 years of age or less. From the first appearance of symptoms, it usually takes about a year to make the correct diagnosis.

A caregiver may feign or produce symptoms in a child by various means:

- Parental description only (such as recounting seizures)
- Parental description plus false specimens or falsified charts
- Poisoning, smothering, or withholding of food or medicine
- Fabrication of psychiatric disorder
- Factitious signs of pregnancy (in adolescents)
- Embellishment of a genuine physical illness

Suspicion may be raised when a parent seems either unconcerned or overly concerned (even to the point of not leaving the bedside) about a seriously ill child; when the child's physician cannot make sense of the symptoms; or when the child remains ill despite apparently adequate treatment. The medical and emotional havoc such a family wreaks may come to light only at the end of a long and frustrating clinical course.

The injurious behaviors usually continue until one of three outcomes occurs: The perpetrator is apprehended; the child's increasing age causes the perpetrator to move on to a younger child; or the child dies (the mortality rate for victims of FDIA is 10%). In one study, nearly one in eight victims were either dead or permanently injured at follow-up, and three of five siblings had had similar experiences. In another survey, over 70% of 117 patients sustained permanent disability or disfigurement.

ESSENTIAL FEATURES OF **FACTITIOUS DISORDER IMPOSED ON {SELF} {ANOTHER PERSON}**

To present a picture of someone who is ill, injured, or impaired, {the patient} {another person acting for the patient} feigns physical or mental signs or symptoms of illness or induces an injury or disease. This behavior occurs even without evident benefits (such as financial gain, revenge, or avoiding legal responsibility).

The Fine Print

The D's: • Differential diagnosis (substance use and physical disorders; psychotic, mood, or anxiety disorders; trauma- or stressor-related disorders; dissociative and neurocognitive disorders; malingering)

Coding Notes

Diagnose:

> **Factitious disorder imposed on self.** The perpetrator is also the patient.
> **Factitious disorder imposed on another.** The perpetrator and victim are separate individuals. The perpetrator receives the factitious disorder code; the victim receives a code reflecting the abuse.

For either type, specify:

> **Single episode.**
> **Recurrent episodes.**

Melissa

It all started with a twisted ankle during soccer practice when she was 8. While driving toward the net, Melissa fell; she had to sit out the rest of the practice session. Her family doctor diagnosed a mild sprain, and recommended ice and a few days of "taking it easy." Though this prescription seemed to help at first, the pain limited her mobility. Eventually, she had to stay in bed and receive home tutoring. But it wasn't until her toes turned blue and she complained of a prickly numbness in her left leg that Melissa was admitted to the hospital. There she was seen by a sports medicine orthopedist and a neurologist.

Despite the devoted attendance of her mother and increasingly heroic therapeutic efforts, the pain became so severe that Melissa couldn't move her foot and wouldn't let anyone touch it but her mother. MRI, EMG, and detailed studies of body chemistry were all normal. The change in the leg's color and temperature alarmed her physicians enough that they transferred her to the intensive care unit. There, separated from her mother, Melissa's improvement seemed almost miraculous. After a week, she had recovered enough that she was returned to the pediatric floor. The day before her scheduled discharge, however, the pain and discoloration returned.

More consultants were called in, but after 2 weeks Melissa's condition again deteriorated. She developed myoclonic jerks of her left leg and spasms of her foot, causing her to kick uncontrollably. Her mother, distraught, begged for more consultants. Increased use of pain medication dulled Melissa's senses so that she slept most of the time; when awake, she was often disoriented and spoke with a thick tongue. The diagnoses ranged from degenerative spinal cord disease to psychogenic myoclonus.

Finally, a neurologist suggested surreptitious video monitoring of Melissa's bedside. The following day, the treatment team watched in horrified fascination as the video showed Melissa's mother soothe her daughter, stroking her hair as she gently tightened a tourniquet around the damaged leg. Before the authorities could be notified and protective measures established, Melissa and her mother stole away from the hospital and disappeared.

Evaluation of Melissa

Other than the identity of the perpetrator, the Essential Features (and DSM-5 criteria) for FDIS and FDIA are exactly the same. In Melissa's case, the video made it crystal-clear that there was deliberate falsification of signs and symptoms (Criterion A). With no evidence of any material gain (C), her mother presented Melissa as ill (B).

Of course, before deciding that any person has FD, we must consider every possible **other medical condition** that can cause the symptoms; just the same as for any other mental disorder, physical (and substance use) etiologies belong at the top of the differential diagnosis. It was only after the members of Melissa's treatment team had considered them all that they suspected foul play. For adults with FDIS, **malingering** should also be considered in the differential diagnosis. However, we know of no instances of young children who have inflicted pain or trauma upon themselves—or even, for that matter, falsified other signs or symptoms of physical or mental disease.

And yet our diagnosis is hung up on one bit of evidence that we do not have: the mother's mental state. Note that in a case of FDIA, it is the perpetrator who receives the diagnosis. Melissa's mother bolted before her motives could be determined and before her daughter's well-being could be safeguarded. The clinicians therefore couldn't rule in or out such conditions as **delusional disorder** or some **other psychotic disorder**, as required by Criterion D. We'll just have to postulate that the mother did not have another mental disorder that better explained the symptoms.

As in most instances where the patient is merely the vehicle for the perpetrator's behavior, we'll also give a Z-code for physical abuse of a child by a parent. Had Melissa herself been the subject of our clinical attention, the code number would be different: Z69.010.)

Of course, due to the lack of information, a **personality disorder** could only be suspected. Similarly, other major mental diagnoses, though possibly warranted, could not be made. We couldn't even guess at a GAF score. We do know that Melissa's mother had assaulted her daughter with the tourniquet on more than one occasion, enabling us to employ the specifier. The full diagnosis for Melissa's mother would therefore be:

F68.10	Factitious disorder imposed on another, recurrent episodes
Z69.011	Perpetrator of physical child abuse by parent
GAF	0 (inadequate information)

Because child abuse is a crime, the treatment team would have a duty to report the situation to the appropriate authorities.

We will never know exactly why Melissa did not herself disclose the reason for her descent into the medical vortex. Her silence undoubtedly hinges on the strength of the family bond and the reluctance of children, even when they suffer the most grievous forms of abuse, to reveal secrets about parents and others who love and harm them.

Had Melissa helped her mother produce false signs or symptoms of a physical disease, she could have received the same diagnosis, more or less: FDIS. Such is sometimes the case for older children, adolescents, and adults who are the nominal victims, but it would rarely be warranted in a child as young as Melissa. Melissa's CGAS score would be relatively high (remember that this score is determined only by mental state, not impairment due to physical or environmental limitations). Melissa's complete diagnosis would be as follows:

Z69.010	Victim of physical child abuse by parent
G25.3	Myoclonus
CGAS	85

ASSESSING FACTITIOUS DISORDER IMPOSED ON ANOTHER

General Suggestions

FDIA taxes the skills of the most experienced interviewers, for the perpetrators are themselves highly experienced—at concealment. And their victims, whether out of fear, love, or simple failure to perceive anything amiss, may remain silent about the maltreatment. When you are faced with possible FDIA, focus on the behaviors and personality characteristics of the principal caregiver, who will almost invariably be the perpetrator. These adults are rarely psychotic, but may have a history of SSD/somatization disorder. They will almost certainly have a personality disorder, with a personality style that may be bizarre, boisterous, demanding, histrionic, or vague. Some of their characteristics include the following:

- Effusive praise of the providers they are attempting to deceive
- In a caricature of good parenting, excessive attentiveness to a sick child, perhaps refusing to desert the bedside for days at a time
- Or rather, lack of appropriate concern for a child who does not respond to treatment and may be desperately ill
- A sometimes remarkable fund of knowledge about a child's medical condition
- Often, a close association with one of the health care professions

Developmental Factors

These children present with all sorts of factitious symptoms, but age helps determine a few basic patterns. Infants and toddlers tend to present with apnea, cyanosis (blue skin), and seizures, whereas older children are likely to have gastrointestinal symptoms such as diarrhea and vomiting. Other symptoms can include ataxia, headache, paralysis, or weakness.

Young children will be able to provide little information about their own health status. Most adolescents and older children will have the knowledge (and perhaps even the judgment) that something is amiss, but will they divulge information that is critical of a parent or other caregiver? For some, an approach that emphasizes truth and trust between patient and clinician may help. You might say, for example, "It is terribly important that we figure out what's happening here. I'm going to ask you some questions about your problem. If you feel you can't answer truthfully, don't lie—that will only confuse us. Just say, 'I'd rather not talk about that right now.' OK?" For others, you will have to rely on covert observation and medical detection.

CHAPTER 19

Feeding and
Eating Disorders

QUICK GUIDE TO THE FEEDING AND EATING DISORDERS

Primary Feeding and Eating Disorders

Each of the primary feeding and eating disorders is defined by behaviors that the world recognizes as abnormal, though the patients themselves regard most of them as normal parts of themselves (ego-syntonic). Some disorders have a number of other features in common. Patients with either anorexia nervosa or bulimia nervosa may binge-eat, purge with laxatives, and exercise excessively. Both conditions are encountered mainly in girls and young women; onset is usually during the teenage years. Both are commonly encountered in adolescent patients.

Pica. The patient eats material that is not food (p. 345).

Rumination disorder. The person persistently regurgitates and rechews food already eaten (p. 347).

Avoidant/restrictive food intake disorder. A child's failure to eat enough leads to weight loss or a failure to gain weight (p. 348).

Anorexia nervosa. Despite being markedly underweight, these patients severely restrict food intake due to intense fear of gaining weight or becoming fat (p. 351).

Bulimia nervosa. These patients eat in binges, then prevent weight gain by self-induced vomiting, purging, and exercise. Although appearance is important to their self-evaluations, they do not have body image distortion (p. 351).

Binge-eating disorder. A person eats in binges but doesn't try to compensate by vomiting, exercising, or using laxatives (p. 355).

Other specified, or unspecified, feeding or eating disorder. These categories cover feeding and eating disorders that do not meet the full criteria for any of the above-named entities (p. 358).

Other Causes of Abnormal Eating

Changes in appetite and weight are characteristic of manic and major depressive episodes (p. 236) and of somatic symptom disorder (p. 328). Patients with schizophrenia or other psychotic disorders may develop bizarre eating habits (p. 218).

INTRODUCTION

Pica has been known for hundreds of years; rumination disorder was introduced as a diagnosis in DSM-III. But binge-eating disorder only became an official diagnosis in DSM-5. Avoidant/restrictive food intake disorder is the DSM-5 diagnosis that replaces the DSM-IV category termed feeding disorder of infancy or early childhood. Overall prevalence rates for these conditions are not known, but they are probably quite low. Also note that the first three disorders mentioned below were formerly included in the first DSM-IV chapter—what we now term the neurodevelopmental disorders.

F98.3 PICA

Derived from the word *magpie* (this bird's scientific genus is *Pica*), pica as a term for abnormal eating behavior dates back at least four centuries—perhaps to a time when someone, watching these large black-and-white birds as they collected clay and mud for nests, assumed that that they were eating it instead. Pica (see the Essential Features for the full criteria) has for centuries been identified with two groups: young children and pregnant women.

Dirt is one of the more common substances these people ingest, but any nonnutritive substance—chalk, wall plaster, soap, burnt matches, or (in extremely rare cases) even feces—will fulfill the definition. In some patients, pica may be a sign of iron deficiency. Others may develop any of a variety of medical complications. Children who eat paint risk lead toxicity; intestinal obstruction can result from ingestion of hair and other bulky, indigestible material.

Individuals with autism spectrum disorder or intellectual disability are especially prone to develop pica, the risk of which increases with the severity of their disorder. Adult women with the condition are likely to have a family history of pica and a personal history of it

ESSENTIAL FEATURES OF **PICA**

The patient persists in eating dirt or something else that isn't food.

The Fine Print

The D's: • Duration and demographics (1+ months in someone who is at least 2 years old) • Differential diagnosis (nutritional deficits, developmentally normal behavior, psychotic disorders, practice endorsed by the person's culture)

Coding Notes

Specify if: **In remission.**

Code by patient's age:

F98.3 Pica in children
F50.8 Pica in adults

when they were children. A background of neglect and low socioeconomic status is common among affected children. The behavior usually begins between the ages of 1 and 2 years, and may remit spontaneously with the onset of adolescence or with the correction of iron deficiency anemia. When it is diagnosed in adults, it carries a different ICD code number (F50.8).

Melanie

Melanie was 12 when both of her parents died in an automobile accident and she went to live with an older sister in Philadelphia. A slender, awkward child who seemed to hunger for friends, Melanie was always hanging about the fringes of a group at school. So, when she was 14 and a freshman in high school, the few who knew her expressed amazement to learn that she was pregnant. "I don't think she's ever even had a period," remarked her sister, "and I've never heard anything about a boyfriend."

Even then, the pregnancy was only discovered when her sister found her one afternoon in the backyard eating potting soil. It had happened several times in the past 2 months, and it was behavior even Melanie couldn't explain. ("I don't know why I do it, I just do it.") She was whisked away to see the pediatrician, who diagnosed anemia and a 4-month pregnancy. Although she had never before eaten dirt, her sister recalled that as a toddler, Melanie would pick up chewing gum and other discarded material from a nearby park and put it into her mouth.

Evaluation of Melanie

Eating material that had no nutritional value (at least for humans) had persisted longer than a month (Criterion A) and was behavior foreign to Melanie's culture (C). She was old enough and mature enough (a freshman in high school at age 14) that her developmental stage could not explain the symptoms (such behavior would be considered due to immaturity in a toddler—Criterion B). Other diagnoses with which pica can co-occur include **schizophrenia** (but Melanie did not explain her behavior with delusions). No information suggested **autism spectrum disorder**, in which unusual eating habits may also be encountered (D).

Although no personality disorder diagnosis should be made, Melanie's relatively poor social relationships suggested avoidant features. The fact that personality traits needed to be further evaluated would be indicated by a sentence or two in the diagnostic summary—DSM-5 has no way to state "diagnosis deferred." For the moment, Melanie's diagnosis would be as follows:

F98.3	Pica in children
Z33.1	Normal pregnancy
CGAS	65 (current)

F98.21 RUMINATION DISORDER

During rumination, an individual regurgitates a bolus of food from the stomach and chews it again. This is a normal part of the digestive process for cattle, deer, and giraffes, which is why they are called *ruminants*. In humans, it is abnormal and can lead to physical complications. When people ruminate, they do not experience nausea or disgust; indeed, in most cases, the food is later swallowed once again to be digested. However, some persons (especially infants and those with intellectual disability) will spit it out instead. Then malnutrition, failure to thrive (in infants), or susceptibility to disease can occur. Mortality rates as high as 25% have been reported.

Rumination disorder is uncommon, though more frequent in males than in females. It most

People with intellectual disability are more often affected by rumination disorder than are persons in the typical range of intellectual ability, though an occasional instance has been reported in a nondisabled adult. Some children with developmental delays may find regurgitation to be stimulating or soothing. In most cases the behavior subsides spontaneously, though it can persist throughout life. Reportedly, Samuel Johnson was one such adult ruminator: Acquaintances of the 18th-century lexicographer noted his "cud-chewing" behavior. (It is also widely believed that he had obsessive–compulsive disorder.) Rumination, if severe enough to justify independent clinical attention, can be diagnosed even in the context of another mental disorder.

ESSENTIAL FEATURES OF **RUMINATION DISORDER**

For at least a month, the patient has been regurgitating food.

The Fine Print

The D's: • Duration (1+ months) • Differential diagnosis (physical disorders, intellectual disability, other eating disorders)

often develops in infants, beginning after solid foods are introduced into the diet. Voluntary regurgitation may not be present initially. Often gastroesophageal reflux precipitates the onset. The act of ruminating may be associated with medical conditions such as hiatus hernia, though DSM-5 Criterion B requires us to dismiss the diagnosis of rumination disorder if such a condition is present. The cause is unknown, though social problems (abnormal parent–child interaction) may be a factor. Intellectual disability is sometimes comorbid.

The criteria (and Essential Features) are descriptive enough that we have provided no clinical vignette.

F50.8 AVOIDANT/RESTRICTIVE FOOD INTAKE DISORDER

Children with avoidant/restrictive food intake disorder (ARFID) essentially take in too little food to provide adequate nutrition. Why they do this is not always clear, but it isn't because they fear gaining weight or looking fat (as in anorexia nervosa). Some patients may dislike a quality (texture, color, taste) of certain foods; others may be concerned that they will repeat an experience of vomiting or choking on food. Or perhaps there's a more general emotional or behavioral problem (for example, an infant too irritable or sleepy to feed). In older individuals—even adults can be diagnosed with ARFID—concern for health consequences of foods may play a role.

Inadequate nutrition can render these children fussy or withdrawn. Neglect, abuse, and parental psychopathology are often described in extreme cases of failure to thrive. Nonorganic failure to thrive has now been linked with a number of conditions besides ARFID, among them rumination disorder, reactive attachment disorder, and breathing-related sleep disorders. Gone, however, is the presumption in earlier DSM editions that the food avoidance behavior was necessarily the result of a failed mother–child bond.

Derek

Deborah had been only 17 when her first child was born. Hours after the delivery, she had left tiny Raymond with relatives, put all the clothes she could carry into a plastic satchel, and headed for San Diego, where she waited on tables. Now Raymond was nearly 13 and lived with his paternal grandmother on the Oregon coast, and it had been years since Deborah had thought about babies. Beyond taking iron tablets and visiting the obstetrician twice, she hadn't prepared at all for another baby. But this one she kept, though Derek was a challenge for a single working mom.

When Deborah was at work, Derek was watched by an immigrant woman from upstairs, who spoke almost no English. "Don't talk foreign to him," Deborah had irritably commanded. "I don't want him growing up with an accent." When she returned from work, she was too tired to pay him much attention. As a result, Derek spent most of his first year staring at the sides of his crib.

When Derek was nearing his first birthday, it was the sitter who, in halting words, pointed out that he still weighed only 14 pounds—in fact, for the past several months he had hardly gained weight at all. She noted that when she tried to feed him, he often cried and turned his head away or pushed back the spoon. "He jus' don' wanna eat," she had said. Those occasions when Deborah herself fed him often ended in tears for both.

When he was finally taken to the well-baby clinic, Derek was pronounced "undernourished and neglected" and was hospitalized for further evaluation.

Evaluation of Derek

Derek's failure to gain weight (Criterion A1) and the sitter's testimony that he failed to eat adequately fulfilled the principal criterion for ARFID. However, this diagnosis could not be made definitively until the appropriate laboratory and radiographic exams had ruled out

ESSENTIAL FEATURES OF
AVOIDANT/RESTRICTIVE FOOD INTAKE DISORDER

With no abnormality of self-image, the patient eats too little to grow or gain weight (for adults, to maintain adequate nutrition or weight). The result can be a need for enteral feeding or interference with personal functioning.

The Fine Print

The D's: • Differential diagnosis (medical conditions; anorexia nervosa; accepted cultural practice; psychotic, mood, or anxiety disorders; factitious disorder)

Coding Notes

Specify if: **In remission.** The patient hasn't met criteria for what DSM-5 calls "a sustained period of time."

other causes of failure to thrive, such as **endocrine**, **gastrointestinal**, and **neurological disorders** (D). We know of no cultural practice that might be involved, and adequate food was available (B). At Derek's age, and minus evidence for problems with body image, anorexia nervosa and bulimia nervosa are not at issue (C).

Although Derek was kept clean, a diagnosis of child neglect was made on the basis of lack of adequate psychological stimulation. Depending on the outcome of medical investigations, in addition to underweight, we might have to code malnutrition. Derek should be watched for symptoms of autism spectrum disorder, which can be comorbid with ARFID; an older child may be at risk for anxiety disorders. His initial diagnosis would be as follows:

F50.8	Avoidant/restrictive food intake disorder
R6251	Failure to thrive (child)
Z69.010	Encounter for mental health services for victim of child neglect by parent
CGAS	65 (on admission)

ASSESSING EARLY CHILDHOOD FEEDING AND EATING DISORDERS

General Suggestions

Although direct observation of parents and child at mealtime may reveal much about early feeding or eating disorders, most of the concrete information about rumination disorder and ARFID will come from the parents. To elicit behaviors associated with pica, you can ask older children: "Do you like to taste things that other people don't eat? Do you ever eat dirt, chalk, soap, that sort of thing?" Of course, children may not be forthcoming about behaviors they perceive adults to frown on, so you might preface your questions with "Sometimes kids eat things that aren't food." On the other hand, pica may only come to light during the investigation of medical problems such as iron deficiency or malnutrition. Watch for other oral behaviors, such as nail biting and thumb sucking. Sometimes ARFID is finally recognized when, upon hospitalization and consistent feeding by sensitive nurses, an underweight child rapidly gains weight.

Developmental Factors

Each of these three disorders occurs early in life; rumination disorder and ARFID usually begin prior to a child's first birthday. Normal toddlers will put nearly anything into their mouths, so the diagnosis of pica should not be made unless the inappropriate eating lasts longer than 1 month in a child developmentally past the toddler stage.

ANOREXIA NERVOSA

F50.2 BULIMIA NERVOSA

Anorexia nervosa (AN), bulimia nervosa (BN), and now binge-eating disorder (BED; discussed separately below) typically arise in middle to late adolescence. They are especially prevalent in young women; males constitute under one-third of patients with either AN or BN. Although case reports of AN have appeared in the literature for at least 200 years, BN has only been recognized in the past few decades. However, the latter is now by far the more common of the two, affecting nearly 2% of adolescent girls in one survey. In the same survey, about 1% had AN. BED prevalence was about 2%.

Patients with AN and BN share a number of features. They have unusual eating habits and place strong emphasis on body weight and shape. They control weight by inappropriate means (purging, fasting, or inappropriate exercising). Either disorder can entail serious consequences for health. Although most cases of AN remit spontaneously or with treatment, about 5% of these patients will eventually succumb to complications of their disease. The prognosis for life is better for patients with BN, who may nonetheless suffer from malnutrition or electrolyte imbalances due to loss of body fluids. The two disorders often occur at different times in the same individual, as illustrated by the history of Camilla.

Camilla

"This thing has gotten beyond me. Even when my weight is normal, I'm still all lumpy."

For the past 4 years, Camilla had had problems with eating. They'd begun in high school during sophomore gym class, where she'd noticed that she seemed fatter than most of the other girls. Even years later, she believed that there had been some truth to this; she still remembered the horror of being teased about "love handles." Whatever the truth of the situation, when she was 15 she resolved never again to risk being called fat. She joined the Health Club, an organization of girls at her school who exchanged diet tips and supported one another for weight loss. Several years earlier, the club had been driven underground after several members were found passing around diet pills. Once the club was banned, parents and teachers had no control at all over what medications and other weight loss aids the girls used.

Camilla had been an extraordinarily successful dieter. From her highest-ever weight of 135 pounds (she stood 5 feet, 3 inches tall), through strict dieting and vigorous exercise she had lost nearly 40 pounds. Even then, she thought the love handles still showed, so she began using laxatives and diuretics supplied by one of her classmates. Although she managed to drop another 10 pounds, her mirror confirmed her worst fears: She still looked fat. By this time, she was eating only about 400 calories a day, and even some of that she would throw up—from the Health Club, she had learned the trick of vomiting at will.

ESSENTIAL FEATURES OF **ANOREXIA NERVOSA**

These patients, usually girls or young women, (1) eat so little that many look skeletal, yet (2) remain fearful of obesity or weight gain and (3) have the distorted self-perception that they are fat.

The Fine Print

Some patients may not admit to fear of overweight, but take steps anyway to avert weight gain.

The D's: • Duration. (Note that the diagnostic criteria don't actually specify duration. However, we are required to specify the subtype that applies to the previous 3 months, which suggests a minimum duration.) • Differential diagnosis (substance use and physical disorders; mood or anxiety disorders; obsessive–compulsive disorder; somatic symptom disorder; bulimia nervosa)

Coding Notes

Specify type that applies to the previous 3 months:

> **F50.02 Binge-eating/purging type.** The patient has repeatedly purged (vomited; misused laxatives, diuretics, or enemas) or eaten in binges.
> **F50.01 Restricting type.** The patient has not recently binged or purged.

Based on body mass index (BMI; kg/meter^2), specify severity (level may be increased, depending on functional impairment). For adults, levels are as follows:

> **Mild.** BMI of 17 or more.
> **Moderate.** BMI of 16–17.
> **Severe.** BMI of 15–16.
> **Extreme.** BMI under 15.

Specify if:

> **In partial remission.** "For a sustained period," the patient is no longer significantly underweight but still is overly concerned about weight or still has misconceptions about body weight/shape.
> **In full remission.** "For a sustained period," the patient has met no criteria for AN.

ESSENTIAL FEATURES OF **BULIMIA NERVOSA**

A patient has lost control over eating, consuming in binges much more food than is normal for a similar time frame. Fasting, vomiting, extreme physical workouts, or the abuse of laxatives or other drugs are used to control weight.

The Fine Print

The D's: • Duration (weekly for 3+ months) • Differential diagnosis (substance use and physical disorders; mood or anxiety disorders; obsessive–compulsive disorder; somatic symptom disorder; anorexia nervosa; traditional Thanksgiving or other ceremonial meal)

Coding Notes

Specify if:

In partial remission. For "a sustained period," the patient meets some, but not all BN criteria.

In full remission. For "a sustained period," no BN criteria have been met.

Based on the number per week of episodes of inappropriate compensatory behavior, specify severity (level may be increased, depending on functional impairment):

Mild. 1–3 episodes/week.
Moderate. 4–7.
Severe. 8–13.
Extreme. 14+.

As Camilla's weight dipped to 85 pounds, her parents finally became sufficiently alarmed to admit her to a hospital. Six months of treatment, education, and fear (while she was there, another patient about her age died of malnutrition) had their effect. She was discharged weighing a healthy 117 pounds, and her periods, absent for nearly a year, started again. To protect her from the adverse consequences of further association with other Health Club members, the family moved to the opposite side of the county. She eventually graduated from the high school there, but she never lost the feeling that something was terribly wrong with the shape of her body.

After high school, Camilla took a business course and went to work in the secretarial pool of an insurance company. As soon as she could afford it, she moved into a tiny studio apartment. Once she was free from the watchful eyes of her parents, her eating habits quickly deteriorated.

About 1 year prior to her present evaluation, she began consuming large quantities of food within a remarkably short period of time. At the movies, she might eat a "family-size" tub of popcorn and a giant cola drink; at home, she would consume a quart of frozen yogurt during a single episode of *Law and Order.* Because she was still morbidly fearful of becoming overweight, she usually regurgitated most of what she had eaten. In recent weeks, these binge episodes had occurred as often as two or three times a week; now they extended beyond snacktime into her regular meals. She told the interviewer, "When I eat alone, I've put away as much as a 1-pound package of spaghetti and two cans of sauce. I don't binge every day, but once I start, I can't seem to stop."

Evaluation of Camilla

When Camilla was 15, she developed the unreasonable and intense fear of being overweight (Criterion B for AN), despite the fact that she was losing so much weight that others worried about her health. At 135 pounds, she had probably been a little overweight for her height, but a drop of 50 pounds—over one-third of her previous weight—clearly far exceeded what was safe (A). When she then refused to regain weight, she had to be hospitalized. Despite pronounced emaciation, she continued to see herself as overweight (C), and her menses ceased for nearly a year. She therefore fulfilled the criteria for AN.

During the later phase of her illness, Camilla became bulimic. No one can doubt that she consumed far more food than normal for a given time period (Criterion A1 for BN), and she admitted feeling that she had lost control of her eating habits (A2). Occurring several times a week, these episodes had persisted throughout the previous year (C). She controlled her weight by vomiting (B); others might exercise excessively or abuse laxatives or other drugs. Although Camilla's view of her own body shape was still unrealistic and dominated her self-perception (D, "still all lumpy"), it no longer had the near-delusional quality that had characterized her anorectic phase. Therefore, at age 19 she had emerged from her episode of AN, and thus fulfilled the final criterion for BN (E).

Disordered appetite occurs in a number of other physical and mental disorders. Some rare **physical disorders** (such as pituitary tumors) are associated with voracious appetite and other abnormalities of eating. Other physical causes of weight loss include diabetes, malignancies, and intestinal malabsorption. Patients with **mood disorders** may eat either too much or too little, but they don't usually have the abnormal self-perception typical of AN. Patients with **schizophrenia** or **other psychoses** can have peculiar eating habits, but usually without fearing weight gain, and patients who have only eating disorders don't have hallucinations or delusions. Camilla's clinician would need to ask further about **anxiety** and **depressive disorders,** as well as about a **personality disorder**—comorbidity is the rule. **Abuse of stimulant medications** should also be suspected in patients who control their weight through misuse of those drugs.

In the coding of Camilla's AN, the subtype would be determined by the fact that she controlled her weight by purging (specifically, forced vomiting). At her lowest weight, Camilla's BMI was 15.1; this would earn her a rating of severe, bordering on extreme. Although we have documented a frequency of bulimic episodes at only 2–3 times a week, they appeared to be increasing, so we'd claim clinicians' privilege and score her BN as moderate. Camilla's full diagnosis at age 15 would thus be the following:

F50.02	Anorexia nervosa, binge-eating/purging type, severe
R634	Abnormal loss of weight
CGAS	41

And at age 19, it would have changed to this:

F50.2	Bulimia nervosa, moderate
GAF	60 (current)

F50.8 BINGE–EATING DISORDER

Binge-eating disorder (BED) has two principal features: A person consumes food at a rate far in excess of what's normal, and, in so doing, experiences a sense of loss of control over the eating behavior. What distinguishes it from BN is that patients with BED do not pursue any of the various attempts at weight control typical of BN—vomiting, laxatives/other medications, dieting, and exercise.

BED behaviors typically begin during adolescence, and occur especially in people who are overweight and sedentary. An episode may commence in response to a sad or gloomy mood. Then, before satiety can set in, the person rapidly consumes vast quantities of food that are typically high in fat, salt, and sugar. The results: the misery of an overstuffed stomach, and a conscience burdened with so much guilt and shame that subsequent binges are likely to be conducted secretly.

Patients don't report craving specific foods; rather, it's the quantity that is key. And what they eat may change with time. Unlike patients with AN and BN, patients with BED don't usually move in and out of other eating disorders. And for BED, dieting typically begins after the bingeing and weight gain, rather than before, as is the case with the other two eating disorders. Weight gain is often a precipitant for investigation of BED; because health care providers may lack familiarity with this disorder, it sometimes takes several visits to make the diagnosis.

BED affects under 2% of adults and perhaps half that many adolescents. Girls predominate by at least a 2:1 ratio, and patients with Type II diabetes may be especially at risk. Not surprisingly, many of these patients are overweight or obese (conversely, about 25% of overweight people have BED). It should come as no surprise that these patients tend to have medical complications as a result of being overweight. There may be a familial component,

ESSENTIAL FEATURES OF **BINGE-EATING DISORDER**

A patient has lost control of eating, consuming in binges much more food than is normal in a similar time frame. During a binge, the patient will eat too fast and too much (until painfully full), yet without actual hunger. The bingeing causes guilt (sometimes depression) and solitary dining (to avoid embarrassment), but it does *not* result in behaviors (such as vomiting and excessive exercise) designed to make up for overeating.

The Fine Print

The D's: • Duration (weekly for 3+ months) • Distress over eating behavior • Differential diagnosis (mood disorders, bulimia or anorexia nervosa, ordinary overweight)

Coding Notes

Specify if:

> **In partial remission.** For "a sustained period," the patient has eaten in binges less often than once a week.
> **In full remission.** "For a sustained period," the patient has met no criteria for BED.

Specify severity (level may be increased, depending on functional impairment):

> **Mild.** 1–3 binges/week.
> **Moderate.** 4–7.
> **Severe.** 8–13.
> **Extreme.** 14+.

but the overall research thus far into risk factors for BED lags far behind that for AN and BN.

Hilty

"Once I get started, I just keep on eating. I don't even think about it—it just slides right down."

For a research project, a lay research interviewer was talking to 15-year-old Hilty about her experience with adolescent eating disorders. "I do it pretty much every time I work at the cart," Hilty explained, "and that's after school Mondays, Wednesdays, and Fridays. It's been going on for the whole school year."

Hilty's family owned and operated a food cart (Dottie's Dumplings), which enjoyed a prime location in the downtown area. Dottie (Dorothy, her mom) made and sold savory and sweet dumplings and other baked goods. She used recipes her grandmother had given her years ago, when Dottie was a girl. "My whole family's foodies," Hilty said with a touch of pride. "And, sad to say, they're all plus-sized. Like me."

Asked when her overeating began, Hilty replied, "Maybe it started when I was working on the cart. I had to be always ready to serve someone who'd walk up, wanting something right now. I'd just stuff down my food—in a few seconds, sometimes."

Most of Hilty's binges were ("Of course!") on dumplings, which she ate right out of the pan, before they'd even cooled. But if those weren't available, she might consume half a pie—savory or fruit, it didn't seem to matter much. "At the time, I can't even say that I'm hungry—I just eat!"

If Hilty wasn't at work when the urge to overeat struck, she might consume a frozen dinner for two "and lick the pan, or I might just clean out the fridge. Afterwards, I'm sometimes so stuffed I feel I need to be burped!" In response to a question, she stated, "No, I never york it up—that'd be too gross for words." She similarly denied using laxatives or pills to try to limit her intake.

When her weight passed 160 pounds, her mother had made an appointment with their family physician. "The doctor had a wrapped sandwich on his desk. I just couldn't talk to him about a problem with eating. I felt so ashamed." Later, she tried going to Overeaters Anonymous. "When I told them what I was doing, everyone looked at me like I was some kind of freak."

Hilty paused to choke back tears. "I feel as though it's someone else who's doing it—it's almost as though I'm not even involved. I've tried having just one, but that's a no-go. I finally just gave up. I feel I'm a total loser. And a gainer at the same time."

Evaluation of Hilty

Several times a week for at least the past half year (Criterion D), Hilty had eaten far more than would be normal for a given meal (A1), to the point that she felt overfull (B2) and ashamed (B5). She'd tried to limit herself (A2; both A criteria are required for diagnosis). Her bingeing was done rapidly (B1) and, to the extent possible, in secret so as to hide her embarrassing behavior (B4); only three of five B criteria are required. When she was telling her story, her distress was palpable (C), but she stoutly denied using any behaviors (such as vomiting or using drugs—Criterion E) to try to keep her weight in check.

Could any other disorder account for her symptoms? People with **atypical depressions** can have increased appetite, but Hilty hadn't expressed feelings of depression, though she was obviously upset about her behavior; furthermore, she didn't experience her eating as hunger, but only felt the desire to eat. She lacked the inappropriate body image that accompanies **anorexia nervosa** (and she certainly wasn't too thin), and she did not engage in compensatory purging or other forms of calorie reduction, as would be the case with **bulimia nervosa**.

The mere counting of episodes seems somehow inadequate to capture the severity of Hilty's binge episodes. If we stuck strictly to this criterion, we would score Hilty's BED as mild because it occurred only three times a week. Using clinicians' prerogative, though, we feel she should be rated a little further along on the severity spectrum. This would make her diagnosis read:

F50.8	Binge-eating disorder, moderate
E66.9	Obesity
CGAS	85

F50.8 OTHER SPECIFIED FEEDING OR EATING DISORDER

F50.9 UNSPECIFIED FEEDING OR EATING DISORDER

Other specified, or unspecified, feeding or eating disorder should be reserved for patients who have problems related to appetite, eating, and weight, but who do not meet the criteria for any of the specific diagnoses included in this chapter. Many such problems (for example, anorexia in which weight is low but remains within the normal range, bulimia with infrequent binges, bulimia without swallowing food) will meet some, but not all, of the criteria for one of these diagnoses; in such a case, you'd use the other specified category. DSM-5 also mentions purging disorder and night eating syndrome within this category; various other syndromes are possible.

ASSESSING EATING DISORDERS

General Suggestions

A patient with AN, whether adult or adolescent, is in denial and may refuse to discuss eating behaviors frankly. You may have better success with questions about mood (which is likely to be depressed), though these patients are often vague about their own feelings. They probably won't perceive themselves as thin—a judgment you should avoid contradicting. They may express disgust at their own physical appearance or reluctance to eat. You can screen for AN by asking, "Have you ever lost so much weight that people said you were too thin?" For suspected BN, ask, "Have you ever eaten so much at one time that it made you sick?"

If possible, observe for suspicious behavior at mealtime: pushing food around on the plate, taking excessively small portions, and using the bathroom immediately after meals. In addition, be alert for vigorous activity in the face of marked weakness and wasting. You will probably encounter denial of behaviors a patient knows are frowned upon, such as self-induced vomiting and purging. Ask about dieting, about frequent weighing, about making and following rules for when and where to eat, and about maintaining lists of forbidden foods. Patients with suspected BN may express a release of tension after vomiting or purging; they and patients with possible BED should also be asked about feelings of loss of control (similar to those experienced in other addictions) over their eating binges. Of course, any child who is overweight should be queried about eating behavior.

Developmental Factors

In patients under the age of 14 with AN, severe weight loss can halt puberty. Indeed, failure to grow to full height may also result. Prepubertal patients are at higher risk for osteopenia as well.

Elimination Disorders

INTRODUCTION

Although encopresis and enuresis usually occur separately, they may occur together, especially in children who have been severely neglected and emotionally deprived. Both bowel and bladder training practices vary with social context and with a family's cultural background, so either disorder must be diagnosed with sensitivity to these practices and the patient's age. DSM-5, using common standards of practice in the United States, has determined that soiling after the age of 4 years or wetting after the age of 5 years qualifies for the respective diagnosis. Criteria of frequency and of social and functional impairment are also mandated, to avoid overdiagnosing the accidents that may occasionally befall any young child.

More often than not, these syndromes first present in the pediatric or primary care setting, where gastrointestinal and genitourinary tract abnormalities (though rare) are often targets of early investigation. The clinical, diagnostic, and economic value of these expensive and intrusive examinations is questionable, especially in view of the fact that a careful medical history is often sufficient to make an accurate diagnosis.

In both encopresis and enuresis, it is important to establish whether the disorder is primary or secondary. A *primary* disorder is one in which symptoms have been present throughout the developmental period (toilet training was never fully successful). In *secondary* disorders, symptoms occur after at least 6 months of successful toilet training. Because these disorders present in primary care settings and because clinicians may use widely varying criteria, it has been difficult to estimate accurately the prevalence of either condition.

F98.1 ENCOPRESIS

Encopresis is usually associated with constipation. Chronic constipation, perhaps related to dietary factors such as intolerance to dairy products, often leads to fissures around the anus that cause pain on defecation. To avoid this pain, children withhold stool. Refusal to eat, weight loss, and dehydration all aggravate the constipation, which in turn hardens the stool and worsens the fissures. Leakage of unformed feces around the impaction in the rectum results in soiling of clothes and bed sheets, necessitating frequent changes of clothes and bedding.

Secrecy and denial are cardinal features of encopresis that is *not* accompanied by constipation. Children hide their formed, soft, normal-sized stools in unusual locations—in bureau drawers, in trash cans, under the bed. When questioned about this behavior, they often claim ignorance of how the stools got there. This form of the disorder is less common than encopresis associated with constipation, and it is often linked with stress and other family psychopathology. Disorganization (a lack of behavioral consistency and structure) characterizes many such households. Some of these children may have been subjected to physical or sexual abuse, though studies with adequate comparison groups are lacking.

With boys predominating, encopresis affects about 1% of elementary-school-age children. Soiling and chronic constipation account for 20% of complaints in pediatric gastroenterology clinics and for 10% of visits to child mental health clinics. Children who present with encopresis should have a thorough cognitive evaluation to rule out the presence of developmental delay.

Kent

"He was murder to toilet-train," said Kent's mother. "I'd sure hate to go through all that again!"

Kent had Down syndrome and a Full Scale IQ (WISC-V) of 68. He had been nearly 4 when he finally stopped wearing diapers. Now, at almost 6, he had started first grade in a special education class. Kent's father, a chief petty officer on a frigate in the Navy, had just deployed for a 6-month cruise in the Mediterranean—his second in the last 4 years. There had been quite a row the evening before he sailed, and Kent had cried himself to sleep. For several nights thereafter, his mother had cried herself to sleep in Kent's bed.

A week or two later, Kent had come home with dirty underpants. He had been spanked and sent to bed with only cereal for supper, but a week later, his mother found feces in one of his father's shoes. "It was at the back of our closet. I'd never have looked there but for the smell," she explained. Over the next several months, this had happened half a dozen times. Each time the feces appeared in a new location—on the front doorstep, in the sandbox of the little girl next door, behind the guest bathroom toilet. Each time, Kent denied knowing how it had happened.

The pediatrician at the naval base hospital took a complete dietary and medical history and performed a rectal examination, but could find nothing physically wrong. Kent's mother denied even keeping laxatives in the house. "I don't know when we'd ever need them—he sure hasn't ever been constipated."

Evaluation of Kent

Kent met the duration and frequency requirements (Criterion B, at least once a month for 3 months) for encopresis; the hiding places were manifestly inappropriate (A). Although he had intellectual disability, his developmental stage was at least the equivalent of a 4-year-old's (C). The history reveals no evidence of any **general medical condition** or a **substance**

ESSENTIAL FEATURES OF **ENCOPRESIS**

The patient repeatedly defecates into clothing or in other inappropriate places.

The Fine Print

The D's: • Duration and demographics (1+ times/month for 3+ months in someone 4 years or older) • Differential diagnosis (laxative use and physical disorders)

Coding Notes

Specify type:

With constipation and overflow incontinence
Without constipation and overflow incontinence

use disorder, including laxative use, that could account for his behavior (D). Although encopresis without constipation and overflow incontinence is the less common type of this disorder, Kent's symptoms fully justify that specifier. There was no evidence for an associated **oppositional defiant disorder** or **conduct disorder** (more commonly reported when a child is intentionally encopretic) or for **enuresis**. Kent's diagnosis would thus be the following:

F98.1	Encopresis without constipation and overflow incontinence
F70	Mild intellectual disability
Q90.9	Down syndrome
Z62.898	Child affected by parental relationship distress (father absent on military duty)
CGAS	55 (current)

F98.0 ENURESIS

Primary enuresis (that is, a child has never been dry) is at least twice as common as the secondary form of this disorder. It is usually limited to nighttime wetting; daytime bladder control is unaffected. By the time such a child is referred to a mental health professional, the common remedies of fluid restriction before bedtime and awakening the child around midnight to use the toilet have usually failed; medical conditions have been ruled out; and bladder function studies have been negative. The child usually wets three to five times weekly and is too embarrassed to risk sleeping over with friends.

In some children, episodes of enuresis may be associated with Stage IV non-rapid eye movement sleep, which occurs especially during the first 3 hours after sleep onset. In other children, episodes occur more than once per night or randomly throughout the period of sleep. Although a child with primary enuresis may explain the episodes by recounting dreams of urinating, awakenings immediately after episodes of bedwetting do not confirm the presence of dream reports. When dreams are elicited, they are not of nightmare quality.

Secondary enuresis, which develops after a child has become dry, most often occurs randomly throughout the night and often appears following a traumatic event such as a hospitalization or separation from parents. Secondary enuresis is also more likely than primary enuresis to be associated with nightmares and with other comorbid disorders, such as ADHD.

Although some children with enuresis have urinary tract infections or anatomical anomalies, the etiology remains unknown in the vast majority of cases. Most authorities cite genetic factors and maturational delay. Approximately 75% of children with enuresis have a first-degree relative with a history of enuresis. When both parents have a positive

ESSENTIAL FEATURES OF **ENURESIS**

Without known cause, a patient repeatedly urinates into clothing or bedding.

The Fine Print

The D's: • Duration and demographics (2+ times/week for 3+ months in someone 5 years or older) • Distress (or frequency as above) • Differential diagnosis (medication side effects and physical disorders)

Coding Notes

Specify the type:

> **Nocturnal only**
> **Diurnal only**
> **Nocturnal and diurnal**

history, three-quarters of their children have enuresis as well. Again, it is strongly associated with ADHD.

At all ages, enuresis is more prevalent in boys than in girls. Although the overall prevalence diminishes with increasing maturation, by age 10 the male–female disparity is about 2:1—despite the fact that urinary tract infections are more common in girls. Overall, nocturnal only is the more common subtype of enuresis, though girls more often have the diurnal-only subtype. Of all 8-year-old children, 7–10% are reported to have enuresis; by early adolescence, the prevalence falls to only about 2–3%. Even a small number of adolescents in their late teens will still wet the bed.

Henry

At age 8, Henry was referred by his pediatrician because of persistent bedwetting, which occurred four or five times a week. Toilet training had been effortless, and he was dry during the day by the time he was 3 years old. His parents, unaware of any psychological problems in the family or in Henry's life, were dismayed at the mental health referral. But they were also concerned that Henry refused invitations to sleepovers with friends; he was equally reluctant to have his friends spend the night with him.

Henry's developmental history and mental status examination were unremarkable. He was an accomplished bicycle rider and enthusiastic participant in Little League baseball. He liked his second-grade classroom teacher and enjoyed playing with his neighborhood friends. In fact, Henry was a happy, well-adjusted boy whose parents were proud of his achievements. His father and his paternal uncle had had enuresis during their school-age years, but both had completely outgrown the problem by age 10.

After a physical exam and urinalysis found no abnormality that could explain his problem, Henry's parents were instructed to keep a sleep diary for 2 weeks. They noted Henry's bedtime, his sleep onset time, and the time of each enuretic episode. The diary revealed that Henry had wet the bed on 9 of the 14 nights of the 2-week period. On seven occasions, the episode occurred within the first 2 hours after sleep onset; twice, Henry wet later at night.

Along with a recommendation for arousing him to use the toilet several hours after he went to sleep, Henry's parents were given a prescription for a bell-and-pad urine alarm. Within 6 weeks, the frequency of Henry's episodes had fallen by 90%. At 6-month follow-up, he was no longer using the alarm and was consistently dry.

Evaluation of Henry

Henry had manifest enuresis (Criterion A). The only significant disorder to be considered in a differential diagnosis for enuresis is **another medical condition** that can explain the symptoms. In that sense, Henry was found to be completely normal (Criterion D: no anomalies of the genitourinary tract, no evidence of diabetes mellitus or diabetes insipidus, no urinary tract infections). He fulfilled diagnostic criteria for age of onset (C), frequency, and duration (B, though some authorities believe that the frequency threshhold of twice a week is too strict).

Because his enuresis occurred only during sleep, the specifier *nocturnal only* was appended. Although children with enuresis may have other mental conditions such as encopresis, delayed development, and sleep disorders, Henry's history gave no reason to suspect an additional diagnosis. His full diagnosis would be this:

Should enuresis even be considered a mental disorder? Although the criteria allow for intentional occurrence, the prevalence of such occurrence must be vanishingly rare. The symptoms are physical, and the pathology is almost exclusively physiological; its treatment is primarily provided by pediatricians, not mental health professionals. Of course, enuresis can have many emotional sequelae—but then the same can be said of obesity, which no authority (certainly not DSM-5) considers to be primarily a mental disorder.

F98.0	Enuresis, nocturnal only
CGAS	81 (current)

OTHER SPECIFIED ELIMINATION DISORDER

Use the other specified elimination disorder category for symptoms of encopresis or enuresis that do not meet the full diagnostic criteria, in cases where you wish to state the reason. Use the following diagnostic codes:

N39.498   With urinary symptoms

R15.9   With fecal symptoms

UNSPECIFIED ELIMINATION DISORDER

Use the unspecified elimination disorder category for symptoms of encopresis or enuresis that do not meet the full diagnostic criteria, in cases where you do not wish to state the reason. Use the following diagnostic codes:

R32   With urinary symptoms

R15.9   With fecal symptoms

ASSESSING ELIMINATION DISORDERS

General Suggestions

Talking about their symptoms may be embarrassing for some children, but you will usually already have the relevant history for a diagnosis of either encopresis or enuresis. Focusing on the involuntary nature of the problem and the hope for improvement will often foster a positive therapeutic alliance. To help build rapport, use the child's own terms (as determined from your interview with the parents) for feces and urine. Ask whether the child has either the sensation of needing to void or of pain with defecation. Can you learn how the child perceives the parents' response—is it warmly supportive, or punitive and cold, or somewhere in between? Try to learn about toilet training for a child with either enuresis or encopresis: What techniques were used, for how long, and with what results?

Colon and rectal segments that lack nerve cells (*aganglionic* segments) represent congenital megacolon (Hirschsprung's disease). During the first year of life, children with Hirschsprung's disease develop symptoms that include abdominal distention, pain, malnutrition, and encopresis with constipation and overflow incontinence. A barium enema and intestinal biopsy are required for evaluation.

Developmental Factors

As with so many other behaviors, just a few years of maturation can separate the pathological from what is developmentally appropriate. By any set of criteria one chooses, the prevalence of enuresis is relatively high (7–33% for boys) at age 5, but it falls off by a factor of two to four by age 10. Encopresis, however, is relatively uncommon (about 1%) throughout childhood, with little reduction until the teenage years.

CHAPTER 21

Sleep–Wake Disorders

QUICK GUIDE TO THE SLEEP–WAKE DISORDERS

Specific sleep–wake disorders are much rarer in children and adolescents than in adults. Here we've focused on those that are most common. This chapter describes three parasomnias, one dyssomnia, and (briefly) one other sleep–wake disorder, in that order. (In many other mental and physical illnesses, sleep problems occur as secondary symptoms rather than as independent disorders.)

And here are the definitions: In a *parasomnia*, the timing, duration, and quality of sleep are essentially normal, but unusual behaviors occur during sleep or when the person is falling asleep or waking up. Three of the parasomnias included in DSM-5 are described in this chapter. Someone with a *dyssomnia* sleeps too little, too much, or at the wrong time of day, though the sleep itself (its architecture, as the sleep experts say) is pretty normal.

Nightmare disorder. Table 21.1 contrasts symptoms of this common and easily identified condition with those of sleep terrors; features are briefly discussed on page 368. For a case example and discussion, see *DSM-5 Made Easy* by James Morrison.

Non-rapid eye movement (non-REM) sleep arousal disorder, sleep terror type. These young people cry out in apparent fear during the first part of the night. Often they don't really wake up at all (p. 369).

Non-REM sleep arousal disorder, sleepwalking type. Persistent sleepwalking usually occurs early in the night (p. 371).

Obstructive sleep apnea hypopnea. Although most patients with breathing problems such as sleep apnea complain of daytime sleepiness, some instead have insomnia (p. 373).

Substance/medication-induced sleep disorder. Most psychoactive substances commonly misused, as well as various prescription medications, can interfere with sleep (p. 376).

DISTINGUISHING AMONG SLEEP–WAKE DISORDERS

DSM-5 describes several disorders that can be categorized as dyssomnias (see the definition above). They include insomnia and hypersomnolence disorders, narcolepsy (in which brief but refreshing sleep intrudes into wakefulness, causing patients to fall asleep abruptly), and circadian rhythm sleep–wake disorders (in which there is a mismatch between a patient's sleep–wake pattern and environmental demands). However, only one dyssomnia, a breathing-related condition called obstructive sleep apnea hypopnea, is found with any frequency in children and adolescents.

Although up to one-quarter of all children experience some sort of problem with sleep, many of these fall under headings that comprise issues not described in DSM-5: (1) behavioral issues that spring from a child's reluctance to go to bed ("limit-setting type," according to the *International Classification of Sleep Disorders* [ICSD] of the American Academy of Sleep Medicine); and (2) activities that distract from sleep, such as eating, watching television, or being rocked ("sleep-onset association type").

Two sleep disorders commonly found in juveniles (especially young children) are sleep terrors and sleepwalking, both of which DSM-5 classifies as arousal parasomnias (and lumbers with much longer names). They are manifestations of central nervous system arousal that usually occur in the first 1–3 hours after sleep onset. Arousal episodes have many features in common: automatic behavior; relative nonreactivity to external stimuli; absent or fragmentary dream recall; mental confusion and disorientation when awakened; and amnesia for the episode the next morning. Arousal parasomnias tend to run in families; children with one type of arousal parasomnia are likely also to have symptoms of another. They are distinguishable by parental report and their typical symptoms, so do not require polysomnography for diagnosis.

Arousal parasomnias, which occur during non-rapid eye movement (non-REM) sleep, must be distinguished from the much more common rapid eye movement (REM) parasomnia, or nightmare disorder. (REM sleep occurs especially during the last part of the night, when most of the dreams we remember occur.) Nightmares are anxiety-laden dreams from which individuals awaken with often detailed recall. Various stressors, especially traumatic experiences, increase the frequency and severity of nightmares. They usually start between the ages of 3 and 6, and they affect a strong minority of children severely enough to worry their parents. Table 21.1 presents a nutshell comparison of sleep terrors and nightmare disorder. However, because nightmares are well known to clinicians (and most parents, for that matter), we do not discuss nightmare disorder further or present a vignette for it.

NON–RAPID EYE MOVEMENT SLEEP AROUSAL DISORDERS

Because they have so much in common, DSM-5 has dragged two sleep disorders, sleepwalking and sleep terror disorders, under the same umbrella and given the umbrella a new name.

TABLE 21.1. Comparison of Sleep Terrors and Nightmares

	Sleep terrors	Nightmares
Occurrence in sleep period	First few hours (non-REM sleep)	Last third (REM sleep)
Arousability	Difficult	Easy
Dream imagery	No	Yes
Episode recalled in morning	No	Yes

However, they are still defined more or less as they have been for years. The new name underscores the fact that they usually occur during the first third of the night—that is, during non-REM sleep.

F51.4 Sleep Terror Type

Approximately 60–90 minutes after falling asleep, a child (the usual age range is 3–10 years) with the sleep terror type of non-REM sleep arousal disorder suddenly sits up, screams, and stares with glassy, unseeing eyes. Signs of autonomic discharge—palpitations, sweating, and irregular respiration—are obvious. The patient is inconsolable and difficult to arouse, but if awakened, is disoriented and confused. Otherwise, after 30 seconds to 5 minutes, the child calms down and drifts back into normal sleep, and in the morning has no recollection of the event.

The condition is common, affecting up to 6% of children (boys and girls equally). It begins early in childhood, There is often a positive family history of sleep terror.

Paul

Paul was a 3-year-old only child brought for evaluation by his parents, who were distraught by the attacks of screaming and agitation that had interrupted his sleep for the past 6 months. Most days, Paul's babysitter cared for him in his own home, but 2 days a week he attended a well-staffed preschool with 30 other toddlers.

His mother described their nightly bedtime routine as follows. After getting ready for bed, she would read him stories for 5–10 minutes. Then Paul would kiss her goodnight, clutch his teddy bear, and fall asleep easily at about 9:00. Two or three times a week, between 11:30 and midnight, Paul would sit bolt upright in bed and begin screaming. His eyes would be open, but he would appear not to see anything. Perspiring, breathing rapidly with pounding heart, he would seem to be in terrible distress. His parents would try unsuccessfully to awaken and console him, but Paul would not speak coherently or respond to questions. After 3–5 minutes, the episode would end spontaneously, and he would quickly slip back into normal sleep. Occasionally, a second attack would occur 60–90 minutes later.

ESSENTIAL FEATURES OF
NON-RAPID EYE MOVEMENT SLEEP AROUSAL DISORDER

The patient repeatedly awakens incompletely from sleep with sleepwalking or sleep terror (see Coding Notes). The attempts of others to communicate or console don't help much. The patient has little if any dream imagery at the time, and tends not to remember the episode the next morning.

The Fine Print

The D's: • Distress or disability (social, educational, occupational, or personal impairment) • Differential diagnosis (substance use and physical disorders; anxiety and dissociative disorders; other sleep disorders)

Coding Notes

Specify type:

F51.3 Sleepwalking type. Without awakening, the patient rises from bed and walks. The patient stares blankly, can be awakened only with difficulty, and responds poorly to others' attempts at communication. Specify if:
With sleep-related eating
With sleep-related sexual behavior (sexsomnia)
F51.4 Sleep terror type. Beginning with a scream of panic, the patient abruptly arouses from sleep and shows intense fear and signs of autonomic arousal, such as dilated pupils, rapid breathing, rapid heartbeat, and sweating.

In the morning, Paul would awaken refreshed and happy, with no recollection of the previous night's event.

Paul was a planned baby whose intrauterine and postnatal development had been normal. He had reached all of his motor, sensory, and social milestones on time. During the day, he was a curious, energetic, bright, happy 3-year-old who brought his parents much pleasure. However, his parents had noted that his episodes seemed more likely to occur after a day in the child care center, and they feared that he was being overwhelmed by his day care experience. The center's staff assured them that Paul was flourishing, though during his days there he usually missed his nap. Those were often the nights when he experienced attacks. Paul's mother also worried that her working away from the home during the day might be responsible. Paul's paternal uncle had had occasional bouts of sleepwalking as a child.

While his mother related the history, Paul explored with curiosity the toys available in the examination room. His attention seemed focused, and he checked in with his mother whenever he moved to a new activity. He formed an appropriate relationship with the examiner, and soon they were comfortably playing together while the examiner continued to question the mother. After requesting Paul's permission, the examiner asked the mother to step out of the room for a few minutes. Paul tolerated the separation without distress; upon her return, he greeted her warmly.

Evaluation of Paul

Paul's arousal 2–3 hours after sleep onset, his agitation, his autonomic arousal (pounding heart and sweating), and his unresponsiveness to his parents' attempts to awaken and console him were all reactions typical of the sleep terror type of non-REM sleep arousal disorder (Criterion A2). Although he was obviously distressed at the time of each episode (D), he expressed no dream imagery (B) and the following day had amnesia for the episode (C). No substance use could explain his symptoms (E). Paul showed no evidence suggesting either **panic disorder** or **psychomotor epilepsy**, either of which can produce fear, even in the middle of the night (F).

Paul played hard at his day care center, and without his usual nap, it was likely that he was more exhausted on those nights (arousal parasomnias are more likely to occur after periods of excessive fatigue). Nightmares are associated with stressful daytime experiences, but episodes of **nightmare disorder** generally occur later, after 4–5 hours of sleep, when REM sleep predominates. Then the patient is wide awake, well oriented, and usually able to relate a vivid and coherent narrative. Paul's diagnosis is unsurprising:

| F51.4 | Non-rapid eye movement sleep arousal disorder, sleep terror type |
| CGAS | 85 (current) |

F51.3 Sleepwalking Type

Sleepwalking usually occurs during the first third of the night, perhaps following excessive fatigue or unusual stresses during the day before. The individual first sits up and makes some sort of random movement (such as picking at the bedclothes). Apparently purposeful behavior (dressing or using the toilet) may follow, but these behaviors are usually poorly coordinated and incomplete. The person's face lacks expression; speech, if it occurs at all, is typically garbled. If the person awakens at all, it is usually to a brief period of disorientation. An episode can last from a few seconds to 30 minutes, and will usually not be remembered later.

This condition affects about 20% of all children (boys outnumber girls), who usually outgrow it by age 15. It is not usually considered pathological in children, though it can be in adults.

George

The examination of 16-year-old George was prompted by his father's concern. At 2:00 one morning earlier that month, George had been discovered sound asleep in his girlfriend's bedroom. Though he had apparently walked more than a mile through suburban streets and used a ladder taken from her garage to climb through the bedroom window, he claimed not to know how he had gotten there. It was unclear whether such episodes had occurred previously. George hadn't had sleep terror attacks when younger; nor was the family history positive for arousal parasomnias.

Contrary to the myth that persons who walk in their sleep never harm themselves, sleepwalking is dangerous. Body movements are clumsy and purposeless, and judgment is abated. Because a person may be injured by falls or by bumping into objects or by venturing outdoors into the cold (or street), once sleepwalking is identified, it is important to make the environment as safe as possible. Locked windows and doors, and alarms that are triggered when the sleepwalker rises from bed may also help prevent injury.

George had had occasional struggles with his parents, who didn't care for some of his recent friends. Until the past year or two he had been a good student, but lately he had put little effort into his studies and had had a number of unexplained absences from school. He admitted to the use of marijuana, which he claimed helped him with his "insight." During the interview, he seemed neither depressed nor anxious.

Evaluation of George

Because individuals are poorly coordinated and disoriented during episodes of sleepwalking, it is highly unlikely that the sleepwalking type of non-REM sleep arousal disorder could explain George's well-organized, goal-directed behavior. Furthermore, to be diagnosable, sleepwalking must also occur repeatedly, not just once (Criterion A1).

Sometimes sleepwalking attacks resemble sleep **seizures,** and an EEG is required to differentiate the two. **Dissociative disorders** may also resemble sleepwalking attacks, but they usually last longer, and the episodes continue into the waking state. George's age of onset was wrong for the **sleep terror type of non-REM sleep arousal disorder**, with which sleepwalking can be associated; the vignette also specifically mentions that he had no previous history of sleep terrors. Although marijuana does not typically cause sleepwalking, further evaluation would be needed to rule out **substance/medication-induced sleep disorder**, which alternatively might be caused by such drugs as psychotropic medications.

The vignette does not permit a definitive DSM-5 diagnosis. Because several possibilities remained to be explored, and because changes in his behavior over the past couple of years suggest that there might be a personality disorder, George's diagnosis would have to be deferred. (With our current information, we cannot be sure that he has a sleep disorder, so even an unspecified diagnosis isn't possible.) The deferred diagnosis would have to be recorded in the case notes, since DSM-5 no longer provides a code for this. We'd give George a current GAF score of 65.

G47.33 OBSTRUCTIVE SLEEP APNEA HYPOPNEA

The principal breathing-related disorder that afflicts children and adolescents is sleep apnea, a condition in which breathing is noisy or discontinuous for periods throughout the night. The cause is usually obstruction of the airway due to mechanical features of the mouth, nose, or throat; hence the complete formal name, obstructive sleep apnea hypopnea (OSAH). The mildest, most obvious symptom of this disorder is snoring, which by itself is a common enough occurrence in childhood and adolescence (10–12% of school-age children snore). But 2–3% of middle school children and perhaps 10% of young children actually stop breathing for brief periods, creating a potential for physical, behavioral, and even cognitive symptoms of varying severity. An even greater risk of OSAH may exist for certain vulnerable patients—black or Hispanic children, and those who are poor or were born prematurely.

Complete apnea for 10 seconds or longer presents a struggle to breathe that is obvious to an observer. The child becomes restless, may sweat, and awakens frequently during the night. Although most children do not suffer from daytime symptoms (common in adults with OSAH), some children may complain of morning sleepiness and headache. Some become hyperactive and oppositional; more severely affected children may experience learning difficulties. At worst, physical consequences can include pulmonary hypertension, developmental delay, short stature, and even death.

OSAH may be especially common in children who have allergies or multiple ear or throat infections. Other risk factors include obesity (which appears to become an important factor only at puberty), abnormalities of the face or cranium, and oral pathology such as large tonsils or tongue. (Indeed, tonsillectomy relieves the symptoms in about 75%.) Clinical history and physical exam alone may not discriminate OSAH from simple snoring. A definitive diagnosis requires an overnight stay in a sleep lab for polysomnography.

OSAH is relatively common even in young children, and its incidence increases in adults. Sex distribution is about equal between boys and girls.

Johann

When Johann was 28 months old, his mother requested an evaluation because he was so small. Although both his height and weight were below the 3rd percentile for his age, a comprehensive endocrine, neurological, metabolic, and gastrointestinal workup had revealed no physical cause for his size. Despite a history of repeated ear infections and upper respiratory

ESSENTIAL FEATURES OF **OBSTRUCTIVE SLEEP APNEA HYPOPNEA**

A patient complains of daytime sleepiness that results from nighttime breathing problems: (often long) pauses in breathing, followed by loud snores or snorts. Polysomnography reveals obstructive apneas and hypopneas.

The Fine Print

At least 5 episodes per hour of sleep are required for diagnosis. If the history doesn't reveal nocturnal breathing symptoms or daytime sleepiness, there must be 15 apnea–hypopnea episodes per hour, as documented by polysomnography.

The D's: None.

Coding Notes

Code severity, based on number of apnea–hypopnea episodes per hour:

Mild. Fewer than 15.
Moderate. 15–30.
Severe. 30+.

illnesses, hearing tests and a chest X-ray were normal. Suspecting stress-related, nonorganic failure to thrive, the pediatrician referred Johann and his mother to the mental health clinic. There the clinician learned the following:

Johann's mother had been 22 and single, and had had few social supports, but she had taken good care of herself throughout an uneventful pregnancy. Johann had weighed 7 pounds, 6 ounces at birth, with Apgar scores of 8 and 10. He and his mother had left the hospital on the second day following his birth. At his first-year checkup, he weighed 19½ pounds; his development seemed on track. Then, because his mother had begun working in a distant city and they'd moved away, the clinic had lost track of Johann until the present.

Johann's mother seemed to be a reliable informant. Parent–child relations appeared warm and appropriately sensitive. Aside from his small stature, Johann seemed perfectly normal; his mental status examination and play interactions with the evaluator were unremarkable. However, a history of snoring spurred a more detailed sleep–wake history. It revealed that he went to bed easily at 8:00 each evening and slept until awakened at 6:30. He didn't appear excessively sleepy during the day, but his mother thought that Johann sometimes lacked energy by the end of the day. At the day care center, he did not nap.

Johann and his mother slept in the same room, so she knew that mouth breathing and expiratory snoring had been present over the past year. At the clinician's request, she made an audio recording of Johann's breathing. On it, mouth breathing, snoring, and repeated, brief sleep apnea episodes were clearly audible. All-night polysomnography revealed an average of 20 episodes per hour of sleep apnea. During the longest of these, Johann's oxygen saturation level dropped as low as 68%.

A careful examination revealed enlarged adenoids, which had not been visible during the earlier examination. Within 2 weeks of a tonsillectomy and adenoidectomy, Johann's apnea–hypopnea ratio and oxygen desaturation improved; his mother reported that his breathing while asleep seemed less labored. Six months after the surgery, his weight and height had increased to the 35th percentile. A year later, Johann's growth and development had returned to normal.

Evaluation of Johann

Johann's mother noted that he snored and had repeated apneic episodes (Criterion A1a). Daytime sleepiness, unrefreshing sleep, and fatigue (A1b) aren't so often noted in children; only one of these is required. Polysomnography then confirmed that he was having apneic (or hypopneic) episodes, thus rounding out the required criteria for diagnosis. With no other medical condition or substance use to explain his condition, an adenoidectomy was performed that completely relieved his symptoms; this was the proof of the pudding.

Although the DSM-5 criteria do not specify any mandatory rule-outs, there are several we should consider anyway. Various other disorders can affect sleep, but none of them was a likely suspect in the case of Johann. **Narcolepsy** and **circadian rhythm sleep–wake disorders** could be ruled out immediately by lack of typical symptoms. At age 3, he exhibited no symptoms of **substance/medication-induced sleep disorder**.

With a mean of 20 apneic episodes an hour, we'd consider Johann's OSAH as in the middle of the moderate range. His complete diagnosis when he was first evaluated would be as follows:

Before antibiotics, fear of chronic infection routinely prompted removal of tonsils and adenoids. Now only about one-fourth as commonplace as it once was, tonsillectomy is performed most often for problems with breathing. Sleeping initially improves in up to 75% of children, who may however not maintain their gains at long-term follow-up. Although only a few controlled outcome studies have been performed to date, these children may experience significant reductions in aggression, hyperactivity, and inattention. The procedure can be helpful in children with underlying conditions as diverse as Down syndrome, asthma, cerebral palsy, and severe obesity.

G47.33	Obstructive sleep apnea hypopnea, moderate
R62.51	Failure to thrive
CGAS	90 (on evaluation)

SUBSTANCE/MEDICATION–INDUCED SLEEP DISORDER

Many psychoactive substances can also produce sleep disturbances. For symptoms, see the Essential Features of Substance Intoxication and Substance Withdrawal (pp. 403 and 404) and the Essential Features of Four Substance/Medication-Induced Mental Disorders (p. 405) in Chapter 24. Table 24.1 can help with wording and code numbers.

ASSESSING SLEEP–WAKE DISORDERS

General Suggestions

The diagnosis of conditions such as the sleep terror and sleepwalking types of non-REM sleep arousal disorder can almost invariably be made on the basis of history. Because these disorders occur sporadically, studies in the sleep lab are unnecessary. In any case where confirmation by observation seems warranted, home videos should prove adequate. Sleep lab studies may be necessary for disorders with greater risk of harm, such as OSAH.

Developmental Factors

Sleep terrors first appear after 18 months of age, whereas sleepwalking first occurs slightly later, during the preschool and school-age years. By adolescence, arousal parasomnias usually either diminish significantly in frequency or disappear altogether.

Over the past several decades, the number of recognized disorders associated with sleep has grown. They include the common and benign sleep start (also known as *hypnic state*, a jerking of the voluntary muscles that occurs at onset of sleep); enuresis (discussed in Chapter 20); sleep paralysis (short-lived inability to move when dropping off to sleep); and bruxism (tooth grinding), which may be associated with anxiety and developmental disabilities. Other benign conditions include sleep talking and hallucinations that occur when a person is falling asleep (*hypnagogic*) or awakening (*hypnopompic*).

Restless legs syndrome is yet another condition that may affect 2% of children and adolescents—as well as adults. It is a nearly indescribable discomfort deep within the lower legs that's relieved only by movement, yielding an irresistible urge to shift leg positions. It tends to begin before bedtime and can delay onset of sleep, resulting in disturbed sleep and reduced sleep time. It is especially common in children with ADHD, and may be related to low stores of iron—which could act through its role in the synthesis of dopamine. Restless legs syndrome is now included in DSM-5, so when it occurs, it should be coded G25.81.

CHAPTER 22

Gender Dysphoria

QUICK GUIDE TO GENDER DYSPHORIA

Primary Gender Dysphoria

Gender dysphoria in adolescents or adults. Patients strongly identify with the gender other than their own assigned gender roles, with which they feel uncomfortable. Some seek resolution in sex reassignment surgery (p. 378).

Gender dysphoria in children. Children as young as 3 or 4 years can be dissatisfied with their assigned gender (p. 378).

Other specified, or unspecified, gender dysphoria. Use one of these categories for a patient who does not meet the full criteria for one of the diagnoses given above. The only example DSM-5 gives for the other specified category is a patient who has met gender dysphoria criteria for less than the 6-month minimum (p. 383).

Other Causes of Cross-Gender Dissatisfaction or Behavior

Schizophrenia spectrum and other psychotic disorders. Some patients with schizophrenia will express the delusion that they actually belong to the other gender from their own (p. 218).

Transvestic disorder. These people have sexual urges related to cross-dressing, but do not wish to be of the other gender. See *DSM-5 Made Easy* by James Morrison for more details.

GENDER DYSPHORIA

To a degree, all diagnoses depend on definitions. But gender dysphoria (GD), whether we're talking about it in children or in adolescents/adults, is unusually definition-driven. To avert confusion, let's get some of these terms under our belts.

Sex and *sexual* are the terms we use here to refer to biological indicators of male and female. *Gender* indicates the role lived in public as a boy or girl, or as a man or woman. *Gender assignment* refers to the initial identification as male or female that occurs at birth (*natal male* and *natal female* sometimes serve as synonyms). And, finally, *gender dysphoria* refers to the misery felt by those who wrestle with the incongruence between their assigned gender and the gender they experience or desire. The intent of DSM-5 is to focus on dysphoria as the clinical problem, not gender identity per se.

Between the ages of 1 and 2 years, children become aware of the physical differences between girls and boys. By age 3, they begin to label themselves as boy or girl. For most children, gender identity is stable by age 4, though *gender role* (oops! another definition: behaving as a male or female) can be influenced by peers, family, the mass media, and perhaps other elements in the environment. At about this time, it is usual for young children to show interest in clothing, toys, or behaviors that are typically regarded as male or female.

But along the way, some children begin to feel uncomfortable with their assigned gender. Indeed, GD begins surprisingly early—often by the age of 2, and usually by the age of 4. These people strongly desire to be of the other gender; they may even insist that they *are* the other gender. And they also have—to be diagnosed with GD, they *must* have—at least five other symptoms* that reveal a strong rejection of their own assigned gender and the desire to embrace characteristics of the one desired. The result is clinically important distress or impairment. The complete list of behaviors is given in the Essential Features below. By definition, GD cannot be diagnosed until a child or adolescent has experienced these symptoms for at least 6 months.

As is true for so many other disorders, no one knows the cause of GD. And as is true for nearly every disorder where this is the case, each possible cause has its adherents. The effects of heredity are surmised from studies that find an excess of brothers in families of boys with GD. A social etiology is suggested by studies that find girls with GD less conventionally attractive, and boys with GD more so, than their respective non-GD-affected peers. It has been associated with abuse, though it remains unclear which factor is cause and which is effect. Findings of depression or borderline personality disorder in over half the mothers of children with GD can be used to support either a biological or a psychological etiology.

---

*Note that for children, diagnosis of GD requires 75% of the possible criteria. This is the strictest requirement of any polythetic criteria set in DSM-5, underscoring the importance of rock-solid ascertainment of a child's strong desire to belong to a different gender.

Clinical populations are heavily weighted toward boys (male–female ratios range from 4:1 to 6:1), but this finding may be skewed by the fact that North American society tolerates effeminate males less well than it does masculine females. Various population estimates put the adult rate of GD at about 1 in 30,000 for men, but half that or even lower for women. Although accurate data are not available, the actual prevalence of GD in children is probably greater. Indeed, a relative minority of children (depending on the study, 2–30% for boys, 12–50% for girls) retain their opposite-sex identification much past puberty. Some studies identify features that may predict outcome, but at this writing, no constellation of symptoms (certainly not cross-dressing or effeminate behavior alone) reliably predicts which children will retain the GD diagnosis through adolescence and into adulthood.

Patients with GD have alarmingly high rates of associated symptoms such as nonsuicide self-harm (perhaps 2 in 5 for adolescents) and suicidal ideas and attempts. Prevalence is also high for anxiety, psychosis, and eating disorders. Recent work has reported GD to be especially prevalent in children with autism spectrum disorder and with ADHD, compared to other children.

Stanley

"I wasn't very comfortable with myself when I was a child, that's for sure," Stanley admitted to the interviewer. "Fact is, I must have been a pretty strange little kid."

At age 19, Stanley was being interviewed for a follow-up research project. He had been evaluated 12 years earlier at a community child guidance center. That information, recorded in neatly checked boxes and tight paragraphs, revealed the following:

Back then, Stanley's mother had reported that he had frequently played dress-up, donning her clothing or that of his older sister. She had noticed that he refused to wrestle or engage in other typical "boy" activities; he usually preferred to play with girls. On one occasion, she heard him and a neighbor girl arguing over which of them would get to be the mother when they were playing house; Stanley's mother had thought it was cute. The year before, he had asked for a doll for his birthday. His father, who worked two jobs and couldn't be present for any of the diagnostic or subsequent therapy sessions, reportedly worried about his son's cross-dressing but had taken no action because his wife assured him that "it would be all right."

"In point of strict fact," Stanley said as he shuffled the papers in front of him, "back then, I truly thought I *was* a girl. It came to me, when I was maybe 6 or 7, that I'd just been born with the wrong equipment. And wasn't *that* weird!"

Stanley had hated team sports and had preferred jacks to baseball. For this and his other mannerisms, he took a merciless ribbing almost from the time he first entered school. During her third interview, his mother admitted that she had been disappointed when Stanley, her fourth and final child, had turned out to be yet another boy.

A physical exam and laboratory tests had been normal, and Stanley had, at that time, been given a DSM-III diagnosis of gender identity disorder of childhood. But at follow-up, the young adult Stanley rejected the notion that he was anything but male. "I outgrew it, that wanting to be a girl, years ago," he told the interviewer. "Maybe it was the therapy, but for quite a while now, I've been happy being a guy. I'm a *gay* guy, you understand, but I am a guy."

ESSENTIAL FEATURES **OF GENDER DYSPHORIA**

In Adolescents or Adults

There is a marked disparity between nominal (natal) gender and what the patient experiences as a sense of self. This can be expressed as a rejection of or wish not to have one's own sex characteristics, or to have those of the other gender. The patient may also express the desire to belong to the other gender and to be treated as though that were the case. Some patients believe that their responses are typical of the other gender.

In Children

The characteristics of GD in children are similar to those in adults, but manifest themselves in age-appropriate ways. So, in their powerful longing to be of the opposite gender, kids may insist that this is what they are; they may prefer clothing, toys, games, playmates, and fantasy roles of the other gender while rejecting their own; and they may say that they hate their own genitalia and want that which they don't have. Note that in children, the number of criteria required (six out of eight) is far greater than for adults (two of six); this is a protective device for persons who have not yet fully matured.

The Fine Print

The D's: • Duration (6+ months, regardless of age) • Distress or disability (social, educational, occupational, or personal impairment) • Differential diagnosis (substance use and physical disorders; psychotic disorders; transvestic disorder, though not in children)

Coding Notes

Specify if: **With a disorder of sex development** (and code the actual congenital developmental disorder).

Specify if: **Posttransition.** The patient is living as a person of the desired gender and has had at least one cross-gender surgical procedure or medical treatment (such as a hormone regimen).

Evaluation of Stanley

As a young child, for far longer than the 6-month minimum (Criterion A), Stanley had been markedly uncomfortable with being a boy; indeed, in retrospect, he admitted that he felt he actually was a girl (A1). He hated team sports and other activities typical for boys (A6). He also clearly, strongly, and persistently identified with girls, as shown by cross-dressing (A2), wanting to assume the mother's role in a game (A3), playing with dolls and jacks (A4), and preferring to play with girls (A5). (The remaining two criteria, dislike of one's own genitalia [A7] and a desire for the anatomy and secondary sex characteristics of the opposite gender [A8], are infrequently encountered in children.) The distress of social ostracism ("merciless ribbing"), in this case administered by peers but sometimes even by family members, completes the requirements for the diagnosis (B).

Apart from the usual substance use and physical disorders (no evidence for these in Stanley's case), we must consider the fact that some kids simply don't conform to our expectations of typical gender role behavior, such as a tomboy girl or a boy who prefers music to sports, reading to toy guns. Some adolescents who cross-dress to achieve sexual arousal may be showing early symptoms of **transvestic disorder**, not GD. And for Stanley, there would be no confusion with **body dysmorphic disorder** or the delusions of a **psychotic disorder**.

If gender identity problems are found in association with adrenal hyperplasia, androgen insensitivity, or other intersex conditions, we would add the specifier *with a disorder of sex development*. That specifier applies to about 1 in 5,000 male babies.

Social isolation is a complication that especially affects boys who maintain effeminate speech or physical mannerisms. In a young child especially, we'd need to be alert for comorbid **anxiety** and **depressive disorders**. Recently, an increased risk of

Although this book intentionally avoids discussing treatment, a diagnosis of GD implies a couple of issues we should mention here. First, the therapy Stanley referred to was supportive, focused on managing his dysphoria and coming to grips with who he was. It was not "conversion therapy"—a discredited (and in some jurisdictions, now illegal) set of coercive techniques to force someone who has shown homosexual inclinations to conform to arbitrary "normative" behavior.

Other complex treatment decisions include hormonal delay of adolescence and possible hormonal or surgical gender reassignment. Each of these is a huge step for a young person, carrying with it implications for permanent anatomical change. Each is rendered especially complex by the finding that, more often than not, childhood GD does not persist past adolescence. Because of the critical role they play, clinicians who evaluate such children must have some knowledge of the ethical issues, treatment options, and local laws pertaining to gender reassignment. And, always, the entire course of therapy (or decision not to provide it) is predicated on a diagnostic process that is both principled and scientific.

eating disorders has also been associated with GD. Stanley's childhood diagnosis (by DSM-5 criteria) would be as follows:

F64.2	Gender dysphoria in children
Z60.4	Social exclusion or rejection
CGAS	71 (age 7)

And here's Stanley at age 19:

Z03.89	No mental disorder
GAF	85 (current)

ASSESSING GENDER DYSPHORIA

General Suggestions

Accurate assessment even of the prevalence of GD is complicated by cultural differences, social stigmatization, inconsistent data collection, and definitional criteria. Complicating matters further is the difficulty of determining whether the gender nonconformity stems from an environmental issue (sexual abuse, bullying, peer pressure) or some emotional state—perhaps a severe depression, an emerging primary psychosis, or a phobia. A prolonged multidisciplinary evaluation may be necessary, especially of adolescent patients, who may be ambivalent or guarded in their presentation. Of course, the possibility of an intersex condition must be evaluated by physical exam and endocrinological tests. As with so many other conditions, the best evaluative tool is a set of comprehensive interviews with parents and the child.

Whether treated or not, the preponderance of children with GD will not retain this diagnosis as adults, as noted in the sidebar (p. 381). Indeed, fluidity of gender identity is common in young people. Focus on the dysphoric symptoms; emphasize to the patient and family that diagnostic certainty may have to wait. Some of the interview instruments for assessing GD are reviewed in the 2010 article by T. Shechner (see Appendix 1).

Developmental Factors

Children age 5 or under may state that they will grow up to be persons of the opposite sex. Older children may display this sort of wish fulfillment in the form of fantasies or play, as well as choice of friends and clothing. Teens can understand and respond to the question "Do you ever feel more like [the opposite gender] than like [the child's actual gender]?"

Although there isn't much objective evidence about its value, some clinicians look to doll play with family figures as a clue to abnormal gender identification in younger children. A child who chooses the opposite-sex doll should be asked to explain the reason for the choice. A girl who indicates neither parent doll when asked which one she would prefer to be might elicit the suspicion of gender identity confusion. An answer couched in terms of a perceived social advantage (for example, "Only men can be firemen") wouldn't indicate difficulty with gender role or identity. Children can also be asked to draw the parent they would like to be. Or you can ask, "What do you like about being a [boy or girl]? What don't you like about it?"

F64.8 OTHER SPECIFIED GENDER DYSPHORIA

You can use the other specified category for a patient who has met the age-appropriate GD criteria for less than the 6-month minimum.

F64.9 UNSPECIFIED GENDER DYSPHORIA

Use unspecified GD for cases of GD symptoms that do not meet full diagnostic criteria and about which you do not wish to be more specific.

CHAPTER 23

Disruptive, Impulse-Control,
and Conduct Disorders

QUICK GUIDE TO THE DISRUPTIVE, IMPULSE-CONTROL, AND CONDUCT DISORDERS

Primary Disruptive, Impulse-Control, and Conduct Disorders

Conduct disorder. A child persistently violates rules or the rights of others (p. 389).

With limited prosocial emotions (specifier for conduct disorder). Use this specifier for children whose disordered conduct is callous and disruptive, showing no remorse and no regard for the feelings of others (p. 390).

Oppositional defiant disorder. Multiple examples of negativistic behavior persist for at least 6 months (p. 386).

Intermittent explosive disorder. With no other demonstrable pathology (psychological or general medical), these patients have episodes during which they aggressively act out—physically or verbally. As a result, they may physically harm others or destroy property. This diagnosis is rarely made in childhood or adolescence, however.

Kleptomania. An irresistible urge to steal things they don't need causes these patients to do so repeatedly. The phrase "tension and release" characterizes this behavior (sidebar, p. 394).

Pyromania. Individuals feel "tension and release" in regard to the behavior of starting fires (sidebar, p. 394).

Antisocial personality disorder. DSM-5 actually includes this disorder in this chapter of the manual, as well as in its chapter on personality disorders. However, though it may have its roots in childhood or adolescence, it cannot be diagnosed until a person is at least age 18.

Other specified, or unspecified, disruptive, impulse-control, and conduct disorder. As usual, use one of these categories for other cases that are not well defined (p. 395).

Other Disorders Characterized by Disruptive, Impulsive, or Conduct-Related Behaviors

Trichotillomania. Pulling hair from various parts of the body is often accompanied by feelings of "tension and release" (p. 289).

Paraphilic disorders. Some people (nearly always males) have recurrent sexual urges involving a variety of behaviors that are objectionable to others; some are illegal. They may act upon these urges in order to obtain pleasure. These disorders are rarely diagnosed before adolescence, however, and not often then.

Substance-related disorders. There is often an impulsive component to the misuse of various substances (Chapter 24).

Bipolar I disorder. Patients with bipolar I disorder may steal, gamble, act out violently, and engage in other socially undesirable behaviors, though this happens only during an acute manic episode (p. 253).

Schizophrenia. In response to hallucinations or delusions, patients with schizophrenia may impulsively engage in a variety of illegal or otherwise ill-advised behaviors (p. 218).

Disruptive mood dysregulation disorder. A child's mood is persistently negative between frequent, severe explosions of temper (p. 246).

Child or adolescent antisocial behavior. This code (Z72.810) is useful when antisocial behavior cannot be ascribed to a mental disorder, such as oppositional defiant disorder or conduct disorder (p. 444).

INTRODUCTION

Any child will misbehave from time to time, but a substantial minority of children have behavior problems that go far beyond the occasional stolen candy bar, schoolyard fist fight, or classroom outburst. The disorders covered in this chapter of DSM-5 constitute a spectrum of disruptive behaviors that exist along the dual continua of age and severity. Some difficult children grow through successive stages of aggressive behavior → oppositional defiant disorder (ODD) → conduct disorder (CD) → antisocial personality disorder (ASPD); far more, of course, do not. Some research seems to demonstrate that those who do progress from one stage to the next have greater family history of psychopathology and are more likely to use psychoactive substances. However, the line of demarcation between CD and ASPD is entirely arbitrary, and no one is entirely sure that any of these stages is a distinct entity. ADHD, though not strictly in the line of succession with these other disorders, is often associated with them.

Although the current definitions may not discriminate disorders with a uniform etiology or prognosis, they do allow clinicians to describe clusters that account for a major portion of any child mental health professional's practice. Specific causes for these disorders are not known, but both genetic and environmental influences are suspected. These conditions may flourish in the aftermath of a bitter divorce or harsh/restrictive parenting; ODD is reported more commonly in families with low socioeconomic status. Parents and other relatives may have other conduct-related disorders, depressive disorders, substance use disorders, and ASPD. ADHD and somatization disorder are often found among relatives of children with ADHD.

DSM-5 has reorganized these disorders: moving into this chapter of the manual some of the conditions that were once included elsewhere in the book; plucking out one (trichotillomania!) and placing it with obsessive–compulsive and related disorders (see Chapter 15 of the present book); and moving still another (gambling disorder) into the substance-related and addictive disorders. Some that are now included in this chapter of DSM-5 aren't usually identified until a person is well past childhood or adolescence; we mention these in the Quick Guide but provide no vignettes for them.

F91.3 OPPOSITIONAL DEFIANT DISORDER

As disruptive behavior disorders go, ODD is relatively mild—despite the severity specifier you choose for a given patient. It occupies an uneasy niche in the broad spectrum of childhood behavioral problems. Here is the source of controversy surrounding these children: Can their persistently defiant, hostile, and uncooperative behavior be adequately differentiated from the behavior of normal toddlers (or adolescents) and from the more severe CD? If it can, what is the prognosis for such individuals? Is ODD then a risk factor for later CD?

The facts known about ODD are sparse. It usually begins early (about age 6), frequently evolving out of a toddler's normal quest for independence. Sometimes implicated have been coercive parenting styles that involve strict, often harsh, and inconsistently applied discipline. The angry and defiant behaviors of these children almost universally disrupt their home lives. Somewhat less often, relationships in the school and in the community are also affected.

Before adolescence, boys are more often affected than girls; thereafter, the sexes are affected about equally. Overall, about 1 in 20 children can be diagnosed with ODD, though researchers have reported a tremendous range (up to 10%). Although many children may have no signs of disorder on follow-up, perhaps 30% of patients with early-onset ODD progress to full-blown CD; some of these will eventually be diagnosed with ASPD, as noted above. When an adult continues to show persistent symptoms of only ODD, it resembles a personality disorder.

Shelly

"Mom can't handle me."

For the 10 or 15 minutes after stating her chief complaint, Shelly was nearly silent. An attractive though immature 13-year-old, she sat with downcast eyes, answering questions with monosyllables or "I don't know." She wore lipstick and eyeshadow, and each of her ears bore multiple piercings.

Colicky as a baby, Shelly had been difficult right from the start. "She never seemed to sleep," her mother had reported during an earlier interview. "She moved from the terrible twos straight through the terrible threes to the terrible fours. She was—and is—the world's pickiest eater. And she always refused to go to bed. The first word she ever learned to say was 'No.'"

ESSENTIAL FEATURES OF **OPPOSITIONAL DEFIANT DISORDER**

These patients are often angry and irritable, tending toward touchiness and hair-trigger temper. They will disobey authority figures or argue with them, and they may refuse to cooperate or follow rules—if only to annoy others. They sometimes accuse others of their own misdeeds; some appear malicious.

The Fine Print

The D's: • Duration and demographics (6+ months—more or less daily for age 5 and under; weekly for older children) • Distress (patient or others) or disability (social, educational, occupational, or personal impairment) • Differential diagnosis (substance use disorders; ADHD; psychotic or mood disorders; disruptive mood dysregulation disorder; ordinary childhood growth and development)

Coding Notes

Specify severity:

> **Mild.** Symptoms occur in only 1 location (home, school, with friends).
> **Moderate.** Some symptoms in 2+ locations.
> **Severe.** Symptoms in 3+ locations.

Almost as soon as she spoke sentences, Shelly had begun to argue. "Now she'll argue about anything. She'll argue until she's grounded. Then she loses her temper, then her allowance, but still she won't give in. She'll just sit in her room and read by the hour."

Although she sometimes became so angry that she slammed doors, Shelly was never destructive or violent toward people. Neither was she dishonest: There had been no history of stealing, and she almost always told the truth. Although in the past few months she had often thrown away homework assignments that she could have completed easily, when questioned she would usually own up to what she had done. But the falling grades were "not my fault."

"She's never willing to take responsibility," her mother commented. "According to her, bad things happen because the teacher has pets or I'm unfair. She says she doesn't have friends because the other girls are jealous. But even when she was in Brownies, I've seen her pick away at another girl till the whole group turned on her."

With shakes of her head, Shelly denied feeling depressed, using drugs or alcohol, and having suicidal ideas. To questions about delusions and hallucinations, she responded, "That's dumb." Only the subject of her parents' divorce produced much interaction or affect. "It really burns me. Sure, Daddy drinks. But he never, like, hit her or anything. And she was always nagging him."

She folded her arms across her chest. "I hate them both."

Evaluation of Shelly

As is typical for this disorder, Shelly's difficulties began when she was tiny; they persisted into early adolescence, far longer than the minimum 6 months required (Criterion A). The extremes to which she would pursue an argument are classic for ODD. Other symptoms included refusing to do her homework (A5), blaming others for her own misconduct (A7), and deliberately annoying another girl in Brownies (A6). She also expressed anger and resentment over her parents' divorce (A3)—but did it really occur more often than we would expect of other kids from broken or battleground homes? However, she often did lose her temper to the point of slamming doors (A1). Only 4 of the Criterion A symptoms are required for diagnosis. Of course, a degree of oppositional behavior is normal at certain developmental stages (toddlerhood, adolescence), but in Shelly it had lasted for years. (For many other children, the issue may be less clear-cut.) Her behavior also caused social and academic problems for her (B).

In a note appended to the diagnostic criteria, DSM-5 states that for a child 5 or older, we'd expect the oppositional behavior to occur at least once a week for a diagnosis of ODD (for younger children, it should be even more frequent). We don't have that information for Shelly, but the degree to which it had affected her life (and that of her family and others) suggests that it certainly occurred often enough to be significant in her life. That's good enough for us. Also note that we would pay far less attention to these behaviors if they occurred only with siblings; of course, this wasn't the case for Shelly, who appears from the vignette to be an only child.

Shelly denied symptoms of a **mood** or **psychotic disorder** (C). Although she had temper outbursts, they occurred in the context of overall argumentativeness and were more or less of a qualitative level you'd expect for Shelly's age, so we would exclude **disruptive mood dysregulation disorder** from our considerations. The vignette includes evidence against aggressive, destructive, or antisocial behavior (she didn't fight or lie) that would suggest the more serious **conduct disorder** or **antisocial personality disorder**. Clinicians should also be on the lookout in some cases for **ADHD**, which may be associated with disruptive behavior and is commonly comorbid with ODD. Another possibility might be **intellectual disability**, which can only be comorbid with ODD if a child's oppositional symptoms are much greater than would be expected for the age and intellectual ability. The inability to understand spoken language caused by **impaired hearing** can also mimic willful disobedience. In some cases (not Shelly's), impaired progress in school may necessitate ruling out a **specific learning disorder** (with impairment in reading or mathematics).

We are asked to judge the severity of Shelly's symptoms based on how many settings (home, school, social) are affected. We have evidence that, beyond her home life, her symptoms affected her (and others) at school and elsewhere. Although severity is to be judged solely on the basis of number of life areas affected, we'll still opt for medium over severe: According to DSM-5, it is used if "some symptoms are present in at least two settings," and this gives us cover to reserve the harsher judgment for someone who is more globally incapacitated:

F91.3	Oppositional defiant disorder, moderate
CGAS	55 (current)

CONDUCT DISORDER

To one degree or other, the behavior of people with CD is persistently antisocial. The behaviors involved have been collected into four categories: aggression toward persons or animals; property destruction; theft or deceit; and other serious rule violations. However, no specific distribution of symptoms is required for diagnosis—any three will fill the bill. Note that most of these symptoms, whether they occur in a juvenile or an adult, can lead to arrest or other legal consequences. In fact, for an adult to be

> In ODD, as in CD (and, indeed, any other mental health disorder), clinicians must keep in mind their duty to protect others from dangers posed even by children who have threatened harm. This principle, formalized as the 1974 *Tarasoff* decision in California, sets forth the duty of health care personnel to directly warn any identifiable persons against whom threats have been made, or to notify law enforcement officials. Although not all jurisdictions have enacted such a statute, good clinical practice suggests that clinicians everywhere should follow the guidelines anyway. Once you do, document your actions!

diagnosed as having ASPD, the exact criteria listed in Criterion A for CD must have been present prior to age 15 (for truancy and staying out at night, prior to age 13).

From the age of 2 or 3, boys are typically more aggressive than girls. Children who are highly aggressive by age 7 or 8 tend to remain so later in life and are three times more likely than other children to have police records as adults. The prevalence of CD in boys is high, ranging from 2% to 10% or more, depending upon the study; the rate for girls is perhaps half as great. DSM-5 is silent as to whether CD should be diagnosed in preschoolers. Although symptoms can begin then, it seems unlikely that such a very young child would be able to demonstrate enough symptoms for diagnosis. That usually doesn't happen until later.

Age of onset, the specifier that determines the actual ICD-10 code number given the patient, is important to the prediction of outcome. The childhood-onset type (beginning before age 10) is more often associated with marked physical aggression; young children who have more serious symptoms are also less likely to do well at follow-up. Patients with childhood-onset CD are far more likely to be male than female, and the contribution of their genetic inheritance is strong. They are especially likely to have ADHD and other mental disorders.

In patients who don't become symptomatic until adolescence (more or less), the sex ratio is less extreme, and the disorder is less likely to result in the adult diagnosis of ASPD. However, even some patients with childhood-onset CD appear to outgrow their conduct problems, becoming adults who are anxious, depressed, or socially isolated—but not anti-social.

With Limited Prosocial Emotions (Specifier for Conduct Disorder)

Predicting outcome for anyone with CD also depends heavily on the presence of certain symptoms that suggest a lack of appreciation for the experience of others. These symptoms, which have for years been called *callous–unemotional*, DSM-5 bundles into the overall term *with limited prosocial emotions* (LPE). Each of the four categories indicates a quality that the individual *lacks*:

- Empathy for the feelings of others, so that the patient appears cold or heartless
- Guilt or remorse for the patient's own misdeeds
- Concern for quality of performance in schoolwork, at home, on the job
- Deep or sincere affect (other than when trying to con or otherwise manipulate others)

Patients with CD and LPE don't recognize fear or sadness in others or respond well to it. They have low levels of fear and anxiety, and are more thrill-seeking and less sensitive to punishment than other people.

For a child or adolescent to qualify for this specifier, a lack of at least two of the four bulleted qualities above must have been manifested in multiple settings and relationships during the preceding year. Up to half of youth with CD meet criteria for the LPE specifier. Those who do have been found to show increased risk for, and greater stability of, antisocial behavior later in life, even after researchers have controlled for number of CD symptoms, age of onset, and presence of ADHD.

> It is noteworthy that although all of the behaviors that constitute criteria for CD are observable, and therefore relatively objective, the criteria for the LPE specifier are deeply subjective—personal constructs that must be inferred.

ESSENTIAL FEATURES OF **CONDUCT DISORDER**

In various ways, these people chronically disrespect rules and other people's rights. Most egregiously, they use aggression against their peers (sometimes elders)—bullying, starting fights, using dangerous weapons, showing cruelty to people or animals, even sexual abuse. They may intentionally set fires or otherwise destroy property; breaking and entering, lying, and theft are well within their repertoires. Truancy, repeated runaways, and refusal to come home at night against a parent's wishes round out their bag of tricks.

The Fine Print

The D's: • Duration (in 1 year, with 1+ symptoms in past 6 months) • Disability (social, educational, occupational, or personal impairment) • Differential diagnosis (ADHD; oppositional defiant disorder; mood disorders; ordinary childhood growth and development; antisocial personality disorder; intermittent explosive disorder)

Coding Notes

Based on age of onset, specify:

F91.1 Childhood-onset type. At least one problem with conduct begins before age 10.
F91.2 Adolescent-onset type. No problems with conduct before age 10.
F91.9 Unspecified onset. Insufficient information about age of onset.

Specify severity:

Mild. Has sufficient symptoms, but not a lot, and harm to others is minimal.
Moderate. Symptoms and harm to others are intermediate.
Severe. Many symptoms, much harm to others.

ESSENTIAL FEATURES OF **WITH LIMITED PROSOCIAL EMOTIONS (SPECIFIER FOR CONDUCT DISORDER)**

Such patients lack important emotional underpinnings. They have a callous lack of empathy (without concern for the emotions or suffering of others). They tend to have shallow affect and little remorse or guilt (other than regret if caught). They are indifferent to the quality of their own performance.

The Fine Print

To receive the specifier, a patient must have experienced these symptoms within the past year.

Jim

The interview with 10-year-old Jim was conducted in juvenile hall, which had been his home for the past 2 weeks. He had taken his penny collection to school for Hobby Day. At lunchtime it went into one of his socks, with which he then bludgeoned a second grader who had refused to surrender the jelly sandwich Jim wanted. The incident was by no means Jim's first attempt at extortion.

"He's been threatening other kids for a couple of years," his mother had said earlier. "We had him down to the child guidance clinic. They said he had a behavior disorder. They're telling me!"

Jim had been a cranky, negative sort of baby, and his temperament hadn't improved by the time he learned to talk. "His first complete sentence was 'I didn't do it,'" his mother remarked. He'd argue about any infraction, even when he was caught red-handed. Beginning in kindergarten, he'd blame the fights he started on his victim. When the other child objected, Jim would sometimes get even by sneaking around to that child's home to destroy a piece of play equipment. He was an angry child who by the age of 8 had cut the tires of more than one bicycle; once he had shredded the awning of a neighbor's sandbox with a pair of scissors he had stolen from a rack at the Safeway.

Repeated shoplifting had prompted his first evaluation 2 years earlier. Twice that same year he had entered neighbors' homes and stolen small items, which he had then tried to sell on the school playground. School reports noted that he was bright and could have been a good student. But repeated truancy and fighting had now earned him expulsion from three different schools.

"He comes by it naturally," his mother explained. "His father's served time twice for armed robbery. I guess you'd say he's a career criminal." She saw a bright spot in Jim's detention: "This is the first time in months I've known where he was at night."

Jim was a chunky, sandy-haired boy, large for his age, who swaggered across the playroom floor in a pair of overalls that had one strap undone. He disdained the various play materials that were offered him; he settled down on a wooden chair with a steady gaze and an air of complete control. For several minutes, he replied to questions with one- or two-word answers. When he finally spoke spontaneously, it was to ask how soon he would be released. He was told that it depended on the results of the evaluation, because he had struck and severely injured the younger child.

Jim gazed steadily at the interviewer. "It wasn't me—I never did nothin' wrong. Besides, the little snot prob'ly had it comin'."

Evaluation of Jim

Of the 15 behavioral symptoms typical of CD, DSM-5 requires only 3 for diagnosis in the mildest cases. For years (Criterion A) Jim had had many symptoms, including bullying (A1), starting fights (A2), using a weapon (A3), property destruction (A9), breaking and entering (A10), lying (A11), truancy (A15), and staying out at night (A13). Some of these behaviors had occurred just recently, and collectively they had greatly affected both Jim and his mother (B). Although lack of empathy is ignored in the basic criteria for CD (partly because it is so hard to measure), Jim's manifest absence of empathy would be regarded by many clinicians as central to the syndrome of CD. It will come up later in the evaluation, when we consider the LPE specifier.

Of course, there are other possible causes of antisocial behavior. **Gross brain pathology**, such as a tumor, an infection, or a seizure disorder, is one such etiology; a **psychotic disorder** or **manic episode** might also qualify. The clinician who saw Jim would have to look carefully for evidence of problems with cognition, hallucinations, delusions, and other symptoms of these conditions.

Besides the symptoms embodied in the criteria, other problems can occur in patients with this diagnosis. Children with CD often begin sexual activity in early adolescence. Some are depressed (they may show evidence of a **major depressive episode** or **persistent depressive disorder [dysthymia]**); many will **abuse substances**. **Specific learning disorder** and other language (oral and written) deficits have been noted in a substantial number of these children, and **ADHD** is comorbid in nearly half. Jim's symptoms (arguments, blaming others, chronic anger, spitefulness) might also qualify him for the diagnosis of **oppositional defiant disorder**—a common precursor to CD. Although DSM-IV did not permit both disorders to be coded simultaneously, DSM-5 does allow it. In our opinion, ODD adds little other than historic perspective to Jim's evaluation; therefore, we've chosen not to mention it further.

Many of Jim's behaviors are what some have called *callous–unemotional*. The claim is that such behaviors portend severe antisocial acting out, delinquency, and recidivism as the patient approaches adulthood. DSM-5 has incorporated these behaviors into criteria for the somewhat clumsily named LPE specifier, described above. To earn it, the patient must have manifested at least two of these attitudes within the previous year. In fact, Jim had more than that: He seemed not to show much affect (other than disdain for the interviewer), and he lacked any sign of remorse for his actions or empathy for his victim. That's three of the criteria. We would have to interview him and his teacher further to learn whether he seemed at all worried about his school performance. In fact, we'd want to interview his mother again and perhaps his teacher, to be certain that he was showing these attitudes in multiple settings.

Because of its grave prognosis and the relative absence of effective treatment, all other possible disorders should be given serious consideration before diagnosing CD, particularly CD with the LPE specifier. However, if any case history justifies the use of CD and LPE, Jim's would appear to be the one. Because he had many more symptoms that the minimum required and he had seriously injured the other child with his homemade sap, we'd judge his CD to be *severe*. We worry that he might be on his way to **antisocial personality disorder**—a diagnosis that cannot be made, however, until the age of 18. At his current age, his complete diagnosis would be the following:

DSM-5 describes three disorders whose titles include the Greek word *mania*, which means "passion." Trichotillomania, the passion for hairpulling, has been dispatched to join the obsessive–compulsive and related disorders (see Chapter 15, p. 289).

The other two, kleptomania (F63.2) and pyromania (F63.1), are characterized by so-called "tension and release," in which the individual feels a mounting sense of pressure to perform the act that builds until the act is, well, performed. Afterward, there is a sort of reward as the tension abates and a sense of pleasure floods the individual. Both of these behaviors occur repeatedly. In neither condition is financial gain the driving force behind the behavior: A person with kleptomania doesn't need to shoplift another pair of jeans; a person with pyromania isn't trying to collect insurance money. Indeed, individuals with pyromania do not limit themselves to the fire-setting act itself, but maintain an active interest in fires and firefighting—including firefighters, fire trucks, and other equipment.

Although persons apprehended for setting fires or for shoplifting may try to claim the irresistible impulse of a *mania*, the disorders are actually highly uncommon. (So little is known about them that together they occupy only 3½ pages in the 900+ pages of DSM-5.) Demographics are as follows: Pyromania is very rare, and much more likely in males. Kleptomania occurs in about 1 in 200 of the general population, with a 3:1 female predominance.

Each of these disorders can start in adolescence. However, there doesn't appear to be much correlation between childhood fire setting and pyromania; in childhood, it is done as a part of conduct disorder, and is not attended by the phenomenon of tension and release.

F91.1	Conduct disorder, childhood-onset type, severe, with limited prosocial emotions
Z65.1	Incarcerated in juvenile hall
CGAS	41 (current)

F91.8 OTHER SPECIFIED DISRUPTIVE, IMPULSE–CONTROL, AND CONDUCT DISORDER

F91.9 UNSPECIFIED DISRUPTIVE, IMPULSE–CONTROL, AND CONDUCT DISORDER

Use the other specified or unspecified category for a child who has clinically important disruptive, impulse-control, or conduct-related behavior that does not fulfill the criteria for any other diagnosis described in this chapter. Use the other specified category when you wish to be specific about a particular presentation; use the unspecified category when you do not wish to do so.

ASSESSING DISRUPTIVE, IMPULSE-CONTROL, AND CONDUCT DISORDERS

General Suggestions

Impulsive and disruptive behaviors can be difficult to assess accurately, in part because they are perceived as shameful or illegal. Some children and adolescents will hide the facts from clinicians, just as they do from school or legal authorities. For reliable data, clinicians may have to rely on other informants—especially parents and teachers—who can report on behaviors such as jumping to another activity without finishing the first one, shouting out in class, or acting rashly without considering the likely consequences.

You may find it useful to interview parent and child separately to assess, for example, just how much of the child's time is unsupervised (this may be correlated with the diagnosis of CD). Accuracy may be improved by noting the earliest instance of a behavior reported by any informant. And here is a good place to ask about the family's television habits: Studies have shown that aggression in children is proportional to the amount of TV they watch—and, to a lesser degree, even to how much time a set is on in their homes.

Asking about unsanctioned behaviors is an invitation to lie. However, if you request an opinion about similar behavior if it was exhibited by a peer or fictional child, you may learn how fully the patient approves of the behavior: "One of the kids who comes in here hit his sister last week because she hid his crayons. Do you think that was OK?" Some children and adolescents may be surprisingly willing to share their exploits—especially if they believe they were justified. Others may be induced to brag about what they've done, though your reaction must not seem to sanction the behavior. All in all, a nonjudgmental attitude and the use of neutral terms for behaviors will probably yield the most information from young people who might have something to hide.

An oppositional child may justify negativistic behavior on the basis that the request was unreasonable. And note that it does not suffice for a diagnosis of ODD merely to observe in an interview that a child is touchy, angry, spiteful, annoying, and prone to blame others—the criteria require the historical evidence that such is *often* the case.

Problematic conduct can easily obscure less dramatic comorbid diagnoses. However, often associated are problems with general intelligence, learning disorders, substance use, anxiety (especially in girls), and language impairment. It is important to consider each of these diagnostic areas in a child or adolescent who presents with disruptive, impulsive, or conduct-related behavior.

Of course, very young children are notoriously negativistic; even defiant behavior may be quite normal in this age range. And toddlers certainly cannot be expected to sustain attention for longer than a few minutes.

Developmental Factors

CD can appear in preschool years; however, it is usually recognized in middle school (or later), when these behaviors bring more serious consequences. It only rarely begins after the age of 16.

Disruptive and impulsive behaviors can produce important social and economic damage. In that sense, though data are sparse, it stands to reason that younger children who shoplift will steal smaller, less expensive items, and that those who tend to be aggressive will present less of a problem at 6 years than at 16. On the other hand, because a fire, once set, can quickly get out of hand, fire setting may present as much of a problem in young children as in teenagers.

In DSM-5, CD is subtyped according to age of onset: childhood versus adolescent. For the former to be diagnosed, a child must have had at least one symptom before age 10. Note that the milder symptoms of CD in younger children will usually become evident first (lying, shoplifting, staying out at night, and truancy will precede robbery at gunpoint, rape, and use of a weapon).

In the half century since the publication of the seminal book *Deviant Children Grown Up* by Lee Robins, the prognostic value of early development of symptoms has been recognized. Robins found that the younger a boy was at first arrest, the greater his risk of a poor outcome. However, over half of even the most disturbed youngsters did not develop ASPD. Those whose symptoms are milder and develop first in adolescence often improve as adults.

CHAPTER 24

Substance–Related

and Addictive Disorders

QUICK GUIDE TO THE SUBSTANCE-RELATED AND ADDICTIVE DISORDERS

Mind-altering substances yield three basic types of disorders: substance intoxication, substance withdrawal, and substance use disorder. Most of these DSM-5 terms apply to nearly all of the substances discussed; exceptions are noted below. Various specific types of substance/medication-induced disorders are also identified by DSM-5.

Substance intoxication. Recent heavy substance use causes this acute clinical state, which can apply to all drugs except nicotine (Essential Features, p. 403).

Substance withdrawal. This class-specific collection of symptoms develops when someone who frequently uses a substance discontinues or markedly reduces the amount used. It applies to all substances except PCP, the hallucinogens, and the inhalants (Essential Features, p. 404).

Substance use disorder. Substance use falling into this category has produced certain behavioral characteristics plus clinically important distress or impaired functioning. Found in all drug classes except caffeine, substance use disorder doesn't have to be intentional; it can develop from medication use, such as the treatment of chronic pain (Essential Features, p. 401).

Other substance/medication-induced disorders. Four other substance/medication-induced disorders are sometimes diagnosed in children and adolescents: substance/medication-induced psychotic disorder, mood disorder, anxiety disorder, and sleep disorder. They can be experienced during intoxication, during withdrawal, or as consequences of substance misuse that endure long after the misuse and withdrawal symptoms have ended (Essential Features, p. 405).

Gambling disorder. Although it isn't discussed in this chapter, and we provide no vignette for it, gambling disorder in adulthood can have its roots in childhood or adolescence. In one study, boys who had been assessed for impulsiveness at age 13 were reassessed in late adolescence for gambling status. The higher a boy's score on impulsiveness was, the more likely the boy was to develop a problem with gambling.

INTRODUCTION

There are several reasons why it's hard to pinpoint the extent of child and adolescent substance misuse:

- *Casual usage.* Many surveys report the percentage of young people who have used a drug, or class of drugs, within a given time period. Yet only a fraction of these children and adolescents may use drugs frequently or develop problems resulting from usage. (Should any degree of substance use by a juvenile be considered "normal"?)

- *Use of specific drugs in particular demographic areas.* "Hard" drugs, such as heroin and cocaine, have traditionally been more prevalent in inner-city areas than in suburban or rural localities (though this situation may be changing). By contrast, some studies show that the more socially acceptable substances—alcohol, tobacco, and marijuana—may be used as frequently in rural as in urban areas.

- *Comorbid diagnoses.* The vast majority of children and adolescents who misuse substances have other disorders, symptoms of which may obscure the evidence of substance misuse. These diagnoses include conduct disorder, ADHD, and mood and anxiety disorders, any of which may be found in a third or more of youth who misuse substances. Multiple comorbid diagnoses are not uncommon.

- *Changing criteria.* For decades, classifications and diagnostic criteria have been revised every few years. This tradition was continued in DSM-5, when the DSM-IV criteria for substance abuse were folded with those for substance dependence into the current criteria for substance use disorder.

- *Multiple points of reference.* Prevalence rates are variously reported for past week, month, year, and lifetime (that is, ever in a person's life), and sometimes in terms of intensity of use (number of drinks, presence of intoxication, daily use). It also matters what we include in the category being discussed: For example, do hallucinogens include phencyclidine (PCP)? Are *narcotics* synonymous with *opioids*? Where do methamphetamines—now so ubiquitous that they must be considered for every demographic—fit into the overall picture? Exactly what medications are considered *tranquilizers?* Finally, reports may focus on different age groups (for example, 8th, 10th, and 12th grades of school; ages 12–17; or sometimes "all students").

With all that said, surveys have identified falling levels of use among children and teenagers for both licit and illegal substances. These reports present many tables and figures; one typical finding is an overall decline in current illicit drug use in teenagers (ages 12–17) from 11.6% in 2002 to 9.5% in 2012. Implications for the future are contained in another report that early use of marijuana (before age 15) was associated with a marked increase in illicit drug dependence as an adult (13%, as compared with only 2% of those adults who had waited until after age 15 to first try marijuana). However, in jurisdictions that allow medical marijuana use, some teenagers are already obtaining marijuana by prescription.

In 2013, lifetime use in 12th-grade students was reported as follows: any illicit substance (including inhalants), 52%; marijuana, 46%; any illicit drug other than marijuana, 25%; inhalants 6.9%; amphetamines, 12%; narcotics other than heroin, 11%; hallucinogens, 7.6%; ecstasy (methylenedioxymethamphetamine or MDMA), 7.1%; PCP, 1.3%; crack cocaine, 1.8%; heroin, 1.0%. For comparison, comparable figures for two legal substances are alcohol, 68%; and cigarettes, 38%.

Decades of research have demonstrated the heavy influence of genetics in creating a problem with substance use, but environmental factors (attitude of peers, setting in which the substance is used) are also important, especially at the novice stage. Comorbid disorders (mood, psychotic, anxiety) may nudge young people to experiment with substances at an earlier age.

THE DSM-5 APPROACH TO DIAGNOSING SUBSTANCE MISUSE

Four Diagnostic Concepts

The foregoing difficulties notwithstanding, DSM-5 takes a giant step toward unifying our understanding of the substance-related disorders. It allows us to make literally hundreds of logical diagnoses according to four diagnostic concepts.

Substance Use Disorder

The generic criteria for substance use disorder (see its Essential Features, p. 401) identify substance-related problems that are mainly issues of control and physiological change. (The hallucinogens, the inhalants, and PCP don't appear to produce clinically significant tolerance or withdrawal symptoms, which therefore do not figure in to the criteria for the substance use disorders involving those substance types.) Children and adolescents are far less likely than adults to receive a diagnosis of substance use disorder, but we should carefully consider it any time it appears appropriate.

ESSENTIAL FEATURES OF **SUBSTANCE USE DISORDER**

These patients use enough of their chosen substance to cause chronic or repeated problems in different aspects of their lives:

- **Personal and interpersonal life.** They neglect family life (relationships with parents, siblings), and even favorite leisure activities, in favor of using their substance of choice; they fight (physically or verbally) with those they care about; and they continue to use the substance despite the realization that it causes interpersonal problems.
- **Employment.** Effort formerly devoted to school (or work or other important activities) now goes into getting the substance, consuming it, and then recuperating from its use. Result: These people are repeatedly absent, suspended, or expelled (or fired).
- **Control.** They often use more of the substance or for longer than they intended; they (unsuccessfully) attempt to eliminate or reduce the usage. Through it all, they desperately crave more.
- **Health and safety.** The individuals engage in behavior that is physically dangerous (usually, operating or riding in a motor vehicle); legal issues can ensue. They continue to use despite knowing that it causes health problems such as cirrhosis, hepatitis C, or HIV.
- **Physiological sequels.** Tolerance develops: The substance produces less effect, so the patients must use more. And once they stop using, patients suffer symptoms of withdrawal characteristic of that substance.

The Fine Print

Tolerance isn't a factor with most hallucinogens, though users may develop tolerance to the stimulant effects of PCP.

Withdrawal isn't a factor in use of inhalants or of PCP and other hallucinogens.

Don't count tolerance or withdrawal that's caused by taking medication as prescribed.

The D's: • Duration (the symptoms you count must have occurred within the past 12 months) • Differential diagnosis (physical disorders; primary mental disorders from nearly every chapter; *truly* recreational use)

Coding Notes

Rate severity by number of symptoms:

Mild (2–3 symptoms).
Moderate (4–5).
Severe (6+).

Add any specifiers that may apply:

In early remission (no criteria met for 1–12 months).
In sustained remission (no criteria met for 1 year or more).
In a controlled environment.
On maintenance therapy (only for opioids and tobacco).

See Table 24.1 for ICD-10 code numbers.

Substance Intoxication

Depending on the amount and rate of intake, anyone can become intoxicated. Substance intoxication is the only substance-related diagnosis you'd make for someone who has used a substance only once. Each of the substance-specific criteria sets (see the Essential Features of Substance Intoxication, p. 403) is applied to patients whose thinking and behavior are currently being influenced by the substance in question.

Substance Withdrawal

Each of the specific criteria sets for substance withdrawal (see its Essential Features, p. 404) is applied to patients who have used enough of a substance that reducing or discontinuing it creates changes in behavior—changes that include physiological and cognitive elements.

Substance/Medication-Induced Mental Disorder

Scattered throughout DSM-5 are criteria sets that describe the effects of medications and other substances on psychosis, mood, anxiety, sleep, cognition, and sex. The Essential Features for the first four of these conditions are given on page 405. The categories of substance/medication-induced neurocognitive disorder and sexual dysfunction rarely if ever apply to children and adolescents. However, substance intoxication and withdrawal can both cause delirium, the Essential Features for which are given in Chapter 25 on page 421.

Classes of Substances That Can Be Misused

DSM-5 lists a total of 11 substance categories plus "other (or unknown)" that can alter behavior, feelings, or perceptions. However, we can condense these 11 into 6 broad categories. Interpret the usage figures cautiously; the rates continually change, and accurate data are not available for some substance classes.

ESSENTIAL FEATURES OF **SUBSTANCE INTOXICATION**

	Alcohol/ sedatives, etc.	Caffeine	Cannabis	Cocaine/ amphetamines
Symptoms	Disinhibition (arguing, aggression, labile mood; impaired attention, judgment, or functioning); neurological impairment (imbalance or wobbly gait, unclear speech, poor coordination, nystagmus, reduced level of consciousness or memory); some patients develop red eyes or flushed face	Increased central nervous system and motor activity (such as fidgeting, increased energy, insomnia, rapid heartbeat, twitching muscles, intestinal upset, excess urination, red face, rambling speech)	Motor incoordination or altered cognition (anxiety or exhilaration, poor judgment, isolation from friends, a sense of slowed time), plus telltale red eyes, dry mouth, rapid heart rate, and hunger	Mood changes; impaired judgment or psychosocial functioning; neurological excitation ($\uparrow$ or $\downarrow$ blood pressure, heart rate, and motor activity; dilated pupils; sweating or chills; nausea; weight loss; weakness, chest pain, respiratory depression, irregular heartbeat; seizures, coma, or perplexity possible)
Other	Distress or impairment; rule out another medical condition or mental disorder			
Specifiers	None	None	With perceptual disturbances	With perceptual disturbances

	PCP	Other hallucinogens	Inhalants	Opioids
Symptoms	Behavioral disinhibition (erratic impulsivity, aggression, poor judgment); neurological impairment and muscle dyscontrol (nystagmus, trouble walking or speaking, stiff muscles, numbness, coma, or seizures); rapid heartbeat; abnormally acute hearing	Dysphoria, misperception, or poor judgment; autonomic overactivity (dilated pupils and blurred vision, sweating, rapid or irregular heartbeat, trembling, reduced muscle coordination)	Poor judgment and aggression, plus symptoms of neuromuscular incoordination (trouble walking, lightheadedness, slow reflexes, trembling, weakness, blurred or double vision, lethargy, nystagmus, unclear speech)	Mood changes (first elation, later apathy); psychomotor activity $\downarrow$ or $\uparrow$; poor judgment; constricted, "pinpoint" pupils with impaired neurological functioning (lethargy, unclear speech, decreased attention or memory)
Other	Distress or impairment; rule out another medical condition or mental disorder			
Specifiers	None	None	None	None

ESSENTIAL FEATURES OF **SUBSTANCE WITHDRAWAL**

	Alcohol/ sedatives, etc.	Caffeine	Cannabis	Cocaine/ amphetamines (stimulants)	Hallucinogens	Opioids	Tobacco
Use	Heavy, prolonged	Heavy, prolonged	Heavy, daily			Several weeks or more	Several weeks or more
Time to onset	Hours to days	Within hours	From 1 to several days	Hours to days		Within several days	Within 1 day
Symptoms	Increased central nervous system and motor activity (tremor, sweating, nausea, rapid heartbeat, high blood pressure, agitation, headache, insomnia, weakness, brief hallucinations or illusions, convulsions)	Symptoms suggesting flu (headache, nausea, muscle pain) and central nervous system depression (fatigue, dysphoria, poor concentration)	Dysphoria and central nervous system overactivity; troubled sleep, poor appetite, depression, anxiety, restlessness; shakiness, sweating, headache, abdominal pain	Dysphoria; central nervous system stimulation or exhaustion (intense dreams; ↓ or sometimes ↑ sleep or motor activity; hunger)	Reexperiencing of one or more misperceptions that occurred during intoxication (hallucinogen persisting perception disorder)[a]	Dysphoria; nausea, diarrhea, muscle aches; tearing (runny nose); yawning, sleeplessness; autonomic symptoms (dilated pupils, hairs standing up, sweating)	Dysphoria (irritability, depression, anxiety); restlessness; trouble concentrating; insomnia; hunger
Other	Distress or impairment; rule out another medical condition or mental disorder						
Specifiers	With perceptual disturbances	None	None	None	None	None	None

[a]Not really a disorder of withdrawal.

ESSENTIAL FEATURES OF
FOUR SUBSTANCE/MEDICATION-INDUCED MENTAL DISORDERS

Psychotic disorder	Bipolar or depressive disorder	Anxiety disorder	Sleep disorder
Delusions or hallucinations	Euphoric or irritable mood; or persistently depressed mood or notably decreased interest in nearly all activities	Prominent anxiety or panic attacks	Prominent and severe sleep problem
Symptoms develop with or after use, *and* the substance is known to be capable of causing the symptoms.			
Non-substance-related causes (such as a delirium) cannot explain the symptoms better.			
The symptoms cause distress or disability.			
Specify: With onset during intoxication or withdrawal	Specify: With onset during intoxication or withdrawal	Specify: With onset during intoxication or withdrawal, or with medication	Specify: With onset during intoxication or withdrawal Specify type: Insomnia, daytime sleepiness, parasomnia, mixed

Central Nervous System Depressants

The two types of substances that are central nervous system depressants have identical DSM-5 criteria sets for substance intoxication and withdrawal.

ALCOHOL. Of course, most adolescents have tried alcohol; the percentage of all teenagers who use it frequently is in the low double digits. With less drinking experience from which to judge, even those young people who do not go on to develop an alcohol use problem may underestimate its effects. As a consequence, when they do drink, they consume far too much. Perhaps for this reason, adolescent alcohol intoxication not infrequently results in stupor or coma.

SEDATIVES, HYPNOTICS, AND ANXIOLYTICS. Readily available in parents' medicine cabinets and on the street, the sedatives, hypnotics, and anxiolytics are reportedly often misused by children and teenagers. Documentary evidence of the extent of this misuse is still lacking, however.

Central Nervous System Stimulants

To one degree or another, each of the substances in the stimulant category increases central nervous system activity, resulting in unusual alertness, elevation of mood and sense of well-being, improved task performance, and decrease in hunger and in the need for sleep. Identical criteria for substance intoxication and withdrawal apply to cocaine and the amphetamines.

AMPHETAMINES. First synthesized over 100 years ago, the powerful amphetamines are reportedly popular with young people, but no one knows to what extent. Although tight government controls on manufacture and distribution probably diminished their use somewhat in past decades, the recent rise in methamphetamine use may have increased it again.

COCAINE. Extracted from coca leaves, which grow in South America and other parts of the world, cocaine is perhaps the most addictive substance ever created. As one of the most widely misused psychoactive substances in the world, cocaine undoubtedly causes problems for some young people. However, there are very few data to draw on.

CAFFEINE. Of course, caffeine presents little danger, certainly as compared with amphetamines and cocaine; in fact, learning to drink coffee is a rite of passage for the vast majority of young people in Europe and the Americas. (Energy drinks, which contain about as much caffeine as a cup of coffee plus a whole lot of sugar, are the latest risk for kids.) Yet, in excess, even this benign substance can cause symptoms of intoxication. Some people go on to experience withdrawal symptoms.

Opioids

Most persons who use heroin get their start through peer pressure when they are in their teens or early 20s. Contributing factors include parental divorce, low socioeconomic status, inner-city residence, relatives who misuse alcohol, and early experimentation with other substances such as marijuana and alcohol. By late adolescence, 5–10% of late adolescents have used opioids in some form.

Perception-Distorting Drugs

As the term indicates, the toxic effect of each of the perception-distorting drugs is to produce hallucinations or illusions (misinterpretations of actual sensory stimuli). None of these drugs has any noteworthy withdrawal syndrome.

INHALANTS. The inhalants include nearly anything that evaporates or can be sprayed from a can. They are cheap, easy to obtain, and (because they are absorbed through the lungs) rapidly effective. These drugs produce changes in the way users see color, size, or the shape of objects. Sometimes they cause actual hallucinations. They can also alter a user's mood, ideas, or sense of time. They are especially popular with young people—about 20% of late adolescents have used them, though mainly when they were younger.

PCP. PCP is cheap, but its (mostly) young male users especially value the euphoria it produces. Some experience psychosis so convincing that, in the absence of adequate history, it cannot be distinguished from schizophrenia.

LSD. LSD (its chemical name, rarely used, is lysergic acid diethylamide) is emblematic of the hallucinogens, which do not usually produce hallucinations at all, but rather illusions. In Canada, they are sometimes called *illusionogens*. At only about 3% past-year prevalence for graduating high school seniors, LSD may be less popular now than it once was; other drugs in the class are probably used more often (an example is MDMA or ecstasy, one of the so-called "designer drugs"). The hallucinogens can affect patients in two ways: intoxication and flashbacks, which DSM-5 somewhat clumsily calls hallucinogen persisting perception disorder.

MARIJUANA. Finally, there is cannabis (marijuana), the illicit drug of choice in the United States—and one that has, by this writing, been legalized in several jurisdictions for both medicinal and recreational use. By graduation, nearly a third of high school students have tried it. Those who use it feel that it sharpens their perceptions or reduces anxiety. Illusions may occur, but hallucinations rarely do.

Tobacco

Here's an oddity: DSM-5 includes tobacco withdrawal, but *still* does not mention tobacco intoxication. Of course, when nicotine is taken in great enough quantity by a naïve user, toxic symptoms are there aplenty (ask any kid who's tried one of Dad's stogies). It is also the most widely used addictive drug in the United States, and perhaps in the world.

Other (or Unknown)

Other mind-altering substances include anabolic steroids (which may be misused by athletes who want to perform better and by others to enhance physical attractiveness). Nitrous oxide ("laughing gas") produces euphoria, and a variety of over-the-counter and prescription drugs (including antihistamines, antiparkinsonian drugs, and cortisone) may be used to produce other states of altered consciousness. Finally, the "unknown" category is used when a patient has obviously ingested a substance, but its exact nature cannot be determined.

APPLICATION OF THE BASIC CONCEPTS IN CLINICAL PRACTICE

The Essential Features of Substance Use Disorder (p. 401) are necessary for the evaluation of any patient suspected of misuse of alcohol or other substances. They can be used with the Essential Features of Substance Intoxication and Substance Withdrawal specific to various drug classes (pp. 403 and 404), and with Table 24.1, which summarizes and codes the mental disorders that can be associated with each class of substance in children and adolescents. Below, we use a single vignette to illustrate the application of the basic DSM-5 concepts in clinical practice.

Rodney

"It was so hard to start, I had no idea it would be harder to stop." Rodney was almost 17, but he looked a lot younger as he lay on his back in a hospital bed, his left arm in a sling and his right leg strung up by pulleys. He didn't recall much about the accident that had put him there. It involved quite a few brandy Alexanders and way too little instruction about hanging onto the passenger bar of the Honda motorcycle driven by his roommate. His only injuries were skeletal, and he was clear-headed enough to realize that he badly needed a smoke.

Rodney was probably the smartest kid ever born in his part of Texas. By the time he was 12, he was already attending high school classes, had won several statewide scholastic contests, and had appeared twice on a popular TV quiz show. When he was 14, his parents reluctantly let him accept a full-tuition scholarship to a small but prestigious liberal arts college several hundred miles from home.

"Of course, I was the smallest one there—except for one guy with some sort of an endocrine disorder," said Rodney. "I didn't really think about it at the time, but I'm sure I started smoking and drinking to compensate for my size." After he had stopped feeling nauseated and dizzy every time he lit up, one of his classmates had taught him to blow one small smoke ring right through the center of another, larger one.

By the time Rodney had been in college 6 months, he was smoking a pack and a half a day of cigarettes. When studying for exams (unless he got the highest grade in the class, he invariably felt that he wasn't "measuring up"), he found himself sometimes lighting one cigarette from another, going through several packs in a day this way—far more than he had intended. The following year, in a mandatory health class, he read the Surgeon General's report on smoking and saw a video about lung cancer ("in living—no, *dying*—color"). Although he swore he'd never smoke again, his resolve lasted exactly 48 hours. For two nights he couldn't sleep, and he noticed that he had become restless, depressed, and "so irritable my roommate begged me to light up again." Over the next year, he had tried twice more to quit. Once he attended Smoke Enders; when that failed, he asked the student health service for nicotine patches. "They wouldn't give them to me without parental consent—I'm going to be a senior in 4 months!"

TABLE 24.1. ICD-10 Code Numbers for Substance Intoxication, Substance Withdrawal, Substance Use Disorder, and Substance/Medication–Induced Mental Disorders

Substance and use disorder (or not)	Substance use/intoxication/withdrawal			Substance/medication-induced disorders										
	Just use	Intoxication	Withdrawal	Psychotic	Mood	Anxiety	OCD	Sleep	Sex	Delirium I	Delirium W	NCD major	NCD mild	Unspecified
				I/W[a]	I/W	I/W		I/W	I/W	I	W	I/W	I/W	I/W
Alcohol F10														
w/mild use dis.	.10	.129		.159	.14	.180		.182	.181	.121	.121			.99
w/mod./severe use dis.	.20	.229	.239 (.232)[b]	.259	.24	.280		.282	.281	.221	.231	.27 (.26)[c]	.288	
No use disorder		.929		.959	.94	.980		.982	.981	.921	.921	.97 (.96)[c]	.988	
Caffeine F15						I		I/W						.99
w/mild use dis.						.180		.182						
w/mod./severe use dis.						.280		.282						
No use disorder		.929	.93			.980		.982						
Cannabis F12				I		I		I/W						.99
w/mild use dis.	.10	.129 (.122)[b]		.159		.180		.188		.121				
w/mod./severe use dis.	.20	.229 (.222)[b]	.288	.259		.280		.288		.221				
No use disorder		.929 (.922)[b]		.959		.980		.988		.921				

(cont.)

Note. Abbreviations in column heads: OCD, obsessive–compulsive and related disorder; Sleep, sleep disorder; Sex, sexual dysfunction; Delirium I, intoxication delirium; Delirium W, withdrawal delirium; NCD, neurocognitive disorder.

[a] I, occurs during intoxication; W, occurs during withdrawal; I/W, occurs during either.

[b] Two numbers in a cell indicate separate codes for intoxication or withdrawal without (or with) perceptual disturbances.

[c] Alcohol NCD can occur without or with confabulation and amnestic syndrome. The number in parentheses is for the amnestic–confabulatory type.

[d] This code is for hallucinogen persisting perception disorder (see Essential Features of Substance Withdrawal, p. 404).

[e] For inhalants and opioids, you can only have depressive mood disorders, not bipolar ones.

[f] Opioid withdrawal delirium has only two numbers after the decimal.

[g] Delirium due to medications taken as prescribed that don't fit one of these drug classes should be coded F19.921.

TABLE 24.1 (cont.)

Substance and use disorder (or not)	Substance use/intoxication/withdrawal			Substance/medication-induced disorders										
	Just use	Intoxication	Withdrawal	Psychotic	Mood	Anxiety	OCD	Sleep	Sex	Delirium I	Delirium W	NCD major	NCD mild	Unspecified
Phencyclidine F16				I	I	I								.99
w/mild use dis.	.10	.129		.159	.14	.180				.121				
w/ mod./severe use dis.	.20	.229		.259	.24	.280				.221				
No use disorder		.929		.959	.94	.980				.921				
Other hallucinogen F16			.983[d]	I	I	I								.99
w/mild use dis.	.10	.129		.159	.14	.180				.121				
w/mod./severe use dis.	.20	.229		.259	.24	.280				.221				
No use disorder		.929		.959	.94	.980				.921				
Inhalant F18				I	I	I						I		.99
w/mild use dis.	.10	.129		.159	.14[e]	.180				.121		.17	.188	
w/ mod./severe use dis.	.20	.229		.259	.24[e]	.280				.221		.27	.288	
No use disorder		.929		.959	.94[e]	.980				.921		.97	.988	
Opioid F11					I/W	W		I/W	I/W					.99
w/mild use dis.	.10	.129 (.122)[b]			.14[e]	.188		.182	.181	.121	.121			
w/mod./severe use dis.	.20	.229 (.222)[b]	.23		.24[e]	.288		.282	.281	.221	.23[f]			
No use disorder		.929 (.922)[b]		.959	.94[e]	.988		.982	.981	.921	.921			
Sed./hyp./anx. F13				I/W	I/W	W		I/W	I/W			I/W	I/W	.99
w/mild use dis.	.10	.129		.159	.14	.180		.182	.181	.121	.121			
w/ mod./severe use dis.	.20	.229	.239 (.232)[b]	.259	.24	.280		.282	.281	.221	.231	.27	.288	
No use disorder		.929		.959	.94	.980		.982	.981	.921	.921	.97	.988	

				I	I/W	I/W	I/W	I/W	I/W	I	I	I/W	I/W	I/W	
Amphetamine F15																
w/mild use dis.	.10	.129 (.122)[b]		.159	.14	.180	.188	.182	.181	.121						.99
w/mod./severe use dis.	.20	.229 (.222)[b]	.23	.259	.24	.280	.288	.282	.281	.221						
No use disorder		.929 (.922)[b]		.959	.94	.980	.988	.982	.981	.921						
Cocaine F14																
w/mild use dis.	.10	.129 (.122)[b]		.159	.14	.180	.188	.182	.181	.121						.99
w/mod./severe use dis.	.20	.229 (.222)[b]	.23	.259	.24	.280	.288	.282	.281	.221						
No use disorder		.929 (.922)[b]		.959	.94	.980	.988	.982	.981	.921						
Tobacco F17																
w/mild use dis.	Z72.0							W								.209
w/mod./severe use dis.	F17.200		.203					.208								
No use disorder																
Other (unknown) F19						I/W	I/W	I/W	I/W	I/W	I/W	I/W	I/W	I/W	I/W	
w/mild use dis.	.10	.129		.159	.14	.180	.188	.182	.181	.121	.121	.17	.188			.99
w/mod./severe use dis.	.20	.229	.239	.259	.24	.280	.288	.282	.281	.221	.231	.27	.288			
No use disorder		.929		.959	.94	.980	.988	.982	.981	.921[g]	.921	.97	.988			

Note. Abbreviations in column heads: OCD, obsessive–compulsive and related disorder; Sleep, sleep disorder; Sex, sexual dysfunction; Delirium I, intoxication delirium; Delirium W, withdrawal delirium; NCD, neurocognitive disorder.

[a] Two numbers in a cell indicate separate codes for intoxication or withdrawal without (or with) perceptual disturbances.

[c] This code is for hallucinogen persisting perception disorder (see Essential Features of Substance Withdrawal, p. 404).

[e] For inhalants and opioids, you can only have depressive mood disorders, not bipolar ones.

[f] Opioid withdrawal delirium has only two numbers after the decimal.

[g] Delirium due to medications taken as prescribed that don't fit one of these drug classes should be coded F19.921.

Rodney's parents worked in the small-town feed and seed store they'd owned for years. Both were hard-working churchgoers who had never touched a drop of alcohol. Growing up in the same small community, both had been appalled at what alcohol had done to their own fathers. Several times in the last few months, when he was so badly hung over he couldn't attend classes, Rodney had vaguely wondered whether he was about to follow in his grandfathers' unsteady footsteps.

The only bright spot, he observed wryly as he shifted uncomfortably in the hospital bed, was that "when I fell off the Honda, I was so drunk I didn't feel a thing." At first it was assumed that he had a concussion, but the blood alcohol level of 0.25 suggested simple intoxication. He had awakened 12 hours later with pins through his femur and a terrific hangover. Now, 2 days later, his vital signs were stable and normal—except for a pulse rate of only 56.

"I don't suppose you could smuggle in some nicotine gum?" Rodney asked.

Evaluation of Rodney

We'll start in this necessarily long discussion with Rodney's smoking. The Essential Features of Substance Use Disorder (p. 401) include behaviors that suggest problems with either physiology or control. Rodney's smoking involved several of the latter, each of which, as the criteria require, had occurred during the preceding 12 months. He had sometimes spent a great deal of time using nicotine (chain-smoking—Criterion A3), and he sometimes smoked more than he intended (A1). He no longer experienced the nausea and dizziness typical of those new to smoking; this, according to DSM-5, was evidence of tolerance (A10b). Later, he had spent much time trying to stop (A2). Right there are four (only two are required) of the criteria for tobacco use disorder.

Should Rodney also be diagnosed with tobacco withdrawal? For evidence, we must look at the specific criteria for tobacco withdrawal (p. 404). He had smoked every day for longer than the minimum of "several weeks" (Criterion A). On at least two occasions, he had suffered from typical withdrawal symptoms: restlessness (B5), depression (B6), irritability (B1), and trouble sleeping (B7). Although these symptoms did not impair his functioning when he was in the hospital, they were distressing, and they had previously caused a social problem with his roommate (C). Assuming that he had no other medical issues that could explain his symptoms (the accident was recent and wouldn't account for symptoms during his previous attempts to quit), we can diagnose tobacco withdrawal and add it to the list of symptoms (A11) supporting a diagnosis of tobacco use disorder; the total of five would earn him a severity specifier of *moderate*. Note that in DSM-5, a patient who is so seriously ill as to be in withdrawal is automatically considered to have a substance use disorder (for whatever substance it is), and one that is either moderate or severe.

At the time of his hospitalization, then, Rodney's diagnosis would read in part:

| F17.203 | Tobacco withdrawal |
| F17.200 | Tobacco use disorder, moderate |

Next, let's consider Rodney's alcohol use. Rodney had never had a lot of trouble with alcohol, but he'd had some. More than once or twice, he'd failed in his obligation to attend school, but DSM-5 requires two or more symptoms for a diagnosis of alcohol use disorder. Sure, riding a motorcycle when intoxicated was also physically dangerous, but he would have had to do it repeatedly to qualify, and this incident was apparently a one-off. (Because experimentation with substances is the rule in young people, making conscientious use of the criteria for substance use disorder is, if anything, even more important than it is for adults.) We would want to make a note in his hospital discharge summary that indicates our concern about Rodney's drinking; we'd also suggest to him that he obtain counseling to address all of his substance use.

Would Rodney meet criteria for alcohol intoxication? They are not demanding—they require only one symptom mentioned in the Essential Features. From Rodney's vignette, we can infer at least two: incoordination and loss of memory. Besides, with a blood alcohol level of 0.25, only a pedant would insist on formal criteria. The code number we would extract from Table 24.1 would be determined by the substance (alcohol), the type of problem (intoxication), and whether the patient also can be diagnosed with a substance use disorder (no).

The differential diagnosis for substance-related disorders spans the mental and physical diagnostic spectrum. Children and adolescents should also be carefully considered for those mental disorders that are often associated with the substance-related conditions, most notably the **mood** and **anxiety disorders**. **Eating disorders** have been reported with particular frequency among substance-misusing girls, and **conduct disorder** and **ADHD** among substance-misusing boys.

Note that the GAF score, which for Rodney would be relatively high at admission, is not supposed to be based on any information concerning a patient's physical condition or environmental situation. (On the other hand, the WHODAS—the World Health Association Disability Assessment Schedule, the system that DSM-5 currently favors—does heavily reflect physical disability.) Rodney's full diagnosis at his admission to the hospital would therefore read as follows:

F17.203	Tobacco withdrawal
F17.200	Tobacco use disorder, moderate
F10.929	Alcohol intoxication
S42.202A	Fractured of left humerus, upper end, closed
S72.301B	Open fracture, shaft (middle third), right femur
GAF 70	(on admission)

Now let's consider what we would say about Rodney at the time of a reevaluation 3 months later. If he had quit smoking, he would probably no longer be in tobacco withdrawal. After no symptoms of substance use disorder other than craving have been experienced for 3 months, a person can be said to be in early remission; after 1 year, it's a sustained remission. So at follow-up, if Rodney was also using a nicotine patch, his diagnosis would be the following:

F17.200   Tobacco use disorder, moderate, in early remission, on maintenance therapy

GAF   75 (current)

ASSESSING SUBSTANCE-RELATED DISORDERS

General Suggestions

Especially with an adolescent patient, obtaining information about substance use often means trying to extract something that is private from someone who wishes to keep it that way. If you encounter an adolescent who is still intoxicated, you may observe classic signs, such as red eyes or slurred speech. It is far more likely, however, that you will have to depend on historical information from a sober patient—and informants. If this is your first contact, you may need multiple sessions to explore this area.

Some young people will be more likely than others to misuse substances: older children and adolescents; those whose parents have had substance use problems; those who have been the victims of physical or sexual abuse; those with other mental disorders (especially mood disorders); and boys, far more than girls. No young patient can be considered completely immune, of course, and the area of substance use is one of four in the pediatric mental health interview that should be considered "must cover." (The others are sex, suicide, and sexual/physical trauma.)

You will probably fare better if you delay asking about this and other sensitive information (misconduct, sex, history of physical or sexual abuse) until well along in the interview, when you have established some rapport. Before you start, it is often wise to set some ground rules, as described in Part I of this book: "If you feel you can't talk about something, please don't lie to me—just say, 'Let's talk about something else.'" You may also want to reemphasize what you have already agreed you will (or won't) relate to parents. Of course, if you've waited to excuse parents from the room until this sensitive topic is broached, you may reduce the amount of relevant information you will collect. If the patient already knows that suspected substance use is the reason for the evaluation, you might acknowledge the fact: "It seems your folks are worried that [type of substance] use may be hurting you. What do you think?"

You might begin by inquiring about alcohol, tobacco, and marijuana, and by assuming that most teens have experimented with some of these socially more acceptable drugs: "What experiences have you had with alcohol [or one of the others]?" With luck, you will get a fair run of information from this open-ended question. Be alert for contradictions and ask frankly for clarification: "I'm confused. First you said . . . , but now you say. . . . Which do you mean?" Watch for body language that suggests prevarication: shifts in posture, lowered gaze, hesitation before answering.

You could also start by asking about peers' involvement with alcohol and drugs. By putting some distance between the teen and the behavior, this device could yield a more truthful account. Another nonthreatening introduction might be to ask about drugs that others use at the patient's school: "How hard would it be for someone to buy pot at your school?" After ascertaining some of these generalities, it is easier to inquire into the teen's own usage. Even then, you might want to start slowly with some history: "How old were you when you had your first beer?"

Of course, the patient can confound any approach at all by simply refusing to talk. Then you may have to invite a discussion of feelings: "I can see that this subject makes you [angry, sad, anxious]. I can't say I blame you . . . " (Similarly acknowledge and accept profanity, which may be used as a shield against unwelcome questions.) Occasionally, an adolescent may try to deflect questions about substances by offering up instances of substance use by parents or other relatives. In such a case, obtain this valuable information about family members, but then use it as a springboard back to the patient: "Now tell me about *your* experience with alcohol." If a patient minimizes (or denies) substance use in the face of evidence to the contrary, you may have to force a confrontation—preferably, after you have established a relationship solid enough to survive one. "Let's see, you say that you've never tried pot, but last week your mom found paraphernalia in your pants pocket. I don't understand that."

The information you need is extensive and varied. For each drug used, try to learn the following:

- Frequency and duration of use
- Average amount of use per episode
- The valued effect of use (for example, to feel high, to ease social awkwardness, to promote introspection)
- The consequences of use (medical problems such as blackouts, or other evidence of substance use disorder)
- The patient's means of financing drug or alcohol use (lunch money, stealing from parents, other illegal activities)

And don't forget to ask about the abuse of prescription and over-the-counter prescriptions.

Developmental Factors

Adolescents are more likely than adults to experience severe toxicity, even to the extent of lapsing into coma. Intoxication in young children suggests child abuse or neglect. Age is also associated with drug of choice: Inhalants and marijuana are more popular among young people than among adults. However, in view of the time required for the development of full-blown substance use disorder, its likelihood increases with advancing age.

The story of substance use treatment might be titled "Too Little, Too Late." Although problem drinking typically starts in early adolescence, we too seldom suspect drinking and drug problems when they first occur. Some writers note that learning disorders and problematic social skills often precede substance use, but recognizing the connection in an individual patient presents a challenge that has yet to be surmounted. Even once substance use issues have been detected, disorders that are typically comorbid—mood disorders, anxiety disorders, conduct disorder, and ADHD—may be missed. The overall outcome is, predictably, vast undertreatment of substance use in American youth.

CHAPTER 25

Cognitive Disorders

QUICK GUIDE TO THE COGNITIVE DISORDERS

Delirium

A delirium is a rapidly developing, fluctuating state of reduced awareness in which a patient has trouble with orientation and shifting or focusing attention; *and* there's at least one defect of memory, orientation, perception, visual–spatial ability, or language; *and* the symptoms aren't better explained by coma or dementia. In young patients, the following types of delirium can be diagnosed:

Delirium due to another medical condition. Delirium can be caused by trauma to the brain, infections, epilepsy, endocrine disorders, and various other diseases throughout the body (p. 418).

Substance intoxication delirium, substance withdrawal delirium, and medication-induced delirium. Alcohol and other sedative drugs of abuse, as well as nearly every class of street drug, can cause delirium. Medications and poisons can also be implicated (p. 418).

Other specified, or unspecified, delirium. Use one of these categories when a patient's delirium doesn't meet the criteria for any of the types described in DSM-5 or when you don't know the cause (p. 422).

Major and Mild Neurocognitive Disorder

From a previous level of functioning, the patient has experienced a decline in at least one of these symptom domains: complex attention, learning and memory, perceptual–motor ability, executive functioning, language, and social cognition. The time course of a neurocognitive disorder (NCD) is usually slow (as compared to delirium), and the cause is usually located within the central nervous system. If there's any impairment in the ability to focus or shift attention, it isn't prominent. One of the following diagnoses will usually apply:

NCD due to traumatic brain injury. Open or closed head injuries can lead to varying degrees of cognitive dysfunction (p. 425).

NCD due to another medical condition. A large number of medical conditions, most of which are rare in children and adolescents, can cause cognitive symptoms. These include brain tumor, Creutzfeldt–Jakob disease, Huntington's disease, Parkinson's disease, HIV disease, and adrenoleukodystrophy.* The most common intermediate paths resulting from medical conditions are kidney and liver failure (p. 424).

Substance/medication-induced NCD. In adults, some 5–10% of NCDs stem from use of alcohol, inhalants, or sedatives, but these are rare in children and adolescents.

Unspecified NCD. This diagnosis is used when the cause for a patient's NCD is not known or the NCD does not meet the criteria for any of the types described in DSM-5 (p. 430).

*Featured in the 1992 Academy Award-nominated film *Lorenzo's Oil.*

INTRODUCTION

Although a specific underlying etiological agent cannot always be identified, cognitive disorders are caused by physical medical conditions or by the use of psychoactive substances. In each case, the result is a defect of brain anatomy, chemistry, or physiology that leads to problems in the domains mentioned above. Two main groups of cognitive disorders have relevance for children and adolescents: delirium, and major and mild neurocognitive disorder (NCD). In this chapter, we discuss these two groups of disorders with two case vignettes. (We also briefly mention unspecified NCD, which is a "catch-all" category for cognitive symptoms that do not meet the criteria for either delirium or NCD.)

Two brief notes on terminology are also in order. Although DSM-5 refers (confusingly, in our view) to this entire group of disorders as the *neurocognitive disorders*, in addition to designating the various forms of major and mild NCD as specific disorders, we are continuing to use the DSM-IV term *cognitive disorders* for the diagnoses covered in this chapter. We also occasionally use the older term *dementia* to refer to major NCD.

DELIRIUM

F05 Delirium Due to Another Medical Condition

Substance Intoxication Delirium, Substance Withdrawal Delirium, and Medication–Induced Delirium

Delirium is the most common cognitive disorder—and, by some accounts, the most common of all mental disorders. Young children, who are easy prey to fever and infection, are especially vulnerable. Other causes in young patients include endocrine dysfunction, drug withdrawal or toxicity (notably anticholinergics), vitamin deficiency, liver or kidney disease, poisons, and anesthesia during surgical operations. Note that most of these causes usually start somewhere in the body other than the brain.

Delirium involves two main sorts of symptoms: (1) difficulty with wandering attention and orientation, and (2) one or more additional cognitive changes. The symptoms develop rapidly, within a period of days or even hours, and are often more pronounced at night. See the Essential Features (p. 421).

In the midst of a conversation or during a favorite activity, a delirious child or adolescent may lapse into the stupor of half-sleep (altered attention) and appear unaware of the surroundings (reduced orientation). Some delirious patients may think less quickly, appear vague, or have difficulty solving problems. You might have to ask questions several times before such a patient answers. Other patients may seem hyperalert and distractible, shifting attention rapidly from one stimulus to another. (Picture a child with high fever who thrashes about in bed and keeps glancing into the corners of the room.) Still other patients, especially those whose delirium is caused by metabolic factors, may instead experience a slowing of physical movement.

The cognitive deficit can manifest itself as one or more problems with language, memory, orientation, or perception:

- The *language* of delirium is rambling; it may be pressured or incoherent. Older children and adolescents may have trouble writing. However, speech that is only slurred, without being incoherent, doesn't indicate delirium.

- *Memory* is nearly always impaired, with recent memory affected first. Retention and recall are also disturbed; patients typically later recall little of their delirious experiences.

- Delirious children and adolescents are often *disoriented*. They may fail to recognize their surroundings; they may misidentify parents or other people familiar to them. Those old enough to be fully aware of dates, months, seasons, and years usually lose orientation to time first. Only in extreme cases does a patient lose awareness of personal identity.

- Distorted *perception* may be experienced in varying degrees of severity. In mild or early delirium, surroundings may appear less clear than usual: Boundaries are fuzzy, colors too bright, images distorted. Adolescents and older children may be able to describe some of these symptoms. As thinking becomes more seriously disordered, patients may experience *illusions*, which are misinterpretations of actual sensory stimuli. Still further advanced across this spectrum are *hallucinations*, which are false perceptions in the absence of an actual sensory stimulus. Younger children are especially likely to respond to illusions or hallucinations with fear or anxiety.

Delirium usually begins suddenly and often fluctuates during the course of the day. Usually this means that patients are more lucid during the morning and less so at night—a characteristic known as *sundowning*. Delirious children are also likely to show emotional lability, suspiciousness, social withdrawal, or oppositional behavior. Most deliriums are relatively short-lived, lasting a week or less, resolving quickly once the underlying cause has been relieved.

Table 24.1 lists the specific types of substance use delirium you could find in children and adolescents. Although the code numbers are specific, the criteria are pretty general. Note that coding depends on the type of substance used, whether the delirium was sustained during intoxication or withdrawal, and whether it was used in the context of a substance use disorder. (Mostly, this is material that will interest the people who code medical records.) The exact name of the substance ingested should be used when a diagnosis is made. Note also that substance intoxication (or withdrawal) *delirium* and just plain substance intoxication (or withdrawal) due to the same substance should not be diagnosed together; whenever symptoms are severe enough to warrant the delirium diagnosis, it should stand alone. Finally, remember that delirium can be induced by the use of a prescribed medication, and that in such cases it is almost always due to toxicity. Such medications are categorized as "other" substances and coded with the exact names of the medications, followed by "-induced" (rather than "intoxication").

Max

Max was 5 when he was brought to the children's ward of the community hospital in a Midwestern university town. Max and Deborah, his 6-year-old sister, lived with their maternal grandparents, who told the clerk in the urgent care unit that Max had been well until that afternoon, when he had come in from play. At first they thought he was just tired; within an hour he appeared drunk. When he intentionally urinated in a corner of the living room, they realized that something was terribly wrong and brought him in for evaluation. A frightened Deborah related that while the two children were playing doctor, Max had swallowed several tablets of their grandfather's medications. The pill bottles she produced contained diazepam and amitriptyline.

During the initial examination that evening, Max seemed lethargic. He did not have toxic blood levels of tricyclics, or an EKG abnormality that would warrant transferring him to the intensive care unit. Though he could be aroused, his gaze drifted off to the curtains at the side of his bed when staff members were trying to talk to him. For a time his mood was euphoric, and he talked about being a doctor—as if he were one already.

Later that evening he seemed fearful and agitated; he moved restlessly in his bed, apparently trying to find a nickel he thought he had lost. He misidentified a nurse as his mother and called a ballpoint pen a gun. Then he volunteered, "I'm not a new skateboard—I'm a Frenchie." At different times he said he was at home and "in a prison for dogs." His agitation prevented a complete reading of the EEG obtained that evening, but "severe disorganization and slowing" were reported.

ESSENTIAL FEATURES OF **DELIRIUM**

Over a short time, a patient develops problems with wandering attention and with orientation, especially to the environment; additional cognitive changes (memory, use of language, disorientation in other spheres, perception, visual–motor capability) set in. Severity fluctuates during the day. The cause can be a physical condition, substance use, toxicity, or some combination.

The Fine Print

The D's: • Duration of onset (hours to days; generally brief, though it can endure) • Differential diagnosis (major neurocognitive disorder, coma, psychotic disorders)

Coding Notes

Specify if:

Hyperactive. Agitation or otherwise increased active.
Hypoactive. Reduced psychomotor activity.
Mixed level of activity. Normal or fluctuating activity levels.

Specify duration:

Acute. Lasts hours to a few days.
Persistent. Lasts weeks or longer.

Code numbers for substance- (and medication-)caused delirium are given in Table 24.1.

Max slept most of the following day, but within 48 hours of admission he was much improved. Now he could name the hospital, identify his grandparents and an already-favorite nurse, and correctly name everyday objects. The following day he was discharged as recovered.

Evaluation of Max

Max's level of consciousness was clearly compromised on the evening of and the day following his admission; he was often drowsy and he could not sustain his attention for longer than a few moments (Criterion A1). Cognitive change (C) was evident in his problems with language (much that he said was gibberish), orientation, and perception. These symptoms had developed within a few hours (B) of ingesting medications known to be toxic (in overdose) to the central nervous system (E).

The most common alternative to consider in the differential diagnosis for delirium is **mild or major NCD,** the likelihood of which we can discount partly by the rapidity of onset, partly by the absence of a candidate etiology (D). The presence of hallucinations might suggest a **psychotic disorder,** which the acute onset would also rule out. Although in any child who presents as Max did, we'd have to consider other **medical conditions** (such as head trauma and infectious disease) that can cause delirium, the vital information obtained from his sister pinpointed the etiology. DSM-5 points out that **malingering** and **factitious disorder** should also be considered when the symptoms are less than classical for delirium and when no causative agent is obvious, but either of these would be rare in a child.

Note that we wouldn't consider Max's condition a medication-induced delirium, which is a diagnosis used when symptoms are side effects of a drug taken as prescribed. Although the drugs involved in Max's delirium would receive exactly the same code number, because each contributed to the intoxication, each would be coded separately as determined from Table 24.1. Living apart from both parents could complicate the care of Max and his sister, so it was coded as specifically as possible. Max's full diagnosis would thus be as follows:

F19.121	Diazepam intoxication delirium, hypoactive
F19.121	Amitriptyline intoxication delirium, hypoactive
Z62.29	Separated from parents (living with grandparents)
CGAS	90 (on discharge)

R41.0 Other Specified Delirium

R41.0 Unspecified Delirium

The other specified and unspecified delirium diagnoses should be reserved for cases that do not meet the criteria for the types of delirium described above, or for any cases where the cause is not known. Use the other specified category when you wish to indicate why a case does not meet criteria for any of the other types.

SYMPTOM DOMAINS

DSM-5 describes six areas (domains) that are central to understanding all cognitive disorders, but especially what is now termed mild or major NCD.

Complex Attention

By *complex attention,* we mean the ability to focus on tasks so that distractions don't derail their completion. More than the simple attention span evaluated by asking a patient to repeat a string of numbers or to spell a word backward, complex attention involves processing speed, keeping items of information in mind, and being able to do more than one thing at a time, such as solving homework problems while watching a music video. In mild NCD, the patient can still perform tasks, though it may require additional effort.

Learning and Memory

Memory exists in many variations. The acronym PEWS provides a simple mnemonic:

- *Procedural memory.* This type of memory allows us to learn a sequence of behaviors and repeat them, without having to expend conscious effort—so that we can exercise skills such as riding a bike and playing the piano.

- *Episodic memory.* This is the memory for the events we experience as personal history—what you got for your 12th birthday, where you spent your last vacation, your dessert choice at supper yesterday. Episodic memory is often visual and always takes the individual's point of view.

- *Working memory.* Here we mean the very short-term storing of data that we are actively processing. We test it by asking a patient to do mental arithmetic or spell words backward. It is often regarded as synonymous with *attention.*

- *Semantic memory.* This is the type of memory that involves general knowledge—in short, facts and figures. It's where most of what we learn ends up, because we no longer associate it with anything concrete in our lives, such as where we were when the learning took place.

Working memory is brief, lasting perhaps a few minutes. In the other divisions, memories may endure for many years, though episodic memories tend to last more briefly than semantic ones.

If memory deteriorates, it takes more time to process information. For instance, a person might have trouble performing mental arithmetic or repeating back a story that was just related, or holding in mind a telephone number long enough to dial it. With advancing NCD, the little assists that once helped out lose their punch.

Perceptual–Motor Ability

Perceptual–motor ability refers to the ability to assimilate and use visual information. Although vision itself is normal, a person has trouble navigating the immediate environment, especially when perceptual cues are reduced (as at twilight or nighttime). Handwork and crafts take extra effort; copying a design onto a sheet of paper may present problems. As with other attributes of neurocognitive functioning, problems in this domain exist on a continuum from nil to mild to major.

Executive Functioning

Executive functioning is the mechanism we use to organize simple ideas and bits of behavior into more complex ones on the way to a goal—getting dressed, following a route, completing homework. Patients with defective executive functioning have trouble interpreting new information and adapting to new situations. Planning and decision making are hard; behavior becomes determined by habit, rather than by reason and feedback-driven error correction.

Language

The category of *language* comprises both receptive and expressive language; the latter includes naming (the ability to state the name of an object such as a fountain pen), fluency, grammar, and syntax (structure of language). Some patients may use circumlocutions to get around words they can't remember. Their speech may become vague, circumstantial, and cliché-ridden; in the end, they may become completely mute.

Social Cognition

By *social cognition*, we refer to the processes that help us recognize the emotions of other people and respond appropriately to them. Social cognition includes decision making, empathy, moral judgment, knowledge of social norms, emotional processing, and *theory of mind*—the ability to imagine that other people have beliefs and desires, and to recognize that others may have ideas different from our own. Someone whose social cognition is deficient may have trouble recognizing the emotion in a facial expression. Some of these people may appear overly friendly; others don't adhere to accepted standards of propriety or conventional social interaction.

MAJOR AND MILD NEUROCOGNITIVE DISORDER

Neurocognitive Disorder Due to Another Medical Condition

On the face of it, childhood NCD seems a contradiction in terms. Childhood is a period of growth, but NCD is actually a decline—as an example, think of NCD due to Alzheimer's disease. Of course, Alzheimer's doesn't affect children or adolescents; nor does substance/medication-induced NCD occur often enough in young patients to warrant more than a mention here. However, children and adolescents can fall prey to some NCD-inducing medical conditions, such as head trauma and HIV disease. Then the Essential Features of NCD (p. 426) can be diagnosed any time after the age of 3 or 4, which is the youngest age at which intelligence can first be reliably measured with objective tests.

In contrast to delirium, the site of underlying pathology in NCD is within the tissues of the brain itself. Although we usually think of dementia as permanent and often progressing inexorably, in some cases it is reversible. Such an outcome is most likely in the case of young children, whose brains are still resilient enough to recover from injuries that would permanently incapacitate an adult.

NCD usually begins gradually. A child may lose interest in school or in recreational activities. Judgment and impulse control begin to suffer. With reduced ability to understand, analyze, and remember, patients of any age must get through the day by relying upon the skeleton of old habits. For children, that is often a fragile structure.

All patients with NCD have the following features in common:

- *Decline.* Regardless of severity (mild or major NCD), there is a regression from a previous level of functioning. Although patients who have always functioned at a low level (such as those with intellectual disability) are not automatically considered to have dementia, such a child can develop NCD, just like anyone else. As is now well known, many patients with Down syndrome develop NCD due to Alzheimer's disease later in life.

- *Formal evaluation.* The decline must be enough to cause a patient to score below accepted norms on standardized testing, or to cause the caregiver to reach the same conclusions based on clinical evaluation.

- *Not a delirium.* If symptoms occur only when a patient is delirious, NCD cannot be diagnosed. The two conditions can occur together, however—as when a child who has NCD due to traumatic brain injury is given a medication that induces a substance intoxication delirium.

- *No better explanation.* Other mental disorders (such as schizophrenia, which was once called *dementia praecox*) don't better account for the symptoms.

- *Impairment.* Finally, the important difference between major and mild NCD is this: In the former, loss of cognitive ability definitely affects the patient's school, work, or social life. In the latter, functioning isn't impaired, but the patient has to try extra hard or rely on special help or reminders to get things done. One way or another, patients with mild NCD can still get along independently; patients with major NCD/dementia cannot.

Neurocognitive Disorder Due to Traumatic Brain Injury

Many children and adolescents develop an NCD that results from a head injury incurred while roller skating or bicycling, climbing a jungle gym, or engaging in some other physical activity.

ESSENTIAL FEATURES OF
{MAJOR} {MILD} NEUROCOGNITIVE DISORDER

Someone (the patient, a relative, the clinician) suspects that there has been a {marked} {modest} decline in cognitive functioning. On formal testing, the patient scores below accepted norms by {2+} {1–2} standard deviations. (Alternatively, a clinical evaluation reaches the same conclusion.) The symptoms {materially} {do not materially} impair the patient's ability to function independently. That is, the patient {cannot} {can} accommodate to such activities of daily life as paying bills or managing medications by putting forth increased effort or using compensatory strategies (for example, keeping lists).

The Fine Print

One standard deviation (1 *SD*) below norms would be at the 16th percentile; 2 *SD* below norms would be at the 3rd percentile.

The D's: • Duration (symptoms tend to chronicity) • Differential diagnosis (delirium, major depressive disorder [pseudodementia], psychosis)

Coding Notes

Specify if:

> **With behavioral disturbance (*specify type*).** The patient has clinically important behaviors such as agitation, apathy, or responding to hallucinations or having mood problems.
> **Without behavioral disturbance.** No such difficulties.

The wording and actual codes are given in Tables 25.1a and 25.1b.

For major NCD, specify:

> **Mild.** The patient requires help with activities of daily living, such as doing chores or managing an allowance.
> **Moderate.** The patient needs help even with such basics as dressing and eating.
> **Severe.** The patient is fully dependent on others.

Karl

When Karl was 10, he fell off his bike. On a Tuesday just after supper, he left his helmet hanging on his bedroom chair and went off with three friends. His mother had no idea where he was until the hospital called at about 8:30 that evening. He'd been admitted to the trauma center.

Karl's parents had been divorced for years. He and his mother lived in subsidized housing near the center of town. When he wasn't drinking, Karl's father was at sea, tending the engine on a fishing boat. Every few months he would turn up, take Karl to the movies or a ball game, then argue with Karl's mother about money and disappear again.

Perhaps it was this most recent visit, which included an afternoon baseball game, that distracted Karl's attention from the road. Even long after he'd recovered, his memory for that entire day was an almost total blank. The police report stated that he swerved his bicycle into the path of a slowly approaching pickup truck and was tossed several yards into some shrubbery. He awakened hours later to the pain of a splitting headache and a broken arm.

That evening, skull X-rays and a CT scan were read as normal. An EEG obtained just after he had awakened showed nonspecific slowing; at follow-up 2 weeks later, it was completely normal.

Karl was released from the hospital on the third day. Though much of the time he seemed his usual self, he would rapidly become irritable and cross. For a few days, he'd awaken at night and roam about the house for 15 or 20 minutes before going back to bed.

The following Monday, he returned to school. He had always been a good student with an excellent attention span, but for several months after the accident his performance

TABLE 25.1a. Coding for Major and Minor NCDs: Five Etiologies

Etiology[a]	Major NCD due to {probable}{possible} [etiology][b]		Mild NCD {with}{without} behavioral disturbance[c]
	With behavioral disturbance	Without behavioral disturbance	
Alzheimer's disease	G30.9 Alzheimer's disease		(No medical disorder code)
	F02.81	F02.80	
Frontotemporal lobar degeneration	G31.09 Frontotemporal disease		—
	F02.81	F02.80	
Lewy body disease	G31.83 Lewy body disease		G31.84 Mild NCD due to [etiology]
	F02.81	F02.80	
Parkinson's disease	G20 Parkinson's disease		
	F02.81	F02.80	
Vascular disease	—		State whether {probable} {possible}, and {with}{without} behavioral disturbance
	F01.51	F01.50	

[a]Only the five Table 25.1a etiologies for NCD include probable and possible levels of certainty.

[b]Under revised rules (not included in the printed version of DSM-5), we must state in words whether the major NCD is due to *probable* or *possible* disease—the numbering is the same.

[c]In mild NCD, you don't include the suspected causative factor (for example, Alzheimer's disease). That's because the level of certainty as regards cause is so much lower in mild than in major NCD. Also, there's no code number for behavioral disturbance, though you should indicate it in the verbiage. Finally, for each Table 25.1a mild NCD, you can add verbiage indicating whether it is probable or possible; again, however, there is no difference in the code number.

TABLE 25.1b. Coding for Major and Minor NCDs: All Other Etiologies

Etiology	Major NCD[a]		Mild NCD[b]
	With behavioral disturbance	Without behavioral disturbance	
Traumatic brain injury	S06.2X9S[c]		(No medical disorder code)
	F02.81	F02.80	
HIV disease	B20 HIV disease		
	F02.81	F02.80	—
Huntington's disease	G10 Huntington's disease		
	F02.81	F02.80	
Prion disease	A81.9 Prion disease		G31.84
	F02.81	F02.80	Mild NCD due to [etiology]
Other medical condition	## ICD-10 name		
	F02.81	F02.80	
Substance/medication-induced	See Table 24.1		(No statement of {probable}{possible})
Multiple etiologies[d]	(Multiple sets of numbers and names)		
	F02.81	F02.80	

[a]Under revised rules (not included in the printed version of DSM-5), we must state in words whether the major NCD is due to *probable* or *possible* disease—the numbering is the same.

[b]In mild NCD, you don't include the suspected causative factor (for example, HIV disease). That's because the level of certainty as regards cause is so much lower in mild than in major NCD. Also, there's no code number for behavioral disturbance, though you should indicate it in the verbiage.

[c]The two code titles for traumatic brain injury were just too long to squeeze into a table: S06.2X9S = diffuse traumatic brain injury with loss of consciousness of unspecified duration, sequela; 907.0 = late effects of intracranial injury without skull fracture.

[d]If a vascular disorder contributes to the multiple causation, list it as one of multiple causes.

suffered. Three months after his return to class, for the first time in his school career, the "doesn't pay attention in class" box was ticked on his report card. His teacher's comment read, "Karl seems restless and distractible; he frequently gets out of his seat and wanders around the room, disturbing other children. He no longer seems to care about completing his assignments."

"Miss Simpson has actually been wonderful with Karl," his mother offered when she brought him for his next evaluation. "She sends his assignments directly to an app on his phone, so he can remind himself what he needs to do." She explained that the phone only used Wi-Fi, and that it had "an ocean" of parental controls. With it, though he was still pretty forgetful about household chores, he managed to complete most of his homework assignments. But the new bike his father had bought him remained unused in storage at their apartment.

Karl was a slightly built boy who appeared a year or so younger than his stated age. There was no evidence of emerging secondary sex characteristics, and his voice had not yet begun to change. He admitted to having had headaches almost daily since the accident, though he thought that recently they might be getting a little better. He spoke clearly and distinctly, and expressed himself in coherent, linear sentences. He emphatically denied any experiences suggestive of hallucinations or delusions. However, loud talking in the hallway and trucks driving outside the office frequently distracted him; several times, the clinician had to redirect his focus to their conversation.

Evaluation of Karl

Karl had suffered head trauma of the sort commonly associated with very serious NCD. He did have a problem sustaining attention while in school, but there was no evidence of the sort of cognitive change (problems with memory, disorientation, language, or perception) required for **delirium**; nor did his symptoms fluctuate with time of day (Criterion C). Nonetheless, for a long time following his accident, Karl's reduced attention span led to difficulty acquiring new information in class (A1); to determine whether his condition would meet Criterion A2, he would need some neuropsychological testing. His cognitive decline was relatively modest, limited to complex attention, which affected his ability to acquire knowledge. However, he was able to use a compensatory strategy (the app on his phone—Criterion B) to help him pursue his studies independently.

The diagnosis of **personality change due to traumatic brain injury** could eventually be warranted (head trauma certainly can precipitate personality change), but Karl had had his symptoms for

> DSM-5 informs us that for mild NCD, we should not list the putative underlying cause. (This blanket proscription supposedly guards against writing down etiologies about which we cannot be certain—and certainty is not a feature of mild NCD.) However, in a case such as Karl's, where we *are* sure about the underlying cause, we feel an obligation to go against the DSM-5 rule and state the cause in writing. We're confident that the hospital neurologist who consulted on Karl's case did this.

only a few months, and for children this diagnosis requires at least 1 year of altered behavior. Karl's symptoms might also suggest the possibility of a **mood disorder** or **anxiety disorder**. As is true whenever a diagnosis is in doubt, both of these categories should be carefully considered; for Karl, however, the data poorly supported such a diagnosis (D). At the time of evaluation, his full diagnosis would be as follows:

S06.2X9S	Diffuse traumatic brain injury with loss of consciousness of unspecified duration, sequela
G31.84	Mild neurocognitive disorder due to traumatic brain injury, with behavioral disturbance
Z63.5	Disruption of family by divorce
CGAS	80 (upon evaluation)

Although we still often prefer the less cumbersome, readily understood *dementia* in place of *major NCD*, Karl's case illustrates the value of the new DSM-5 terminology. The less pejorative *mild NCD* is often more appropriate for a child or adolescent. It has the ability to describe a condition without the connotation of no treatment options and a lifetime that must be spent with limited cognitive abilities.

R41.9 Unspecified Neurocognitive Disorder

The diagnosis of unspecified NCD should be reserved for either situations where symptoms do not meet the criteria for any of the conditions described elsewhere in this chapter of DSM-5, or (more often) patients for whom there is insufficient evidence to confirm an etiology.

ASSESSING COGNITIVE DISORDERS

General Suggestions

Like most DSM-5 diagnoses, the cognitive disorders can present in a variety of ways, depending on a patient's age and developmental stage (see below). In younger children, behavioral changes may be the most obvious. Especially in delirium, diminished attention span often appears as trouble concentrating. A delirious child may doze off during an interview. Alternatively, a child's difficulty in maintaining focus may show itself as marked, often irritable restlessness. In such a case, if even the parents are unable to soothe their child, delirium may be the cause. Also, picking at bedclothes suggests delirium.

As with every DSM-5 diagnosis, a complete history is vital. Changes in cognitive ability can only be evaluated with respect to previous levels of development. For example, did a child who now has difficulty constructing sentences or remaining continent ever possess these capabilities? The answer spells the difference between a cognitive disorder and developmental delay. Sexual abuse and other psychological problems can also mimic symptoms of NCD.

Careful and repeated observation and assessment are especially important in children who have sustained a traumatic brain injury, whether or not they have been unconscious. Metabolic imbalances or structural brain malfunction may be suggested by physical findings such as tremor, seizures, abnormal posture, or poor visual acuity. Children with cognitive disorders other than delirium may appear slow at study or in initiating play. They have trouble planning activities and are sometimes thought lazy. They may be concrete in their responses, suggesting low intelligence that belies their actual innate ability.

Frontal lobe disinhibition can produce a variety of changes in the personality of a child, who may become oppositional, outspoken, overly talkative, impulsive, careless in grooming, or given to making inappropriate personal comments. Emotions may be described as moody (labile) or irritable.

Developmental Factors

The themes expressed in delirious hallucinations reflect the age of the patient: A young child may dream of peanut butter sandwiches or scenarios featuring abandonment.

The assessment of attention and concentration is particularly difficult in young children, whose cooperation and understanding of tasks are still immature. A diagnosis of NCD requires a demonstration of retreat from a previous cognitive level, so it cannot be made until a child's intellect can be reliably assessed (at about the age of 4 or 5).

The age of the child is a far less important determinant of psychopathology than are the nature, location, and severity of the underlying medical condition. Nonetheless, here are two general principles: (1) The effects of a traumatic brain injury are especially severe in children under the age of 2, who are prone to subdural hematomas; and (2) adolescents, by virtue of their boisterousness, experimentation, activity level, and often faulty judgment, are especially vulnerable to car crashes and other accidental causes of traumatic brain injury.

Head injuries were once the most frequent cause of NCD in children, but a number of other disorders usually encountered in adults may be etiological: Wilson's disease, Huntington's disease, metachromatic leukodystrophy, normal-pressure hydrocephalus, hypothyroidism, brain tumor, and chronic lead exposure. In the 21st century, HIV/AIDS encephalopathy may become the single most frequent cause of NCD in children and adolescents.

CHAPTER 26

Personality Disorders

INTRODUCTION

DSM-5 lists 10 specific personality disorders, divided into three clusters, plus 1 other condition. Because these 11 conditions are so seldom diagnosed in children or adolescents, we do not discuss them individually in this chapter; neither do we provide a Quick Guide. However, we outline them here very briefly for the sake of differential diagnosis.

- *Cluster A.* Generally withdrawn, cold, suspicious, or irrational, patients with Cluster A disorders typically have few friends or close associates. Cluster A includes paranoid, schizoid, and schizotypal personality disorders.

- *Cluster B.* Cluster B disorders are characterized by behavior that is dramatic, emotional, and attention-seeking; by labile, shallow moods; and by intense interpersonal conflicts. Covered here are antisocial, borderline, histrionic, and narcissistic personality disorders.

- *Cluster C.* Patients in Cluster C are often anxious, tense, or overcontrolled. Cluster C includes avoidant, dependent, and obsessive–compulsive personality disorders.

- Another cause of long-standing character disturbance is *personality change due to another medical condition*, in which a physical illness affects how a patient deals with other people. Because it originates in somatic disease, may not be pervasive, and may begin when the patient is no longer young, it does not qualify as a personality disorder.

A number of other mental disorders can distort the way a person behaves and relates to others. Such effects are especially likely in the mood disorders (see Chapter 13), the psychotic disorders (Chapter 12), and the cognitive disorders (Chapter 25).

ISSUES IN DIAGNOSING PERSONALITY DISORDERS IN YOUNG PATIENTS

Although some authorities believe that personality disorders can be reliably diagnosed in adolescents, few would make that claim for children. With the relationships among child disorders, adult disorders, and adult personality disorders still not well worked out, the study of childhood personality disorders is yet in its infancy. Several features of personality disorders limit their application to juveniles, especially young children:

- The DSM-5 criteria for personality disorders require a lifelong pattern of experiences and behaviors. Children (especially younger children) simply haven't lived long enough to attain this standard.

- When personality disorder diagnoses are made in adolescents, they tend to be unstable.

- Changing diagnostic standards promote uncertainty in the diagnostic process. (DSM-5 very nearly abandoned the traditional categorical diagnostic scheme for personality disorders in favor of a dimensional scheme; this move still may occur in a later edition. Meanwhile, the dimensional scheme is included in Section III of DSM-5, "Emerging Measures and Models.")

- In fact, as personality disorder diagnoses fall out of favor (consider the case of passive–aggressive personality disorder), even less stability in this diagnostic process can be assumed.

- Many teenagers and adults qualify for several personality disorder diagnoses.

- According to DSM-5 criteria, the best-validated personality disorder, antisocial personality disorder (ASPD), cannot be diagnosed before the age of 18.

Consider the behavioral symptoms that constitute the attention-deficit and disruptive, impulse-control, and conduct disorders (see Chapters 11 and 23). Over the past several decades, it has been well documented that these behaviors often predict pervasive social difficulties in later life. (These difficulties will not necessarily be severe ones, however; nor do they imply that individuals will continue to act out in an antisocial manner. In fact, fewer than half of teenagers who qualify for a diagnosis of conduct disorder will eventually be rediagnosed as having ASPD.) Nonetheless, it is uncommon for children with conduct problems to become adults who have no diagnosable mental pathology at all. It is also unusual to the point of rarity for adult personality disorders to develop from a background of normal childhood or adolescent behavior.

Considering all of these factors, we recommend avoiding specific personality disorder diagnoses for all children and for most adolescents. Rather, we prefer to use the generic criteria for personality disorders (see the Essential Features, below), and to indicate in the body of the evaluation a level of uncertainty that avoids labeling young patients with pejorative diagnoses and biasing future clinicians' judgments about such patients.

Further Evaluation of Jim

Jim, as we have already seen in Chapter 23 (p. 392), amply met the criteria for conduct disorder. Which, if any, personality disorder diagnosis might be appropriate? Reading through the Essential Features of a Generic Personality Disorder suggests the following assessment:

Jim presented with a lifelong pattern of behavior problems and a way of perceiving the world that was strikingly different from the expectations of his mother and teachers. At least three life areas were affected: cognitive (he perceived the faults in others, not himself); affective (at a minimum, he showed an inappropriate emotional response when the interviewer mentioned the injury to the other child); and interpersonal (he had a history of bullying and extortion). Any evidence for deviant impulse control would have to be sought by the interviewer. These behaviors were present in a variety of situations (home, school, social) and impaired his personal and social functioning.

Could other diagnoses better account for Jim's symptoms? In addition to those we've already discarded (see the Chapter 23 discussion of Jim's case), the vignette provides no evidence in support of a **physical** or **substance-related disorder**. He presented no symptoms suggestive, even vaguely, of an **anxiety disorder**; although we don't know that he had been abusing any substances, his clinician would have to inquire specifically. Indeed, a personality disorder would seem a more parsimonious explanation.

However, Jim's vignette also provides far too few symptoms to define any of the 10 currently sanctioned DSM-5 personality disorders. The one that seems most likely, ASPD,

ESSENTIAL FEATURES OF A **GENERIC PERSONALITY DISORDER**

There is a lasting pattern of behavior and inner experience (thoughts, feelings, sensations) that is markedly different from the patient's culture. This pattern manifests itself as problems with *affect* (type, intensity, lability, appropriateness); *cognition* (how the patient sees and interprets self and the environment); *control of impulses*; and *interpersonal relationships*. This pattern is fixed and applies broadly across the patient's personal and social life.

The Fine Print

The D's: • Duration (lifelong, with roots in adolescence or childhood) • Diffuse contexts • Distress and disability (social, educational, occupational, and personal impairment) • Differential diagnosis (substance use, physical illness, other mental disorders, other personality disorders, personality change due to a physical disorder) specifically cannot be diagnosed until the age of 18. For a patient who meets the criteria for this disorder except for age, the appropriate diagnosis would be other specified or unspecified personality disorder, and even one of these "catch-all" diagnoses cannot be used unless the clinician believes that some such diagnosis is warranted. That would not be the case for Jim: Although he might well grow up to have a defined personality disorder, he might turn out to have something else—or, improbably, nothing at all. We therefore advocate a written indication of uncertainty about any future personality diagnosis; this would keep clinicians thinking until more information (or the passing of time) could settle the problem. Jim's complete current diagnosis would therefore remain as given in Chapter 23:

F91.1	Conduct disorder, childhood-onset type, with limited prosocial emotions, severe
Z65.1	Incarcerated in juvenile hall
CGAS	41 (current)

ASSESSING PERSONALITY DISORDERS

General Suggestions

Of course, in the quest for personality disorders, the most important information remains that which comes from other people and previous evaluations. Some of the material gathered on the history of the present illness may provide information about character—stealing, repeated suicide attempts, chronically making excuses. With this acknowledged, what techniques are useful in evaluating the possibility of a personality disorder in a teenager?

Consider observation of affect: Does the patient's mood match the content of the discussion? (For example, patients with borderline personality disorder may show inappropriate anger.) Does it seem of approximately normal intensity? (In the absence of a substance-related disorder or manic episode, a mood that is too bright and eager suggests histrionic personality disorder.) Is the mood stable? (Histrionic and borderline personality disorders are associated with marked lability.)

Be alert for behaviors that can tip you off to personality characteristics; flirtation, inappropriate dress, and arrogance are just a few of a wide variety. Sometimes spontaneous statements may provide a guide to attitudes about self, others, and events: "Most people think I'm pretty strange," "I don't have any close friends," "I have trouble staying out of trouble," or "The kids are always making fun of me behind my back."

Perhaps a good screening question for personality disorders doesn't exist, but it is certainly fair to request a self-evaluation: "What sort of a person do you think you are?" or "How would you describe yourself?" A follow-up appropriate for an adolescent might be this: "Have you always been that way? When did you begin to be different?" Children and adolescents—for that matter, all of us—may not readily admit to attitudes or behaviors that society frowns upon. Questions about personal attributes can be softened with a prefatory statement that "some kids are this way."

Apart from the difficulty of making personality disorder diagnoses in young patients, there's a lot of opportunity for confusion with major mental disorders. Consider the following:

- Histrionic personality disorder has been found in up to half of patients with DSM-IV somatization disorder; many clinicians consider them to be nearly synonymous.
- Schizotypal personality disorder often precedes schizophrenia.
- Autism spectrum disorder shares a number of features with schizoid and schizotypal personality disorders.
- It can be hard to define the line between paranoid personality disorder and chronic depressive (delusional) disorder.
- Many patients officially cross the border between conduct disorder and ASPD on their 18th birthday.
- Although their criteria make them quite distinct, the similarities between obsessive–compulsive personality disorder and obsessive–compulsive disorder are obvious.
- Many patients with social anxiety disorder also have avoidant personality disorder; should they therefore really be considered as separate conditions?

As if these issues weren't enough, note also that:

- Cyclothymic disorder used to be a personality disorder (in DSM-II).
- Passive–aggressive personality disorder was included in DSM-III and DSM-III-R, but was remanded to an appendix of DSM-IV to await further study. In DSM-5, it's missing in action completely.
- Borderline personality disorder, introduced in DSM-III, is so popular with some mental health professionals that other clinicians mistrust the diagnosis whenever they encounter it in a patient's records.
- Finally, many patients qualify for two or more personality disorder diagnoses.

We cannot state too forcefully that personality disorder diagnoses should rarely if ever be made before late adolescence. It is true that all adult personality disorders but one, ASPD, are theoretically permissible; in practice, however, the younger the patient, the less willing we should be to make any such definitive diagnosis.

CHAPTER 27

Other Diagnostic Issues

In the field of child and adolescent mental health, many problems that are not themselves mental illnesses can become the focus of clinical attention. For a number of these, such as abuse, neglect, and difficulty in dealing with other people, DSM-5 provides codes for our use; we list some of them here. At the end of the chapter are some administrative codes that may be applied to patients for whom no clear diagnosis is immediately apparent.

RELATIONAL PROBLEMS

We call it a *relational problem* when two or more people have difficulty dealing with one another—and a mental illness is not responsible. These problems are especially common in a child or adolescent mental health practice. There are no actual criteria for relational problems, but if there were, they would probably be something like the Hypothetical Essential Features we're providing (p. 439). These are brief and appropriately generic, yet they cover a lot of territory; they would be appropriate for parent–child, partner, or sibling relational problems. A little later, the case vignette of Scott provides an example of the process for identifying a relational problem.

Z62.820 Parent–Child Relational Problem

Use parent–child relational problem when clinically important symptoms or negative effects on functioning are associated with the ways a parent and child interact. The problematic interaction may involve overprotection, faulty communication, or ineffective or inconsistent discipline. However, when the conflict results in physical abuse, also use the code Z69.010 (encounter for mental health services for victim of child abuse by parent).

Z63.0 Relationship Distress with Spouse or Intimate Partner

Of course, most adolescents will not have a partner (spouse), but when a teen is married or living with a partner, clinically important symptoms or negative effects on functioning may be caused by the way the patient and partner interact. The problematic interaction pattern may be faulty communication or an absence of communication. Note that this category does *not* include partner neglect or abuse.

Z62.891 Sibling Relational Problem

Use sibling relational problem when clinically important symptoms or negative effects on functioning are associated with the ways brothers and sisters interact.

Z62.898 Child Affected by Parental Relationship Distress

In some cases, help for children is sought when the real problems lie with the parents. These can include marital conflicts, personal mental disorder, and the like. The diagnosis of parental and interparental disorders is beyond the scope of this book, but you need to be alert to all possible causes of a young patient's troubles.

Z62.29 Upbringing Away from Parents

Use upbringing away from parents for problems that arise because a child is living in foster care or with relatives or friends, but not in residential care or boarding school.

Z63.5 Disruption of Family by Separation or Divorce

Z63.4 Uncomplicated Bereavement

It is natural to grieve when a relative or close friend dies. When the symptoms of the grieving process are a reason for the clinical attention, DSM-5 allows a diagnostic code of uncomplicated bereavement—provided that the symptoms are relatively brief and relatively mild. The problem is that grief can closely resemble the sadness associated with a major depressive episode. DSM-5 mentions certain symptoms that can help us discriminate the difference.

Symptoms that point to a major depressive episode, even in a grieving child or adolescent, include the following:

- Guilt feelings (other than about actions that might have prevented the death)
- Death wishes (other than the survivor's wishing to have died with the loved one)

- Reduced level of psychomotor activity
- Marked preoccupation with worthlessness
- Severely impaired functioning for an unusually long time
- Hallucinations (other than of seeing or hearing the deceased)

The presence of any of these suggests that we consider major depressive disorder. In addition, people who are "only" bereaved typically regard their emotion as normal. Traditionally, a diagnosis of depressive illness was withheld in these cases unless the symptoms had lasted longer than 2 months. With DSM-5, we are encouraged to make the diagnosis of major depressive disorder whenever the symptoms warrant, regardless of bereavement.

Scott

"Scott, come on! It's our turn to go in. The doctor wants to see both of us." Scott didn't look up at his mother, who stood in the doorway of the interviewer's office. He slouched deeper into his chair and turned a page of the magazine he was holding. "Scott, come on!" He still didn't move. With a palms-up gesture of exasperation, she disappeared inside the office alone.

"He's always this way with me," she told the therapist when they were seated. "His teachers seem to like him, and he minds his grandfather just fine. I'm the only one who has trouble with him."

His mother's difficulties with Scott had begun 4 years earlier, when he was 12. His father, who had been the family disciplinarian, had been killed in a skydiving accident, and she and Scott had had to move in with her in-laws. Scott's behavior had been acceptable for a year, until she won a product liability suit against the parachute supplier and they moved back to California to be near her parents. She got a boyfriend and a job—and, she admitted, probably hadn't spent as much time with Scott as he needed. "And for the last year, life's

HYPOTHETICAL ESSENTIAL FEATURES FOR **RELATIONAL PROBLEMS**

Two or more individuals have a problem getting along with one another. This problem is the focus of clinical attention or treatment.

The Fine Print

The D's: • Duration (the symptoms do not last longer than 6 months after the end of the stressor—or its consequences) • Differential diagnosis (no physical, mental, substance use, or personality disorder better explains the behavior)

been nothing but hell. He hasn't been in trouble, and he isn't violent or anything, but we're always arguing, and I never seem to win. I think he's actually brighter than I am."

Scott was very bright. Even without studying, he'd maintained above-average grades, and none of his teachers had complained about his classroom behavior. Whenever his mother would suggest that he do his homework, he would smile and continue watching TV or reading a book. Sent to his room, he would listen to music, draw, or just look out the window—in short, he'd do just about anything but study.

When his mother emerged from the office, the interviewer invited Scott to enter. Pleasant and cooperative, he responded fully to all questions and volunteered other information about his relationship with both of his parents. He had worshiped his father and deeply resented it when his mother eventually began dating again. "I don't care much what she does," Scott said, leaning forward in his chair. "Why should I? She doesn't really care what I do."

Scott denied feeling either anxious or depressed. In fact, his mood was pretty good most of the time. He acknowledged that his mother thought him irritable and angry, but denied that this was so. "If I feel anything, it's contempt," he said. "I can twist her around my little finger."

Evaluation of Scott

The focus of Scott's evaluation was an important interpersonal problem, thereby fulfilling the main requirement of the Hypothetical Essential Features. Before parent–child relational problem could be listed as the *principal* diagnosis, however, all other possible mental and physical causes for his behavior would have to be ruled out.

The attention-deficit and disruptive, impulse-control, and conduct disorders would be important to consider on two counts: They are the disorders most commonly encountered in child and adolescent mental health clinics, and they cover at least some of the symptoms of which Scott's mother complained. However, Scott's attention span and activity level were normal (ruling out **ADHD**), and his problematic conduct, directed only toward his mother, did not violate the boundaries of person, property, or truth (as would be true for **conduct disorder**). Although several of the interactions with his mother could be construed as consistent with **oppositional defiant disorder**, he did not show the typical anger, spite, or loss of temper. Aberrant behaviors are encountered in the **impulse-control disorders** (such as **intermittent explosive disorder**), but Scott's behavior was planned, not impulsive.

Of course, ample academic evidence ruled out **intellectual disability,** all of the **specific learning disorders**, and **autism spectrum disorder**. No speech problems were reported or noted, eliminating **selective mutism** and any of the **communication disorders**. (Although the history includes no mention of problems involving **eating** or **elimination**, a review of systems should include questions about these.) There were no motor problems reported or noted, rejecting **developmental coordination disorder**, **tic disorders**, and **stereotypic** movement disorder. Scott certainly did have a problem in relating to his mother, but not to other adults (including his grandfather, teachers, and the interviewer), ruling out **reactive attachment disorder.**

What about all the *other* major mental disorders? Scott specifically denied any symptoms of anxiety or worry, eliminating any **anxiety disorder** (including **separation anxiety disorder**). There was a similar lack of support for a **mood disorder** or **cognitive disorder.** Of course, almost any behavior imaginable can be encountered in the course of **substance use,** and the clinician would need to ask both Scott and his mother about this possibility. An **adjustment disorder** would have had to occur within 3 months of and in response to a stressor (could his mother's dating be considered a legitimate stressor?). The death of his father had occurred too long ago for **uncomplicated bereavement** to be applicable. Finally, a **personality disorder** (even if there were sufficient symptoms to diagnose one) would have to affect more than one aspect of Scott's life, not just his relationship with his mother—and besides, we'd discourage that diagnosis prior to any patient's late teens.

Perhaps some might argue for an other specified or unspecified diagnosis, but what would it be? **Other specified or unspecified disruptive, impulse-control, and conduct disorder** might be a possibility, but any such "catch-all" diagnosis should be used only when it seems clear that the symptoms place the diagnosis within the general category; Scott's presentation was far too atypical.

Finally just as for adjustment disorder, no one can be positive about causation of symptoms attributed to a relational problem until the problem has resolved and the symptoms abate. That is why we'd add the cautious term *provisional* to the Z-code for Scott (and his mother—the code could be applied to any family member who was under consideration):

Z62.820   Parent–child relational problem (provisional)
CGAS   75   (current)

The history of Tonya in Chapter 13 (p. 254) presents another example of parent–child relational problem.

PROBLEMS RELATED TO ABUSE OR NEGLECT

Although precise information is difficult to obtain, some estimates place the number of children in the United States who are abused or neglected by their parents or other adults at 3 million—or more. As compared with nonabused children, those abused as infants tend to become much more avoidant, resistant, and noncompliant. In addition to the simple fact of abuse, it is vital to assess its possible consequences, especially including depression, substance misuse, posttraumatic stress disorder, and conduct and other behavioral disor-

TABLE 27.1. Code Numbers to Use for Different Forms of Child Maltreatment

Form of maltreatment	Abuse confirmed	Abuse suspected
Child physical abuse	T74.12	T76.12
Child sexual abuse	T74.22	T76.22
Child neglect	T74.02	T76.02
Child psychological abuse	T74.32	T76.32

ders—as well as physical sequelae such as traumatic brain injury. Table 27.1 gives the code numbers for various forms of child maltreatment. If clinical attention is focused on the perpetrator rather than on the victim, or if the emphasis is on the encounter for mental health services in cases of parental versus nonparental maltreatment, many different Z-codes are used to make these distinctions—but that's an issue for a different text.

One problem with studies of the effects of childhood abuse is that they often conflate physical and sexual abuse, rather than reporting their effects separately. Perhaps this is because the two types of abuse often go together. In general, more severe abuse and earlier abuse are more likely to produce psychopathology. However, most studies don't carefully assess the cause–effect relationship (does the risk factor of abuse clearly antedate the behavior in question?). Abuse in children or adolescents has been associated with substance use problems (alcohol, marijuana, other drugs); sexual acting out and teen pregnancy; depression and low self-esteem; anxiety symptoms; running away; sleep problems (trouble initiating and maintaining sleep); eating disorders (especially anorexia nervosa); or conduct disorder. Adults may develop dissociation; decreased satisfaction with sexual relationships; posttraumatic stress disorder symptoms; eating disorders (especially bulimia nervosa); and physical conditions such as back pain. Perhaps 20% of female children may be sexually abused in some way; 5–6% of girls suffer severe abuse involving actual or attempted intercourse. Comparable rates for boys are about one-fourth of those for girls.

Ongoing collaborative research called the Adverse Childhood Experiences (ACE) Study identifies adult health risk attributable to early child trauma. In brief, instances of abuse (physical, sexual, emotional) and neglect are summed to arrive at a total score that then can be used to predict such adult problems as alcoholism, depression, ischemic heart disease, chronic obstructive pulmonary disease, and liver disease, as well as health-related quality-of-life issues.

Of course, we have only touched the surface of this issue. Interested readers should consult the references in Appendix 1 for further information about the ACE study and the National Child Traumatic Stress Network's 12 core concepts for understanding children's response to traumatic stress.

OTHER CONDITIONS THAT MAY NEED CLINICAL ATTENTION

Z91.19 Nonadherence to Medical Treatment

Nonadherence to medical treatment (we used to call it noncompliance) identifies a patient who has ignored or thwarted attempts at treatment for a mental disorder or a general medical condition, and therefore now requires attention. An example would be a teenager with schizophrenia who requires repeated hospitalization for refusal to take medication. And yes, it could also be (somewhat more precisely) listed as a psychological factor affecting a medical condition (p. 334).

Z76.5 Malingering

Malingering is the intentional production of the signs or symptoms of a physical or mental disorder. The purpose is some sort of gain: obtaining something desirable (money, drugs, insurance settlement) or avoiding something unpleasant (punishment, work, military service [back when there was a draft], jury duty). Malingering is sometimes confused with factitious disorder, for which the criteria describe no underlying motive, though external gain does not appear to be a feature. It is also sometimes confused with other somatic symptom disorders, in which the symptoms are not intentionally produced at all.

Malingering should be suspected when a patient:

- Has legal problems or the prospect of financial gain.

- Tells a story that does not accord with informants' accounts or with other known facts.

- Does not cooperate with the evaluation.

- Has traits suggestive of antisocial personality disorder.

Malingering is easy to suspect and difficult to prove. If we don't observe an overt instance of malingering behavior (such as someone placing sand in a urine specimen or holding a thermometer over a glowing light bulb), it may be almost impossible to detect a resolute and clever individual. When malingering involves symptoms that are strictly mental or emotional, detection may not be possible at all. Because the consequences of using this diagnostic code are dire (it can alienate patients from their clinicians), use it only in the most obvious and imperative of circumstances. Remember that frank malingering is rare to the point of nullity in children, and probably extremely uncommon even in late adolescence.

Z72.810 Childhood or Adolescent Antisocial Behavior

The diagnostic code for childhood or adolescent antisocial behavior might be used in an isolated example of criminal activity in which an adolescent has followed the lead of an older person.

R41.83 Borderline Intellectual Functioning

With the change in how intellectual disability is defined (DSM-5 no longer uses IQ score as a criterion), the definition of borderline intellectual functioning has been thrown into disarray. It used to be reserved for patients whose IQ and level of functioning fell within the range of 71–84. DSM-5 says that differentiating between borderline intellectual functioning and mild intellectual disability requires careful assessment, but it doesn't state how they are to be differentiated. You might consider for this diagnostic code a patient who functions pretty well overall, despite relatively low intelligence.

Z55.9 Academic or Educational Problem

A child or adolescent whose problem is related to schoolwork, and who does not have a learning disorder or other mental disorder that accounts for the problem, may be given the Z-code for academic or educational problem. Even if another disorder can account for the problem, the academic problem itself may be so severe that it independently justifies clinical attention. Then you would list both the Z-code and the clinical disorder.

Z59.3 Problem Related to Living in a Residential Institution

The code for problem related to living in a residential institution can be used for a child or adolescent who attends boarding school or is receiving residential care—and has specific issues that result from it.

Z56.9 Other Problem Related to Employment

Other problem related to employment is the work-related equivalent of academic or educational problem; examples might include choosing a career and job dissatisfaction. Of course, use of this Z-code will be rare until late adolescence.

Z65.8 Religious or Spiritual Problem

Patients who require evaluation or treatment for issues pertaining to religious faith (or its lack) may be coded as having a religious or spiritual problem.

Z60.3 Acculturation Problem

Acculturation problem may be useful for children or adolescents whose problems center on a move from one culture to another; many immigrants in contemporary Western society may qualify for this diagnostic code.

Z60.0 Phase of Life Problem

You can use phase of life problem for a young patient whose problem is due not to a mental disorder but to a life change (such as entering school or leaving home for college).

MEDICATION-INDUCED DISORDERS

Medication-induced movement (and other) disorders are important in mental health settings because (1) they may be mistaken for mental disorders (such as tics, schizophrenia, and anxiety disorders); or (2) they can affect the management of patients who are receiving neuroleptic medications. Although these disorders are very infrequently encountered in children or adolescents, the following codes may occasionally be appropriate:

G21.0	Neuroleptic malignant syndrome
G24.01	Tardive dyskinesia
G24.02	Medication-induced acute dystonia
G25.1	Medication-induced postural tremor
G21.11	Neuroleptic-induced parkinsonism
G21.19	Other medication-induced parkinsonism
G25.71	Medication-induced acute akathisia
G25.79	Other medication-induced movement disorder
T43.205	Antidepressant discontinuation syndrome
T50.905	Other adverse effects of medication

ADDITIONAL CODES

Several other codes are useful for administrative purposes. Some of these codes state that a patient has no mental disorder diagnosis. Others provide ways to indicate that you don't know what's wrong, if anything. Not all of these are stated in DSM-5; we've borrowed a few from ICD-10.

F48.9 Unspecified Nonpsychotic Mental Disorder

Unspecified nonpsychotic mental disorder may serve as a useful placeholder if (1) the diagnosis you want to give is not contained in DSM-5; or (2) you have too little information to make a definitive diagnosis when a child or adolescent is clearly ill, but lacks psychotic symptoms, and no other unspecified category seems appropriate. Once you have obtained more information, you should be able to substitute a more specific diagnosis.

F09 Other Specified Mental Disorder Due to Another Medical Condition

F09 Unspecified Mental Disorder Due to Another Medical Condition

Use one of these two codes in cases where mental symptoms due to another medical condition are present, but the criteria are not met for any other disorder due to such a condition. As usual, the other specified code should be used in a situation in which you wish to indicate the reason why criteria are not met.

Z03.89 Encounter for Observation for Other Suspected Diseases and Conditions Ruled Out

This is the (rather clumsy) ICD-10 way of saying "No diagnosis." It means that no major mental disorder or personality disorder is the focus of clinical attention.

F99 Other Specified Mental Disorder

F99 Unspecified Mental Disorder

The other specified and unspecified mental disorder codes mean that there is not currently enough information to permit any specific DSM-5 diagnosis to be made. The code will be changed once enough further information becomes available.

APPENDICES

Reference Materials

Structured and semistructured interviews have both advantages and disadvantages. Whereas they prompt the clinician to cover all the material required by a given set of diagnostic criteria, they may not reveal material that is unusual, complex, or unexpected in a given context. Structured interviews are at their best in selecting a relatively homogeneous group of patients for mental health research purposes; they can also help establish baseline data for individual patients—an especially valuable point for patients whose care may be shared by a number of clinicians. We hasten to point out that often the best test of all remains an interview by a sensitive, experienced clinician.

This appendix consists of two sections. First, we provide brief descriptions of interviews, schedules, and tests that may prove useful in assessing children and adolescents, along with addresses and references for the instruments themselves or for further information about them. Second, we present an annotated bibliography of books and articles relevant to the different chapters of this book.

INTERVIEWS, SCHEDULES, AND TESTS

In compiling this section, we have tried to focus on what is easily available in conventionally published form or online. References marked with a dagger (†) contain the full test text; otherwise, we give authors' or publishers' addresses and, where available, websites or e-mail addresses. For further information about individual tests, consult the websites given below or standard texts. These are the three most cited websites (with their "short form" names in parentheses):

  Psychological Assessment Resources (PAR)
  16204 North Florida Avenue
  Lutz, FL 33549
  www4.parinc.com

- Western Psychological Services (Western)
  625 Alaska Avenue
  Torrance, CA 90503
  www.wpspublish.com

- Pearson Clinical Assessment (Pearson)
  P.O. Box 599700
  San Antonio, TX 78259
  www.pearsonclinical.com

General

The **Schedule for Affective Disorders and Schizophrenia for School-Age Children (K-SADS)** is probably the most widely used semistructured interview for patients ages 6–17. Affectionately termed the "Kiddie-SADS," it uses probe questions and DSM criteria to assess current and past episodes of psychopathology in children and adolescents. The clinician adjusts the interview to the developmental level of the patient and uses the patient's (or parent's) language. The K-SADS covers many of the commonly experienced DSM-IV-TR diagnoses, including major depressive disorder, the bipolar disorders, and dysthymic and cyclothymic disorders; schizophrenia, schizoaffective disorder, schizophreniform disorder, and brief psychotic disorder; panic disorder, agoraphobia, separation anxiety disorder, specific and social phobias, generalized anxiety disorder, obsessive–compulsive disorder, and posttraumatic stress disorder; attention-deficit/hyperactivity disorder, conduct disorder, oppositional defiant disorder, enuresis, encopresis, transient tic disorder, Tourette's disorder, and chronic motor or vocal tic disorder; anorexia nervosa and bulimia nervosa; alcohol and other substance abuse; and adjustment disorder. [†The K-SADS-PL (Present and Lifetime version) is available online in its entirety, at no charge: *www.psychiatry.pitt.edu/sites/default/files/Documents/assessments/ksads-pl.pdf*]

    The **Diagnostic Interview Schedule for Children (DISC)** has over 200 items that capture information regarding the onset, duration, severity, and associated impairment of behaviors and symptoms for children ages 9–17. Disorders covered by the DISC are organized into five sections: Anxiety, Mood, Behavior, Substance-Use, and Miscellaneous. It can be administered by either clinicians or lay interviewers. There are paper and electronic versions for both the identified patient and a parent. [Prudence Fisher, MS, NIMH-DISC Training Center at Columbia University/New York State Psychiatric Institute Division of Child and Adolescent Psychiatry, 722 West 168th Street, Unit 78, New York, NY 10032; telephone, 212-543-5357; e-mail, *nimhdisc@appchild.cpmc.columbia.edu*]

    The **Child Behavior Checklist (CBCL)** is actually part of the Achenbach System of Empirically Based Assessment (ASEBA), a group of assessments that collect data on general functioning from a variety of respondents. Its subscales assess internalizing and externalizing behaviors, including aggression, anxiety/depression, attention, delinquency, sex, social problems, somatic problems, and withdrawal. Separate forms of the CBCL are available for children ages 1½ –5 years and 6–18 years. There are teacher, parent, and youth self-report versions as well. [ASEBA, 1 South Prospect Street, St. Joseph's Wing (Room 3207), Burlington, VT 05401; *www.aseba.org*]

The **Global Assessment of Functioning (GAF)** and the **Children's Global Assessment Scale (CGAS)** both reflect the current overall occupational (academic), psychological, and social functioning of a patient—but not environmental problems or physical limitations. The score on each instrument is recorded as a number on a 100-point scale. The scale for the CGAS is roughly as follows:

81–100: Functions well at home, at school, with friends. At lower end of this range, may have mild but temporary problems.
61–80: Some problems in some of the areas above, but still has friends even at the lower end of this range.
41–60: Mild to moderate levels of difficulty.
21–40: Severe difficulty with functioning in most areas.
1–20: Much supervision required to prevent harm to self or others.

Both instruments specify symptoms and behavioral guidelines to help determine the score for an individual patient. The GAF is designed for adults and may be useful with adolescents and older children; the CGAS is designed for patients ages 4–16 and is couched in terms more appropriate for children. Both scales are inherently subjective, so that their most effective use may be in tracking changes in a level of functioning across time, as assessed by a single examiner. [The GAF may be found in DSM-IV-TR and in James Morrison's *DSM-IV Made Easy;* †it is also widely available online. The CGAS may be found in its original source: Shaffer D, Gould MS, Brasic J, Ambrosini P, Fisher P, Bird S, et al. A Children's Global Assessment Scale (CGAS). *Archives of General Psychiatry* 1983; 40:1228–1231. It is also available in the first edition of the present book, *Interviewing Children and Adolescents* by James Morrison and Thomas F. Anders, and †widely available online.]

Additional measures relevant to assessment of various areas are reviewed in a series published in the *Journal of the American Academy of Child and Adolescent Psychiatry* by K. M. Myers and colleagues:

Overview, psychometric properties, and selection. 2002; *41*:114–122.
Suicidality, cognitive style, and self-esteem. 2002; *41*:1150–1181.
Trauma and its effects. 2002; *41*:1401–1422.
Attention-deficit/hyperactivity disorder. 2003; *42*:1015–1037.
Externalizing behaviors. 2003; *42*:1143–1170.
Functional impairment. 2005; *44*:309–338.

Intellectual Disability; Autism Spectrum Disorder

The **Wechsler Intelligence Scale for Children—Fifth Edition (WISC-V)**, intended for ages 6 years, 0 months–16 years, 11 months, is a revision of a test that has been in use for more than 50 years. The WISC-V offers five index scores: Verbal Comprehension, Visual Spatial, Fluid Reasoning, Working Memory, and Processing Speed. [Pearson]

The **Bayley Scales of Infant and Toddler Development, Third Edition (Bayley-III),** is a battery assessing the developmental functioning of children ages 1–42 months. It yields information in five domains: Social-Emotional Behavior, Adaptive Behavior, Cognitive, Motor, and Language. [Pearson]

In the **Peabody Picture Vocabulary Test, Fourth Edition (PPVT-4),** the patient chooses a picture that best represents a word spoken by the examiner. The score generated equates to IQ, though the publishers discourage the use of the term *verbal intelligence.* This test can be used from ages 2½ to 90+ years. [Pearson]

The **Beery–Buktenica Developmental Test of Visual–Motor Integration (VMI), Sixth Edition,** assesses visual–motor skills in young people ages 2–18. A child or adolescent copies geometric figures that are arranged in ascending order of difficulty. The 24 culture-free items require about 15 minutes to complete. The test is used to screen children who may need special assistance or services. [Pearson]

The **Modified Checklist for Autism in Toddlers (M-CHAT)** is a 23-item checklist that can spur a more definitive interview for those who score high (3–6 items); higher scores should prompt immediate referral. [Robins DL, Fein D, Barton ML, Green JA. The Modified Checklist for Autism in Toddlers: An initial study investigating the early detection of autism and pervasive developmental disorders. *Journal of Autism and Developmental Disorders* 2001; *31*:131–144. †A revised version, the M-CHAT-R, is available at *www.autismspeaks.org/what-autism/diagnosis/screen-your-child*]

The 15 items of the well-validated **Childhood Autism Rating Scale, Second Edition (CARS-2),** help to identify children, adolescents, and adults with autism spectrum disorder and to distinguish them from those who have developmental delays but not ASD. It also discriminates severe ASD from mild to moderate ASD. Based on direct observation as well as historical information, the CARS-2 is suitable for use with any child 2 years of age or over. [Western]

Learning Disorders

The **Wide Range Achievement Test 4 (WRAT4)** is easy to administer and assesses reading, spelling, and math skills from ages 5 to adult. It is normed by age and grade level. [Western]

Communication Disorders

The **Multilingual Aphasia Examination, 3rd Edition (MAE),** provides a brief (40-minute) evaluation of articulation, oral expression, oral verbal understanding, reading, spelling, and writing. It is suitable for ages 6 to adult. [PAR]

Attention–Deficit/Hyperactivity Disorder

The **Conners 3rd Edition** is a group of relatively brief instruments (20 minutes or less administration time) for assessing ADHD and reporting results in terms of DSM-5. [Pearson]

Tic Disorders

For any age, the **Yale Global Tic Severity Scale** provides an overall evaluation of complexity, frequency, intensity, interference, and number of motor and vocal tics, including those found in patients with Tourette's disorder. [†Leckman JF, Riddle MA, Hardin MT, Ort SI, Swartz KL, Stevenson J, et al. The Yale Global Tic Severity Scale: Initial testing of a clinician-rated scale of tic severity. *Journal of the American Academy of Child and Adolescent Psychiatry* 1989; 28:566–573. †Also available at *www.cappcny.org/home/images/TIC-YGTSS-Clinician.pdf*]

Mood Disorders

Mood disorders can be evaluated with the K-SADS and the DISC (discussed above). Here are some additional instruments:

The **Mania Rating Scale (MRS)** was developed to evaluate manic behavior in prepubertal children; its use may discriminate between manic behavior and hyperactivity due to ADHD. The MRS may also help distinguish severity of mania. [†Fristad MA, Weller EB, Weller RA. The Mania Rating Scale: Can it be used in children? A preliminary report. *Journal of the American Academy of Child and Adolescent Psychiatry* 1992; 31(2):252–257. †Also available at *https://psychology-tools.com/young-mania-rating-scale*]

The **Children's Depression Inventory 2 (CDI 2)** is a self-report, symptom-oriented scale that requires young patients (ages 7–17) to score the severity of their own symptoms over the past 2 weeks. Its 28 items yield two scales (Emotional Problems and Functional Problems) and four subscales (Negative Mood/Physical Symptoms, Interpersonal Problems, Ineffectiveness, and Negative Self-Esteem). [Pearson]

The **Suicide Probability Scale (SPS)** measures suicidal ideation, hopelessness, and social isolation to predict subsequent suicide attempts, suicide verbalizations, and minor self-destructive behaviors. It can be administered in under 10 minutes; it is suitable for ages 14 and over. [Western]

Anxiety Disorders; Trauma– and Stressor–Related Disorders

The **State–Trait Anxiety Inventory for Children (STAIC)** consists of two scales, each made up of 40 self-administered items, assessing how children feel at a particular moment and how they generally feel. The STAIC is useful for ages 9–12 years; administration time is about 20 minutes. [PAR]

The **Screen for Adolescent Violence Exposure (SAVE)** assesses the exposure of adolescents to violence in the school, home, and community, with excellent reliability and validity. This 32-question screening instrument correlates significantly with objective data on crime and with constructs that are theoretically relevant, such as anger and posttraumatic stress symptoms. [†Hastings TL, Kelley ML. Development and validation of the Screen for Adolescent Violence Exposure (SAVE). *Journal of Abnormal Child Psychology* 1997; 25:511–520. †Also available at *https://mospace. umsystem.edu/xmlui/bitstream/handle/10355/4148/research.pdf?sequence=3*]

Dissociative Disorders

The **Child Dissociative Checklist (CDC)** is a reliable and valid observer report measure of dissociation in children that can be used in research or in screening individual patients. It discriminated well among four test samples: typical girls, girls who had been sexually abused, boys and girls with dissociative disorders, and children with DSM-III-R multiple personality disorder. [†Putnam FW, Helmers K, Trickett PK. Development, reliability, and validity of a child dissociation scale. *Child Abuse and Neglect* 1993; 17(6):731–741. †Also available at *https://secure.ce-credit.com/articles/102019/ Session_2_Provided-Articles-1of2.pdf*]

Somatic Symptom Disorder with Predominant Pain

An excellent review of childhood pain assessment is available. [Cohen LL, Lemanek K, Blount RL, Dahlquist LM, Lim CS, et al. Evidence-based assessment of pediatric pain. *Journal of Pediatric Psychology* 2008; 33:939–955. †The full text is available free online at *http://jpepsy.oxfordjournals.org/cgi/ reprint/33/9/939*]

Eating Disorders

The **Eating Disorder Inventory–3 (EDI-3)** is a 91-item self-report instrument useful as a screening tool for specific cognitive and behavioral dimensions of persons ages 13–53 with eating disorders, as well as a means of distinguishing them from persons who engage in typical dieting. Twelve subscales yield six composite scores: Affective Problems, Eating Disorder Risk, General Psychological Maladjustment, Interpersonal Problems, Overcontrol, and Ineffectiveness. [Western]

The **Anorectic Behavior Observation Scale** queries parents about specific eating behaviors and attitudes in their children. With a cutoff score of 19, its sensitivity and specificity were 90%. [†Vandereycken W. Validity and reliability of the Anorectic Behavior Observation Scale for parents. *Acta Psychiatrica Scandinavica* 1992; 85(2):163–166]

The **Contour Drawing Rating Scale**, a body image assessment tool, consists of nine male and nine female contour drawings that can be used to measure ideal and perceived body sizes and the discrepancy between the two. The drawings can be split at the waist to compare perceptions of the upper and lower body. [†Thompson MA, Gray JJ. Development and validation of a new body-image assessment scale. *Journal of Personality Assessment* 1995; 64:258–269]

Substance Use

Many tools for assessing substance use, several of which can be downloaded free of charge, are described on a National Institute on Drug Abuse webpage. [*www.drugabuse.gov/nidamed-medical-health-professionals/tool-resources-your-practice/additional-screening-resources*]

The **CAGE** questionnaire is a simple screening device for alcoholism that is widely used because it is easy to remember and quick to administer. However, it may lack sufficient specificity and sensitivity for use in teen populations. [†Ewing JA. Detecting alcoholism: The CAGE questionnaire. *Journal of the American Medical Association* 1984; 252:1905–1907. †Also widely available online.]

The semistructured **Comprehensive Adolescent Severity Inventory (CASI)** can be administered on paper or by computer in 45–90 minutes, and is intended to guide treatment planning and assess outcome. It assesses symptoms, known risk factors, and consequences of alcohol or drug use within seven main areas of functioning: education status, alcohol/drug use, family relationships, peer relationships, legal status, mental distress, and use of free time. Sponsored by the National Institute on Alcohol Abuse and Alcoholism, the Index is free, but training is mandatory—and expensive. [†*http://pubs.niaaa.nih.gov/publications/AssessingAlcohol/InstrumentPDFs/21_CASI.pdf*]

The 30-item **Drug and Alcohol Problem Quick Screen** is a useful office screening tool for the detection of serious problems in adolescents. [†Schwartz RH, Wirtz PW. Potential substance abuse: Detection among adolescent patients. *Clinical Pediatrics* 1990; 29:38–43. †Also available at *www.emcdda.europa.eu/html.cfm/index4381EN.html*]

Cognitive Disorders

For older children and adolescents, **the Mini-Mental State Exam (MMSE)** offers a rapid, reproducible way to conduct and score a brief evaluation of the cognitive state. [†Folstein MF, Folstein SE, McHugh PR. Mini-Mental State: A practical method of grading the cognitive state of patients for the clinician. *Journal of Psychiatric Research* 1975; 12:189–198. †Also available at *https://www.mountsinai.on.ca/care/psych/on-call-resources/on-call-resources/mmse.pdf*]

Personality Disorders

Many children age 12 or older can complete questionnaires themselves. Similar to the adult version, the adolescent version (ages 14–18) of the **Minnesota Multiphasic Personality Inventory (MMPI-A)** contains 478 true–false items, some of which directly target adolescent concerns. The resulting clinical profile resembles the psychopathology scales of the MMPI-2. [Pearson]

The 150 true–false items in the **Millon Adolescent Personality Inventory (MAPI)** yield information about impulse control, rapport, personality style, school functioning, self-esteem, and more. A great deal of research has been published about this increasingly venerable measure for ages 13–18. [Pearson]

Abuse and Parental Stress

The 120 items on the **Parenting Stress Index, Fourth Edition** (36 items to screen) yield percentile scores in two domains: Child (Adaptability, Acceptability, Demandingness, Mood, Distractibility/Hyperactivity, Reinforces Parent) and Parent (Depression, Attachment, Role Restriction, Competence, Isolation, Spouse/Parenting Partner Relationship, Health). [PAR]

BOOKS AND ARTICLES

For reviews of specific topics in child and adolescent mental health, you can search PubMed (*www.ncbi.nlm.nih.gov/pubmed*) for articles that have appeared in professional journals worldwide. Type in the disorder name you want to explore and click "Enter"; then scroll down and check "Abstracts" under "Text availability," and "Review" under "Article types." You can also click "Show additional filters" and select "Child: birth–18 years" under "Ages." Then click "Search."

General Books and Articles

Ainsworth M, Blehar M, Waters E, Wall S. *Patterns of Attachment: A Psychological Study of the Strange Situation.* Hillsdale, NJ: Erlbaum, 1978.

American Psychiatric Association. *Diagnostic and Statistical Manual of Mental Disorders,* 5th ed. Arlington, VA: Author, 2013. The famous DSM-5 is the standard of current American diagnostic thinking in mental health.

Cheng K, Myers KM (eds). *Child and Adolescent Psychiatry: The Essentials,* 2nd ed. Philadelphia: Lippincott Williams & Wilkins, 2011.

Chess S, Thomas A. Issues in the clinical application of temperament. In G Kohstamm, J Bates, M Rothbart (eds), *Temperament in Childhood,* pp. 377–386. New York: Wiley, 1989.

Dulcan MK. *Dulcan's Textbook of Child and Adolescent Psychiatry,* 2nd ed. Arlington, VA: American Psychiatric Publications, 2016.

Eaton, DK, Kann L, Kinchen S, Shanklin S, Flint KH, Hawkins J, et al. Youth risk behavior surveillance—United States, 2011. MMWR *Surveillance Summaries* 2012; 61:1–162.

Gadermann AM, Alonso J, Vilagut G, Zaslavsky AM, Kessler RC. Comorbidity and disease burden in the National Comorbidity Survey Replication (NCS-R). *Depression and Anxiety* 2012; 29:797–806.

Gould MS, Marrocco FA, Kleinman M, Thomas JG, Mostkoff K, Cote J, et al. Evaluating iatrogenic risk of youth suicide screening programs: A randomized controlled trial. *Journal of the American Medical Association* 2005; 293:1635–1643.

Lieberman A, Wieder S, Fenichel E (eds). *The DC 0–3 Casebook.* Washington, DC: National Center for Infants, Toddlers, and Families, 1997. An alternative diagnostic classification system for very young patients; includes plenty of examples.

Mash EJ, Barkley RA (eds). *Child Psychopathology,* 3rd ed. New York: Guilford Press, 2014. Contains a wealth of information concerning childhood mental illness.

Merikangas KR, He JP, Burstein M, Swanson SA, Avenevoli S, Cui L, et al. Lifetime prevalence of mental disorders in US adolescents: Results from the National Comorbidity Survey—Adolescent Supplement (NCS-A). *Journal of the American Academy of Child and Adolescent Psychiatry* 2010; 49:980–898.

Morrison J. *DSM-5 Made Easy.* New York: Guilford Press, 2014. A simplified approach to understanding DSM-5 diagnoses of adults.

Ollendick T, Hersen M (eds). *Handbook of Child and Adolescent Assessment.* Boston: Allyn & Bacon, 1993. A valuable, though older, reference that covers basic issues underlying assessment strategies, the strategies themselves, and specific child disorders.

Ozonoff S, Rogers S, Hendren R (eds). *Autism Spectrum Disorders: A Research Review for Practitioners.* Washington, DC: American Psychiatric Press, 2003. An overview of screening, diagnosis and treatment of children with ASD.

Petresco S, Anselmi L, Santos IS, Barros AJD, Fleitlich-Bilyk B, Barros FC, et al. Prevalence and comorbidity of psychiatric disorders among 6-year-old children: 2004 Pelotas birth cohort. *Social Psychiatry and Psychiatric Epidemiology* 2014; 49:975–983.

Robins E, Guze SB. Establishment of diagnostic validity in psychiatric illness: Its application to schizophrenia. *American Journal of Psychiatry* 1970; 126:983–987.

Rush AJ, First M, Blacker D (eds). *Handbook of Psychiatric Measures,* 2nd ed. Washington, DC: American Psychiatric Press, 2008. A comprehensive review of structured assessment, with several chapters devoted to instruments used with children and adolescents.

Sadock BJ, Sadock VA, Ruiz P (eds). *Kaplan and Sadock's Comprehensive Textbook of Psychiatry,* 9th ed. New York: Lippincott Williams & Wilkins, 2009.

Schalock RL, Borthwick-Duffy SA, Bradley VJ, Buntinx WHE, Coulter DL, Craig EM, et al. *Intellectual Disability: Definition, Classification, and Systems of Support,* 11th ed. Washington, DC: American Association on Intellectual and Developmental Disabilities, 2010. Clinicians who assess and treat children with ID should become familiar with this competing classification system.

Strauss E, Sherman EMS, Spreen O. *A Compendium of Neuropsychological Tests,* 3rd ed. New York: Oxford University Press, 2006. This compendium includes descriptions of tests of cognition, intelligence, achievement, attention, memory, language, motor, and other attributes.

Thapar A, Pine D, Leckman JF, Scott S, Snowling MJ, Taylor E (eds). *Rutter's Child and Adolescent Psychiatry,* 6th ed. Ames, IA: Wiley-Blackwell, 2015.

Winnicott DW. *Therapeutic Consultations in Child Psychiatry.* London: Hogarth Press, 1971. Source of the famous Squiggles game.

Zeanah CH Jr. (ed). *Handbook of Infant Mental Health,* 3rd ed. New York: Guilford Press, 2009. Interdisciplinary analysis of clinical, developmental, and social aspects of infant mental health.

Books and Articles Related to Specific Topics and Chapters

Over one-third of these articles are available to anyone, without payment. We've labeled these as [free].

Interviewing

Anglin TM. Interviewing guidelines for the clinical evaluation of adolescent substance abuse. *Pediatric Clinics of North America* 1987; 34:381–398.

Barker P. *Clinical Interviews with Children and Adolescents*. New York: Norton, 1990. This (now older) work deals with the interviewing process from a largely theoretical perspective (no examples).

Coupey SM. Interviewing adolescents. *Pediatric Clinics of North America* 1997; 44:1349–1364.

Cox A, Holbrook D, Rutter M. Psychiatric interviewing techniques: A second experimental study. *British Journal of Psychiatry* 1988; 152:64–72. Provides references to a series of seminal papers.

Greenspan SI, with Greenspan NT. *The Clinical Interview of the Child*, 3rd ed. Washington, DC: American Psychiatric Press, 2003. The authors' own developmental perspective, presented with a number of very detailed (though not verbatim) examples.

Havighurst SS, Downey L. Clinical reasoning for child and adolescent mental health practitioners: The mindful formulation. *Clinical Child Psychology and Psychiatry* 2009; 14:251–271. Reviews use of the "four P's" in constructing a formulation.

Hughes JN, Baker DB. *The Clinical Child Interview*. New York: Guilford Press, 1990. A detailed (though older) guide to the interview process that focuses on school-age children and young adolescents.

Morrison J. *The First Interview*, 4th ed. New York: Guilford Press, 2014. Discusses the interview process in adults.

Peterson C, Biggs M. Interviewing children about trauma. *Journal of Trauma and Stress* 1997; 10:279–290.

Pinegar C. Screening for dissociative disorders in children and adolescents. *Journal of Child and Adolescent Psychiatric Nursing* 1995; 8:5–14.

Saywitz K, Camparo L. Interviewing child witnesses: A developmental perspective. *Child Abuse and Neglect* 1998; 22:825–843.

Trad PV. *Conversations with Preschool Children*. New York: Norton, 1990. Focuses on the developmental process.

Neurodevelopmental Disorders

Alm PA. Stuttering in relation to anxiety, temperament, and personality: Review and analysis with focus on causality. *Journal of Fluency Disorders* 2014; 40:5–21.

Brentani H, de Paula CS, Bordini D, Rolim D, Sato F, Portolese J, et al. Autism spectrum disorders: An overview on diagnosis and treatment. *Revista Brasileira de Psiquiatria* 2013; 35:S62–S72. [free]

Chapman C, Laird J, Ifill N, KewalRamani A. *Trends in High School Dropout and Completion Rates in the United States: 1972–2009* (NCES 2012-006). Washington, DC: National Center for Education Statistics, 2012. Retrieved from *https://nces.ed.gov/pubs2012/2012006.pdf* [free]

Conti-Ramsden G, Botting N, Simkin Z, Knox E. Follow-up of children attending infant language units: Outcomes at 11 years of age. *International Journal of Language and Communication Disorders* 2001; 36:207–219.

Cortiella C, Horowitz SH. *The State of Learning Disabilities: Facts, Trends and Emerging Issues*, 3rd ed. New York: National Center for Learning Disabilities, 2014. Retrieved from *www.ncld.org/wp-content/uploads/2014/11/2014-State-of-LD.pdf* [free]

Devlin JT, Jamison HL, Gonnerman LM, Matthews PM. The role of the posterior fusiform gyrus in reading. *Journal of Cognitive Neuroscience* 2006; *18*:911–922. [free]

Einfeld SL, Ellis LA, Emerson E. Comorbidity of intellectual disability and mental disorder in children and adolescents: A systematic review. *Journal of Intellectual and Developmental Disability* 2011; *36*:137–143.

Iverach L, Rapee RM. Social anxiety disorder and stuttering: Current status and future directions. *Journal of Fluency Disorders* 2014; *40*:69–82.

King BH, de Lacy N, Siegel M. Psychiatric assessment of severe presentations in autism spectrum disorders and intellectual disability. *Child and Adolescent Psychiatric Clinics of North America* 2014; *23*:1–14.

Knight T, Steeves T, Day L, Lowerison M, Jette N, Pringsheim T. Prevalence of tic disorders: A systematic review and meta-analysis. *Pediatric Neurology* 2012; *47*:77–90.

Lauritsen MB. Autism spectrum disorders. *European Child and Adolescent Psychiatry* 2013; *22*(Suppl 1):S37–S42.

Martino D, Mink JW. Tic disorders. *Continuum* (Minneapolis) 2013; *19*:1287–1311.

Matthews M, Nigg JT, Fair DA. Attention deficit hyperactivity disorder. *Current Topics in Behavioral Sciences* 2014; *16*:235–266. [free]

Moll K, Kunze S, Neuhoff N, Bruder J, Schulte-Köme G. Specific learning disorder: Prevalence and gender differences. *PLoS ONE* 2014; *9*(7):e103537. [free]

Rakhlin N, Cardoso-Martins C, Kornilov SA, Grigorenko EL. Spelling well despite developmental language disorder: What makes it possible? *Annals of Dyslexia* 2013; *63*:253–273. [free]

Shaw ZA, Coffey BJ. Tics and Tourette syndrome. *Psychiatric Clinics of North America* 2014; *37*:269–286.

Smeets EEJ, Pelc K, Dan B. Rett syndrome. *Molecular Syndromology* 2011; *2*:113–127. [free]

Stein DJ, Woods DW. Stereotyped movement disorder in ICD-11. *Revista Brasileira de Psiquiatria* 2014; *36*:S65–S68. [free]

Stothard SE, Snowling MJ, Bishop DVM, Chipchase BB, Kaplan CA. Language impaired preschoolers: A follow up into adolescence. *Journal of Speech, Language and Hearing Research* 1998; *41*:407–418.

Swineford LB, Thurm A, Baird G, Wetherby AM, Swedo S. Social (pragmatic) communication disorder: A research review of this new DSM-5 diagnostic category. *Journal of Neurodevelopmental Disorders* 2014; *6*:41. [free]

Tarver J, Daley D, Sayal K. Attention-deficit hyperactivity disorder (ADHD): An updated review of the essential facts. *Child: Care, Health and Development* 2014; *40*:762–774.

Thomas R, Sanders S, Doust J, Beller E, Glasziou P. Prevalence of attention-deficit/hyperactivity disorder: A systematic review and meta-analysis. *Pediatrics* 2015; *135*:e994-e1001. [free]

Volkmar FR, McPartland JC. From Kanner to DSM-5: Autism as an evolving diagnostic concept. *Annual Review of Clinical Psychology* 2014; *10*:193–212.

Wilson PH, Ruddock S, Smits-Engelsman B, Polatajko H, Blank R. Understanding performance deficits in developmental coordination disorder: A meta-analysis of recent research. *Developmental Medicine and Child Neurology* 2013; *55*:217–228.

Yairi E, Ambrose N. Epidemiology of stuttering: 21st century advances. *Journal of Fluency Disorders* 2013; 38:66–87.

Zeanah CH, Gleason MM. Annual research review: Attachment disorders in early childhood—clinical presentation, causes, correlates, and treatment. *Journal of Child Psychology and Psychiatry* 2015; 56:3207–3222.

Zwicker JG, Missiuna C, Harris SR, Boyd LA. Developmental coordination disorder: A review and update. *European Journal of Paediatric Neurology* 2012; 16:573–581.

Schizophrenia Spectrum and Other Psychotic Disorders

Cak HT, Cengel Kültür SE, Pehlivantürk B. Remitting brief psychotic disorder in a 15-year-old male. *European Child and Adolescent Psychiatry* 2007; 16:281–285.

Castro-Fornieles J, Baeza I, de la Serna E, Gonzalez-Pinto A, Parellada M, Graell M, et al. Two-year diagnostic stability in early-onset first-episode psychosis. *Journal of Child Psychology and Psychiatry* 2011; 52:1089–1098.

Frazier JA, McClellan J, Findling RL, Vitiello B, Anderson R, Zablotsky B, et al. Treatment of early-onset schizophrenia spectrum disorders (TEOSS): Demographic and clinical characteristics. *Journal of the American Academy of Child and Adolescent Psychiatry* 2007; 46:979–988.

Kelleher I, Connor D, Clarke MC, Devlin N, Harley M, Cannon M. Prevalence of psychotic symptoms in childhood and adolescence: A systematic review and meta-analysis of population-based studies. *Psychological Medicine* 2012; 42:1857–1863.

Kelleher I, Keeley M, Corcoran P, Lynch F, Fitzpatrick C, Devlin N, et al. Clinicopathological significance of psychotic experiences in non-psychotic young people: Evidence from four population-based studies. *British Journal of Psychiatry* 2012; 201:26–32. [free]

McClellan J, Stock S. Practice parameter for the assessment and treatment of children and adolescents with schizophrenia. *Journal of the American Academy of Child and Adolescent Psychiatry* 2013; 52:976–990. [free]

Okkels N, Vernal DL, Jensen SO, McGrath JJ, Nielsen RE. Changes in the diagnosed incidence of early onset schizophrenia over four decades. *Acta Psychiatrica Scandinavica* 2013; 127:62–68.

Tandon R, Heckers S, Bustillo J, Barch DM, Gaibel W, Gur RE, et al. Catatonia in DSM-5. *Schizophrenia Research* 2013; 150:26–30.

Tiffin PA, Welsh P. Practitioner review: Schizophrenia spectrum disorders and the at-risk mental state for psychosis in children and adolescents—evidence-based management approaches. *Journal of Child Psychology and Psychiatry* 2013; 54:1155–1175.

Mood Disorders

Clark MS, Jansen KL, Cloy A. Treatment of childhood and adolescent depression. *American Family Physician* 2012; 86:442–448. [free]

Copeland WE, Angold A, Costello EJ, Egger H. Prevalence, comorbidity and correlates of DSM-5 proposed disruptive mood dysregulation disorder. *American Journal of Psychiatry* 2013; 170:173–179. [free]

Copeland WE, Shanahan L, Egger H, Angold A, Costello EJ. Adult diagnostic and functional outcomes of DSM-5 disruptive mood dysregulation disorder. *American Journal of Psychiatry* 2014; *171*:668–674. [free]

DeFilippis MS, Wagner KD. Bipolar depression in children and adolescents. *CNS Spectrums* 2013; *18*:209–213.

Dinya E, Csorba J, Grósz Z. Are there temperament differences between major depression and dysthymic disorder in adolescent clinical outpatients? *Comprehensive Psychiatry* 2012; *53*:350–354.

Dougherty LR, Smith VC, Bufferd SJ, Carlson GA, Stringaris A, Leibenluft E, et al. DSM-5 disruptive mood dysregulation disorder: Correlates and predictors in young children. *Psychological Medicine* 2014; *44*:2339–2350. [free]

Gould MS, Marrocco FA, Kleinman M, Thomas JG, Mostkoff K, Cote J, et al. Evaluating iatrogenic risk of youth suicide screening programs. A randomized controlled trial. *Journal of the American Medical Association* 2005; *293*:1635–1643.

Harrington R, Rutter M, Weissman M, Fudge H, Groothues C, Bredenkamp D, et al. Psychiatric disorders in the relatives of depressed probands: I. Comparison of prepubertal, adolescent and early adult onset cases. *Journal of Affective Disorders* 1997; *42*:9–22.

Jonsson U, Bohman H, von Knorring L, Olsson G, Paaren A, von Knorring A-L. Mental health outcome of long-term and episodic adolescent depression: 15-year follow-up of a community sample. *Journal of Affective Disorders* 2011; *130*:395–404.

Kessler RC, Avenevoli S, Costello EJ, Georgiades K, Green JG, Gruber MJ, et al. Prevalence, persistence, and sociodemographic correlates of DSM-IV disorders in the National Comorbidity Survey Replication Adolescent Supplement. *Archives of General Psychiatry* 2012; *69*:372–380. [free]

Kessler RC, Avenevoli S, Costello J, Green JG, Gruber MJ, McLaughlin KA, et al. Severity of 12-month DSM-IV disorders in the National Comorbidity Survey Replication Adolescent Supplement. *Archives of General Psychiatry* 2012; *69*:381–389. [free]

Leibenluft E. Severe mood dysregulation, irritability, and the diagnostic boundaries of bipolar disorder in youths. *American Journal of Psychiatry* 2011; *168*:129–142. [free]

Lochman JE, Evans SC, Burke JD, Roberts MC, Fite PJ, Reed GM, et al. An empirically based alternative to DSM-5's disruptive mood dysregulation disorder for ICD-11. *World Psychiatry* 2015; *14*:30–33. [free]

Margulies DM, Weintraub S, Basile J, Grover PJ, Carlson GA. Will disruptive mood dysregulation disorder reduce false diagnosis of bipolar disorder in children? *Bipolar Disorders* 2012; *14*:488–496.

Mayes SD, Mathiowetz C, Kokotovich C, Waxmonsky J, Baweja R, Calhoun SL, et al. Stability of disruptive mood dysregulation disorder symptoms (irritable-angry mood and temper outbursts) throughout childhood and adolescence in a general population sample. *Journal of Abnormal Child Psychology* 2015; *43*:1543–1549.

Merikangas KR, Cui L, Kattan G, Carlson GA, Youngstrom EA, Angst J. Mania with and without depression in a community sample of US adolescents. *Archives of General Psychiatry* 2012; *69*:943–951. [free]

Nardi B, Francesconi G, Catena-Dell'osso M, Bellantuono C. Adolescent depression: Clinical features and therapeutic strategies. *European Review for Medical and Pharmacological Sciences* 2013; *17*:1546–1551. [free]

Rapkin AJ, Mikacich JA. Premenstrual dysphoric disorder and severe premenstrual syndrome in adolescents. *Pediatric Drugs* 2013; *15*:191–202.

Roy AK, Lopes V, Klein RG. Disruptive mood dysregulation disorder: A new diagnostic approach to chronic irritability in youth. *American Journal of Psychiatry* 2014; *171*:918–924. [free]

Swedo SE, Pleeter JD, Richter DM, Hoffman CL, Allen AJ, Hamburger SD, et al. Rates of seasonal affective disorder in children and adolescents. *American Journal of Psychiatry* 1995; *152*:1016–1019.

Tonetti L, Barbato G, Fabbri M, Adan A, Natale V. Mood seasonality: A cross-sectional study of subjects aged between 10 and 25 years. *Journal of Affective Disorders* 2007; *97*:155–160.

Van Meter A, Youngstrom EA, Youngstrom JK, Feeny NC, Findling RL. Examining the validity of cyclothymic disorder in a youth sample. *Journal of Affective Disorders* 2011; *132*:55–63. [free]

Anxiety Disorders

Asmundson GJG, Taylor S, Smits JAJ. Panic disorder and agoraphobia: An overview and commentary on DSM-5 changes. *Depression and Anxiety* 2014; *31*:480–486.

Bagnell AL. Anxiety and separation disorders. *Pediatrics in Review* 2011; *32*:440–446.

Beesdo K, Knappe S, Pine DS. Anxiety and anxiety disorders in children and adolescents: Developmental issues and implications for DSM-V. *Psychiatric Clinics of North America* 2009; *32*:483–524. [free]

Copeland WE, Angold A, Shanahan L, Costello EJ. Longitudinal patterns of anxiety from childhood to adulthood: The Great Smoky Mountains study. *Journal of the American Academy of Child and Adolescent Psychiatry* 2014; *53*:21–33. [free]

Creswell C, Waite P, Cooper PJ. Assessment and management of anxiety disorders in children and adolescents. *Archives of Disease in Childhood* 2014; *99*:674–678. [free]

Klein RG. Anxiety disorders. *Journal of Child Psychology and Psychiatry* 2009; *50*:153–162.

Lewinsohn PM, Holm-Denoma JM, Small JW, Seeley JR, Joiner TE Jr. Separation anxiety disorder in childhood as a risk factor for future mental illness. *Journal of the American Academy of Child and Adolescent Psychiatry* 2008; *47*:548–555. [free]

McBride ME. Beyond butterflies: Generalized anxiety disorder in adolescents. *The Nurse Practitioner* 2015; *40*:28–36.

Mesa F, Beidel DC, Bunnell BE. An examination of psychopathology and daily impairment in adolescents with social anxiety disorder. *PLoS ONE* 2014; *9*:e93668. [free]

Mohr C, Schneider S. Anxiety disorders. *European Child and Adolescent Psychiatry* 2013; *22*(Suppl 1):S17–S22.

Silverman WK, Moreno J. Specific phobia. *Child and Adolescent Psychiatric Clinics of North America* 2005; *14*:819–843.

Viana AG, Beidel DC, Rabian B. Selective mutism: A review and integration of the last 15 years. *Clinical Psychology Review* 2009; *29*:57–67.

Waite P, Creswell C. Children and adolescents referred for treatment of anxiety disorders: Differences in clinical characteristics. *Journal of Affective Disorders* 2014; *167*:326–332. [free]

Obsessive–Compulsive and Related Disorders

Boileau B. A review of obsessive–compulsive disorder in children and adolescents. *Dialogues in Clinical Neuroscience* 2011; *13*:401–411. [free]

Harrison JP, Franklin ME. Pediatric trichotillomania. *Current Psychiatry Reports* 2012; *14*:188–196. [free]

Ivanov VZ, Mataix-Cols D, Serlachius E, Lichtenstein P, Anckarsäter H, Chang Z, et al. Prevalence, comorbidity and heritability of hoarding symptoms in adolescence: A population based twin study in 15-year olds. 2013; PLoS ONE 8:e69140. [free]

Krebs G, Heyman I. Obsessive–compulsive disorder in children and adolescents. *Archives of Disease in Childhood* 2015; *100*:495–499. [free]

Leibovici V, Murad S, Cooper-Kazaz R, Tetro T, Keuthem NJ, Hadayer N, et al. Excoriation (skin picking) disorder in Israeli University students: Prevalence and associated mental health correlates. *General Hospital Psychiatry* 2014; *36*:686–689.

Murphy TK, Patel PD, McGuire JF, Kennel A, Mutch PJ, Parker-Athill EC, et al. Characterization of the pediatric acute-onset neuropsychiatric syndrome phenotype. *Journal of Child and Adolescent Psychopharmacology* 2015; *25*:14–25.

Schieber K, Kollei I, de Zwaan M, Martin A. Classification of body dysmorphic disorder: What is the advantage of the new DSM-5 criteria? *Journal of Psychosomatic Research* 2015; *78*:223–227.

Snorrason I, Stein DJ, Woods DW. Classification of excoriation (skin picking) disorder: current status and future directions. *Acta Psychiatrica Scandinavica* 2013; *128*:406–407.

Storch EA, Rahman O, Park JM, Reid J, Murphy TK, Lewin AB. Compulsive hoarding in children. *Journal of Clinical Psychology: In Session* 2011; *67*:507–516.

Trauma- and Stressor-Related Disorders

Casey P. Adjustment disorder: New developments. *Current Psychiatry Reports* 2014; *16*:451.

Pelkonen M, Marttunen M, Henriksson M, Lönnqvist J. Adolescent adjustment disorder: Precipitant stressors and distress symptoms of 89 outpatients. *European Psychiatry* 2007; *22*:288–295.

Rosenberg AR, Postier A, Osenga K, Kreicbergs U, Neville B, Dussel V, et al. Long-term psychosocial outcomes among bereaved siblings of children with cancer. *Journal of Pain Symptom Management* 2015; *49*:55–65. [free]

Schmid M, Petermann F, Fegert JM. Developmental trauma disorder: Pros and cons of including formal criteria in the psychiatric diagnostic systems. *BMC Psychiatry* 2013; *13*:3. [free]

Stoddard FJ Jr. Outcomes of traumatic exposure. *Child and Adolescent Psychiatric Clinics of North America* 2014; *23*:243–256.

Dissociative Disorders

Bernier M-J, Hébert M, Collin-Vézina D. Dissociative symptoms over a year in a sample of sexually abused children. *Journal of Trauma and Dissociation* 2013; *14*:455–472.

Boysen GA. The scientific status of childhood dissociative identity disorder: A review of published research. *Psychotherapy and Psychosomatics* 2011; *80*:329–334.

Li J, Vestergaard M, Cnattingius S, Gissler M, Bech BH, Obel C, et al. Mortality after parental death in childhood: A nationwide cohort study from three Nordic countries. *PLoS Medicine* 2014; *11*:e1001679. [free]

Sar V, Onder C, Kilincasian A, Zoroglu SS, Alyanak B. Dissociative identity disorder among adolescents: Prevalence in a university psychiatric outpatient unit. *Journal of Trauma and Dissociation* 2014; *15*:402–419.

Wolf MR, Nochajski TH. Child sexual abuse survivors with dissociative amnesia: What's the difference? *Journal of Child Sexual Abuse* 2013; *22*:462–480.

Somatic Symptom and Related Disorders

Ani C, Reading R, Lynn R, Forlee S, Garralda E. Incidence and 12-month outcome of non-transient childhood conversion disorder in the UK and Ireland. *British Journal of Psychiatry* 2013; *202*:413–418. [free]

Bass C, Glaser D. Early recognition and management of fabricated or induced illness in children. *Lancet* 2014; *383*:1412–1421.

El-Metwally A, Halder S, Thompson D, Macfarlane GJ, Jones GT. Predictors of abdominal pain in schoolchildren: A 4-year population-based prospective study. *Archives of Disease in Childhood* 2007; *92*:1094–1098. [free]

Fava GA, Fabbri S, Sirri L, Wise TN. Psychological factors affecting medical condition: A new proposal for DSM-V. *Psychosomatics* 2007; *48*:103–111.

Patel H, Dunn DW, Austin JK, Doss JL, LaFrance WC Jr, Plioplys S, et al. Psychogenic nonepileptic seizures (pseudoseizures). *Pediatrics in Review* 2011; *32*:e66–e72.

Schulte IE, Petermann F. Somatoform disorders: 30 years of debate about criteria! What about children and adolescents? *Journal of Psychosomatic Research* 2011; *70*:218–228.

Feeding and Eating Disorders

Allen KA, Byrne SM, Oddy WH, Crosby RD. DSM-IV-TR and DSM-5 eating disorders in adolescents: Prevalence, stability, and psychosocial correlates in a population-based sample of male and female adolescents. *Journal of Abnormal Psychology* 2013; *122*:720–732.

Bucchianeri MM, Ariklan AJ, Hannan PJ, Eisenberg ME, Neumark-Sztainer D. Body dissatisfaction from adolescence to young adulthood: Findings from a 10-year longitudinal study. *Body Image* 2013; *10*:1–7. [free]

Campbell K, Peebles R. Eating disorders in children and adolescents: State of the art review. *Pediatrics* 2014; *134*:582–592. [free]

Föcker M, Knoll S, Hebebrand J. Anorexia nervosa. *European Child and Adolescent Psychiatry* 2013; *22*(Suppl 1): S29–S35.

Herpertz-Dahlmann B. Adolescent eating disorders: Update on definitions, symptomatology, epidemiology, and comorbidity. *Child and Adolescent Psychiatric Clinics of North America* 2015; *24*:177–196.

Kelly NR, Shank LM, Bakalar JL, Tanofsky-Kraff M. Pediatric feeding and eating disorders: Current state of diagnosis and treatment. *Current Psychiatry Reports* 2014; *16*:446.

Elimination Disorders

Fritz G, Rockney R, Bernet W, Arnold V, Beitchman J, Benson RS, et al. Practice parameter for the assessment and treatment of children and adolescents with enuresis. *Journal of the American Academy of Child and Adolescent Psychiatry* 2004; *43*:1540–1550.

Robson WL. Clinical practice: Evaluation and management of enuresis. *New England Journal of Medicine* 2009; *360*:1429–1436.

Von Gontard, A. The impact of DSM-5 and guidelines for assessment and treatment of elimination disorders. *European Child and Adolescent Psychiatry* 2013; *22*(Suppl 1):S61–S67.

Sleep–Wake Disorders

American Academy of Sleep Medicine. *International Classification of Sleep Disorders*, 3rd ed. Darien, IL: Author, 2014.

Barclay NL, Gregory AM. Sleep in childhood and adolescence: Age-specific sleep characteristics, common sleep disturbances and associated difficulties. *Current Topics in Behavioral Neurosciences* 2014; *16*:337–365.

Byars KC, Yolton K, Rausch J, Lanphear B, Beebe DW. Prevalence, patterns, and persistence of sleep problems in the first 3 years of life. *Pediatrics* 2012; *129*:e276–e284. [free]

Carter KA, Hathaway NE, Lettieri CF. Common sleep disorders in children. *American Family Physician* 2014; *89*:368–377. [free]

Stores G. Aspects of parasomnias in childhood and adolescence. *Archives of Disease in Childhood* 2009; *94*:63–69.

Gender Dysphoria

Holt V, Skagerberg E, Dunsford M. Young people with features of gender dysphoria: Demographics and associated difficulties. *Clinical Child Psychology and Psychiatry* 2016; *21*:108–118.

Shechner T. Gender identity disorder: A literature review from a developmental perspective. *Israel Journal of Psychiatry and Related Sciences* 2010; *47*:132–138. [free]

Spack NP, Edwards-Leeper L, Feldman HA, Leibowitz S, Mandel F, Diamond DA, et al. Children and adolescents with gender identity disorder referred to a pediatric medical center. *Pediatrics* 2012; *129*:418–425. [free]

Zucker KJ, Wood H. Assessment of gender variance in children. *Child and Adolescent Psychiatric Clinics of North America* 2011; *20*:665–680.

Disruptive, Impulse-Control, and Conduct Disorders

Aboujaoude E, Gamel N, Koran LM. Overview of kleptomania and phenomenological description of 40 patients. *Primary Care Companion to the Journal of Clinical Psychiatry* 2004; *6*:244–247. [free]

Blair RJJ. The neurobiology of psychopathic traits in youths. *Nature Reviews Neuroscience* 2013; *14*:786–799. [free]

Burke JD. An affective dimension within ODD symptoms among boys: Personality and psychopathology outcomes into early adulthood. *Journal of Child Psychology and Psychiatry* 2012; 53:1176–1183. [free]

Chan LG, Bharat S, Dani DK. Pattern of psychiatric morbidity among theft offenders remanded or referred for psychiatric evaluation and factors associated with reoffence. *Singapore Medical Journal* 2013; 54:339–342. [free]

Fairchild G, van Goozen SH, Calder AJ, Goodyer IM. Research review: Evaluating and reformulating the developmental taxonomic theory of antisocial behavior. *Journal of Child Psychology and Psychiatry* 2013; 54:924–940. [free]

Frick PJ, Ray JV, Thornton LC, Kahn RE. Can callous–unemotional traits enhance the understanding, diagnosis, and treatment of serious conduct problems in children and adolescents?: A comprehensive review. *Psychological Bulletin* 2014; 140:1–57.

Grant JE, Kim SW. Clinical Characteristics and associated psychopathology of 22 patients with kleptomania. *Comprehensive Psychiatry* 2002; 43:378–384.

Grant JE, Potenza MN, Krishnan-Sarin S, Cavallo DA, Desai RA. Stealing among high school students: Prevalence and clinical correlates. *Journal of the American Academy of Psychiatry and the Law* 2011; 39:44–52. [free]

Herpers PC, Rommelse NN, Bons DM, Buitelaar JK, Scheepers FE. Callous–unemotional traits as a cross-disorders construct. *Social Psychiatry and Psychiatric Epidemiology* 2012; 47:2045–2064. [free]

Lambie I, Randell I. Creating a firestorm: A review of children who deliberately light fires. *Clinical Psychology Review* 2011; 31:307–327.

McLaughlin KA, Green JG, Hwang I, Sampson NA, Zaslavsky AM, Kessler RC. Intermittent explosive disorder in the National Comorbidity Survey Replication Adolescent Supplement. *Archives of General Psychiatry* 2012; 69:1131–1139. [free]

Robins L. *Deviant children grown up: A sociological and psychiatric study of sociopathic personality.* Baltimore, Williams & Wilkins, 1974.

Shelleby EC, Kolko DJ. Predictors, moderators, and treatment parameters of community and clinic-based treatment for child disruptive behavior disorders. *Journal of Child and Family Studies* 2015; 24:734–748.

Steiner H, Remsing L, The Work Group on Quality Issues. Practice parameter for the assessment and treatment of children and adolescents with oppositional defiant disorder. *Journal of the American Academy of Child and Adolescent Psychiatry* 2007; 46:126–141.

Vaughn MG, Fu Q, DeLisi M, Wright JP, Beaver KM, Perron BE, et al. Prevalence and correlates of fire-setting in the United States: Results from the National Epidemiological Survey on Alcohol and Related Conditions. *Comprehensive Psychiatry* 2010; 51:217–223. [free]

Substance-Related and Addictive Disorders

Bukstein OG, Bernet W, Arnold V, Beitchman J, Shaw J, Benson RS, et al. Practice parameter for the assessment and treatment of children and adolescents with substance use disorders. *Journal of the American Academy of Child and Adolescent Psychiatry* 2005; 44:609–621.

Johnston LD, O'Malley PM, Bachman JG, Schulenberg JE, Miech RA. *Monitoring the Future:*

National Survey Results on Drug Use, 1975–2013. Vol 1. Secondary School Students. Ann Arbor: Institute for Social Research, University of Michigan, 2014. Retrieved from *http://monitoringthefuture.org//pubs/monographs/mtf-vol1_2013.pdf* [free]

McCabe SE, West BT, Veliz P, Frank KA, Boyd CJ. Social contexts of substance use among U.S. high school seniors: A multicohort national study. *Journal of Adolescent Health* 2014; 55:842–844.

Simkin DR. Adolescent substance use disorders and comorbidity. *Pediatric Clinics of North America* 2002; 49:463–477.

Windle M, Spear LP, Fuligni AJ, Angold A, Brown JD, Pine D, et al. Transitions into underage and problem drinking: Developmental processes and mechanisms between 10 and 15 years of age. *Pediatrics* 2008; 121(Suppl 4):S273–S289. [free]

Cognitive Disorders

Kelly P, Frosch E. Recognition of delirium on pediatric hospital services. *Psychosomatics* 2012; 53:446–451.

Max JE. Neuropsychiatry of pediatric traumatic brain injury. *Psychiatric Clinics of North America* 2014; 37:125–140. [free]

Nilsson L-G. Memory function in normal aging. *Acta Neurologica Scandinavica* 2003; 107(Suppl 179):7–13.

Smith HAB, Brink E, Fuchs DC, Ely EW, Pandharipande PP. Pediatric delirium: Monitoring and management in the pediatric intensive care unit. *Pediatric Clinics of North America* 2013; 60:741–760.

Personality Disorders

Kaess M, Brunner R, Chanen A. Borderline personality disorder in adolescence. *Pediatrics* 2014; 134:782–793. [free]

Larrivée M-P. Borderline personality disorder in adolescents: The He-who-must-not-be-named of psychiatry. *Dialogues in Clinical Neuroscience* 2013; 15:171–179. [free]

Other Diagnostic Codes

The Centers for Disease Control has a webpage on violence prevention: *www.cdc.gov/violenceprevention/overview/index.html*

National Child Traumatic Stress Network's 12 core concepts for understanding children's response to traumatic stress. *http://nctsn.org/resources/audiences/parents-caregivers/what-is-cts/12-core-concepts* [free]

Felitti VJ, Anda RF, Nordenberg D, Williamson DF, Spitz AM, Edwards V, et al. Relationship of childhood abuse and household dysfunction to many of the leading causes of death in adults: The Adverse Childhood Experiences (ACE) Study. *American Journal of Preventive Medicine* 1998; 14:245–258. (More information at *www.acestudy.org*)

Harrison AG, Edwards MJ, Parker KC. Identifying students faking ADHD: Preliminary findings and strategies for detection. *Archives of Clinical Neuropsychology* 2007; 22:577–588. [free]

Walker JS. Malingering in children: Fibs and faking. *Child and Adolescent Psychiatric Clinics of North America* 2011; 20:547–556.

Wamboldt M, Kaslow N, Reiss D. Description of relational processes: Recent changes in DSM-5 and proposals for ICD-11. *Family Process* 2015; 54:6–16.

Outline of DSM-5 Diagnoses

$\mathbf{A}$ppendix 2 is an overview of the specific DSM-5 diagnoses likely to be useful for juvenile patients. Not every disorder or other diagnostic code covered in Part II of this book is included in this appendix. To save space, we have chosen to omit all of the "catch-all" diagnoses (the ones beginning with the words *other specified* or *unspecified*). We have also omitted the medication-induced disorders and additional administrative codes listed in Chapter 27, and a few disorders that are extremely rare in children and adolescents.

We have made use of the following typographical conventions. Names of diagnosis groups within sections are given in *italics*. Names of individual diagnoses for which we provide Essential Features sets in this book are given in **boldface;** names of other diagnoses are given in roman type. Diagnoses illustrated by case presentations are marked with an asterisk (*); a few disorders are illustrated by more than one case example; and more than one disorder is sometimes represented in a single case example. When known, relative frequency by gender is stated.

This appendix also states the presence of disorders in various age groups, according to the code given below. In some cases, it is not known when the diagnosis is most likely to be first encountered; in others, a bimodal distribution has been reported.

> 0 = Diagnosis is inappropriate at this age
> + = Diagnosis can apply to age group
> ++ = Diagnosis is likely to be first encountered in this age group

Finally, the abbreviation AMC is used throughout for *another medical condition*.

Section, Group, or Disorder	Code Number	Page Number	Male–Female Ratio	Infancy	Toddler	Preschool Age	School Age	Early Adolescence	Late Adolescence	Adulthood
Neurodevelopmental Disorders										
Intellectual disability		164	M > F							
Mild*	F70			+	++	+	+	+	+	+
Moderate	F71			+	++	+	+	+	+	+
Severe	F72			++	+	+	+	+	+	+
Profound	F73			++	+	+	+	+	+	+
Global developmental delay	F88	172		0	+	++	0	0	0	0
Language disorder*	F80.2	172	M > F	0	+	++	+	+	+	+
Speech sound disorder*	F80.0	175	M > F	0	+	++	+	+	+	+
Childhood-onset fluency disorder (stuttering)	F80.81	176	M > F	0	+	++	+	+	+	+
Social (pragmatic) communication disorder	F80.89	177		0	0	+	++	+	+	+
Autism spectrum disorder*	F84.0	181	M > F	+	++	+	+	+	+	+
Attention-deficit/hyperactivity disorder*	F90.x	192	M > F	0	+	+	++	+	+	+
Predominantly inattentive presentation	F90.0									
Predominantly hyperactive/impulsive presentation	F90.1									
Combined presentation	F90.2									
Specific learning disorder*	F81.xx	197								
With impairment in reading	F81.0	198	M = F	0	0	0	++	+	+	+
With impairment in mathematics	F81.2	201		0	0	0	++	+	+	+
With impairment in written expression	F81.81	202		0	0	0	++	+	+	+
Developmental coordination disorder*	F82	203	M > F	0	0	+	++	+	+	+
Stereotypic movement disorder*	F98.4	207		0	+	+	+	+	+	+
Tourette's disorder*	F95.2	209	M > F	0	+	+	++	++	+	+
Persistent motor or vocal tic disorder	F95.1	209	M > F	0	+	+	++	++	+	+
Provisional tic disorder	F95.0	209	M > F	0	+	+	++	++	+	+
Schizophrenia Spectrum and Other Psychotic Disorders										
Schizophrenia*	F21	218	M > F	0	0	0	+	+	++	++
Delusional disorder	F22	225	M = F	0	0	0	+	+	+	++
Schizophreniform disorder*	F20.81	223	M > F	0	0	0	+	+	+	++

Section, Group, or Disorder	Code Number	Page Number	Male–Female Ratio	Infancy	Toddler	Preschool Age	School Age	Early Adolescence	Late Adolescence	Adulthood
Schizophrenia Spectrum and Other Psychotic Disorders *(cont.)*										
Schizoaffective disorder	F25.x	223	F > M	0	0	0	+	+	+	++
Brief psychotic disorder	F23	223	F > M	0	0	0	+	+	+	++
Psychotic disorder due to [AMC]	F06.x	224	F > M?	0	0	+	+	+	+	++
[Substance/medication]-induced psychotic disorder	—.—	225	M > F?	0	0	0	+	+	+	++
Catatonia associated with another mental disorder (catatonia specifier)	F06.1	223		0	0	0	+	+	+	++
Mood Disorders										
Bipolar and Related Disorders										
Bipolar I disorder*	F31.xx	253	F > M	0	0	0	0	+	+	++
Bipolar II disorder	F31.81	253	F > M	0	0	0	0	+	+	++
Cyclothymic disorder	F34.0	254	M = F	0	0	0	0	+	+	++
Depressive Disorders										
Disruptive mood dysregulation disorder*	F34.8	246								
Major depressive disorder, single episode*	F32.xx	239	F > M	0	0	+	+	+	+	++
Major depressive disorder, recurrent episode	F33.xx	239	F > M	0	0	0	+	+	+	++
Persistent depressive disorder (dysthymia)*	F34.1	241	F > M	0	0	+	+	+	+	++
Premenstrual dysphoric disorder	N93.4	247	F	0	0	0	0	+	+	++
Other Mood Disorders										
{Depressive} {Bipolar} disorder due to [AMC]	F06.3x	258		0	0	0	+	+	+	++
[Substance/medication]-induced {depressive} {bipolar} disorder	—.—	258		0	0	0	+	+	+	++
Anxiety Disorders										
Separation anxiety disorder*	F93.0	262	F > M	0	0	+	++	+	+	+
Selective mutism*	F94.0	266	F > M	0	+	+	++	+	+	+
Specific phobia*	F40.2xx	270	F > M	0		++	+	+	+	++
Social anxiety disorder*	F40.10	272		0	0	+	+	++	+	+
Panic disorder*	F41.0	275	F > M	0	0	+	+	+	++	++
Agoraphobia*	F40.00	275	F > M							
Generalized anxiety disorder*	F41.1	279	F > M	0	0	+	++	++	+	+

Section, Group, or Disorder	Code Number	Page Number	Male–Female Ratio	Infancy	Toddler	Preschool Age	School Age	Early Adolescence	Late Adolescence	Adulthood
Anxiety Disorders (*cont.*)										
[Substance/medication]-induced anxiety disorder	—.–	283		0	0	0	+	+	+	++
Anxiety disorder due to [AMC]	F06.4	283		0	0	+	+	+	+	++
Obsessive–Compulsive and Related Disorders										
Obsessive–compulsive disorder*	F42	285	M = F	0	0	+	++	+	+	++
Body dysmorphic disorder	F45.22	291	M = F	0	0	0	+	++	++	+
Hoarding disorder	F42	291								
Trichotillomania*	F63.3	291	F > M	0	0	0	+	+	+	++
Excoriation (skin-picking) disorder	L98.1	291								
[Substance/medication]-induced obsessive–compulsive and related disorder	—.–	294		0	0	0	+	+	+	++
Obsessive–compulsive and related disorder due to [AMC]	F06.8	294		0	0	+	+	+	+	++
Trauma- and Stressor-Related Disorders										
Reactive attachment disorder*	F94.1	297		++	++	+	+	+	+	+
Disinhibited social engagement disorder*	F94.2	297								
Posttraumatic stress disorder*	F43.10	303	F > M	0	+	+	+	+	+	++
Acute stress disorder	F43.0	303		0	+	+	+	+	+	++
Adjustment disorder*	F43.2x	311	M = F	0	0	+	+	+	+	++
Dissociative Disorders										
Dissociative identity disorder	F44.81		F > M	0	0	0	+	+	+	++
Dissociative amnesia*	F44.0	319		0	0	0	+	+	+	++
With dissociative fugue	F44.1			0	0	0	0	+	+	++
Depersonalization/derealization disorder	F48.1			0	0	0	+	+	+	++
Somatic Symptom and Related Disorders										
Somatic symptom disorder*	F45.1	328	F > M	0	0	0	0	+	+	++
With predominant pain*		332	F > M	0	0	+	+	+	+	++
Illness anxiety disorder	F45.21		M = F	0	0	0	+	+	+	++
Conversion disorder*	F44.x	324	F > M	0	0	+	+	+	+	++
Psychological factors affecting other medical conditions	F54	334		0	0	0	+	+	+	++
Factitious disorder*	F68.10	338	M > F	0	0	+	+	+	+	++

Section, Group, or Disorder	Code Number	Page Number	Male–Female Ratio	Infancy	Toddler	Preschool Age	School Age	Early Adolescence	Late Adolescence	Adulthood
Feeding and Eating Disorders										
Pica (in children)*	F98.3	345			+	++	+	+	+	+
Rumination disorder	F98.21	347	M > F	++	+	+	+	+	+	+
Avoidant/restrictive food intake disorder*	F50.8	348		++	+	0	0	0	0	0
Anorexia nervosa*	F50.0x	351	F > M	0	0	0	+	+	++	+
Bulimia nervosa*	F50.2	351	F > M	0	0	0	+	+	++	+
Binge-eating disorder*	F50.8	355								
Elimination Disorders										
Encopresis*	F98.1	361	M > F	0	0	+	++	+	+	+
Enuresis*	F98.0	363	M > F	0	0	+	++	+	+	+
Sleep–Wake Disorders										
Insomnia disorder	F51.01		F > M	0	0	0	+	+	+	++
Hypersomnia disorder	F51.11		M > F	0	0	0	+	+	++	++
Narcolepsy	G47.4xx		M = F	0	0	0	0	+	+	++
Obstructive sleep apnea hypopnea*	G47.33	373	M > F	0	+	+	++	+	+	++
Circadian rhythm sleep–wake disorder	G47.2x							+	++	++
Non-REM sleep arousal disorder										
Sleepwalking type*	F51.3	371	M = F	0	0	+	++	+	+	+
Sleep terror type*	F51.4	369	M > F	0	0	++	+	+	+	+
Nightmare disorder	F51.5			0	+	+	+	+	+	+
REM sleep behavior disorder	G47.52									
[Substance/medication]-induced sleep disorder	—.—	376		0	0	0	+	+	+	++
Gender Dysphoria										
In children*	F64.2	378	M > F	0	0	+	+	+	0	0
In adolescents or adults	F64.1		M > F	0	0	0	0	+	+	++
Disruptive, Impulse-Control, and Conduct Disorders										
Oppositional defiant disorder*	F91.3	386	M > F	0	0	+	++	+	+	+
Intermittent explosive disorder	F63.81		M > F	0	0	0	0	0	+	++
Conduct disorder*	F91.x	389	M > F	0	0	+	++	+	+	+
Pyromania	F63.1	394	M > F	0	0	0	0	0	+	++
Kleptomania	F63.2	394	F > M	0	0	0	0	0	+	++

Section, Group, or Disorder	Code Number	Page Number	Male–Female Ratio	Infancy	Toddler	Preschool Age	School Age	Early Adolescence	Late Adolescence	Adulthood
Substance-Related and Addictive Disorders										
[Substance] use disorder*	—.—	400	M > F	0	0	0	+	+	+	++
[Substance] intoxication*	—.—	402	M > F	0	0	0	+	+	+	++
[Substance] withdrawal*	—.—	402	M > F	0	0	0	+	+	+	++
Gambling disorder	F63.0		M > F	0	0	0	0	+	++	++
Cognitive Disorders										
Delirium										
[Substance] intoxication delirium*	—.—	418		0	0	0	+	+	+	++
[Substance] withdrawal delirium	—.—	418		0	0	0	+	+	+	++
Medication-induced delirium	—.—	418								
Delirium due to [AMC]	F05	418		+	++	++	+	+	+	+
Major and Mild Neurocognitive Disorder (NCD)[a]										
NCD due to Alzheimer's disease	F02.8x		F > M	0	0	0	0	0	0	++
Vascular NCD	F01.5x		M > F	0	0	+	+	+	+	++
NCD due to traumatic brain injury*	F02.8x	425	M > F	0	0	+	+	+	+	++
NCD due to HIV infection	F02.8x		M > F	0	0	+	+	+	+	++
NCD due to prion disease	F02.8x			0	0	+	+	+	+	++
NCD due to Huntington's disease	F02.8x		M = F	0	0	0	0	+	+	++
NCD due to [AMC]	F02.8x	424		0	0	+	+	+	+	++
[Substance/medication]-induced NCD	—.—			0	0	+	+	+	+	++
Personality Disorders*										
Paranoid personality disorder	F60.0		M > F	0	0	0	0	+	+	++
Schizoid personality disorder	F60.1		M > F	0	0	0	0	+	+	++
Schizotypal personality disorder	F21			0	0	0	0	+	+	++
Antisocial personality disorder	F60.2		M > F	0	0	0	0	0	+	++
Borderline personality disorder	F60.3		F > M	0	0	0	0	+	+	++
Histrionic personality disorder	F60.4		F > M	0	0	0	0	+	+	++
Narcissistic personality disorder	F60.81		M > F	0	0	0	0	+	+	++
Avoidant personality disorder	F60.6		M = F	0	0	0	0	+	+	++
Dependent personality disorder	F60.7		M = F	0	0	0	0	+	+	++
Obsessive–compulsive personality disorder	F60.5		M > F	0	0	0	0	+	+	++
Personality change due to [AMC]	F07.0			0	0	0	+	+	+	++

[a]Code numbers are given for major NCD (dementia); all etiologies of mild NCD are coded G31.84. For major NCD, the fifth digit (x) is 1 for *with behavioral disturbance* and 0 for *without behavioral disturbance.*

Section, Group, or Disorder	Code Number	Page Number	Male–Female Ratio	Infancy	Toddler	Preschool Age	School Age	Early Adolescence	Late Adolescence	Adulthood
Other Conditions That May Be a Focus of Clinical Attention										
Relational Problems										
Parent–child relational problem*	Z62.820	437		0	+	+	+	+	+	+
Sibling relational problem	Z63.891	438		0	+	++	+	+	+	+
Upbringing away from parents	Z62.29	438		+	+	+	+	+	+	+
Child affected by parental relationship distress	Z62.898	438		+	+	+	+	+	+	+
Uncomplicated bereavement	Z63.4	438		0	+	+	+	+	+	+
Problems Related to Abuse or Neglect[b]										
Child physical abuse, confirmed	T74.12	441		+	+	+	+	+	+	0
Child sexual abuse, confirmed	T74.22	441		+	+	+	+	++	+	0
Child neglect, confirmed	T74.02	441		+	+	+	+	+	+	0
Child psychological abuse, confirmed	T74.32	441		+	+	+	+	+	+	0
Additional Conditions That May Be a Focus of Clinical Attention										
Nonadherence to medical treatment	Z91.19	443		0	0	0	+	+	+	++
Malingering	Z76.5	443					+	+	+	+
Child or adolescent antisocial behavior	Z72.810	444		0	0	0	+	+	+	0
Borderline intellectual functioning	R41.83	444		0	0	+	+	+	+	+
Academic or educational problem	Z55.9	444		0	0	0	+	+	+	+
Other problem related to employment	Z56.9	444		0	0	0	0	0	+	++
Extreme poverty	Z59.5			+	+	+	+	+	+	+
Homelessness	Z59.0			+	+	+	+	+	+	+
Religious or spiritual problem	Z65.8	444		0	0	0	+	+	+	+
Acculturation problem	Z60.3	445		0	0	+	+	+	+	++
Phase of life problem	Z60.0	445		0	0	0	+	+	+	+
Social exclusion or rejection	Z60.4				+	+	+	+	+	+
Personal history of self-harm	Z91.5						+	+	+	+
Target of (perceived) adverse discrimination or persecution	Z60.5			+	+	+	+	+	+	+
Other problem related to psychosocial circumstances	Z65.8			+	+	+	+	+	+	+

[b]Different codes are used for the four child maltreatment categories when the maltreatment is suspected (see Table 27.1), and numerous Z-codes are used for an encounter for mental health services: for victim versus perpetrator, and for parental versus nonparental abuse/neglect (see DSM-5).

A Questionnaire for Parents

Name of child	
Child's current age/date of birth	
Was child adopted? If so, details?	
Who lives in the home with the child?	
Who is the legal guardian?	
Who referred your child for evaluation?	

What problem or concerns do you have about your child at this time?

_____

_____

_____

Has your child had problems or been diagnosed with any of the following? (If so, note details below.)

❑ Feeling sad or hopeless; frequent crying

❑ Irritability

❑ Often thinking about death/loss

❑ Thoughts of suicide

❑ Feeling anxious/nervous/worried

❑ Having panic attacks

❑ Vision/hearing problems

❑ Seeing/hearing/feeling things that aren't real

❑ Change in appetite

❑ Picky eating

❑ Weight loss or concern with body image

❑ Binge eating/purging or restricting diet

❑ Difficulty falling asleep or staying asleep

❑ Nightmares/night terrors/sleepwalking

❑ Snoring or difficulty breathing while asleep

❑ Excessive daytime sleepiness

❑ Bedwetting

❑ Daytime toileting accidents

❑ Tics/Tourette's, involuntary movements

❑ Language/speech delay

❑ Learning disorder (reading/math/writing)

❑ Pulling out hair/eyelashes or picking at skin

❑ Having few friends

❑ Being bullied (physically, verbally, online)

❑ Victim of neglect or physical/sexual abuse

❑ Excessively rigid adherence to routine

❑ Problems transitioning between activities

❑ Social withdrawal

❑ Hyperactivity

❑ Impulsivity

❑ Being disorganized/forgetful

❑ Difficulty finishing tasks/projects

❑ Temper outbursts

❑ Aggressive behavior at home

❑ Aggressive behavior at school

❑ Truancy

❑ Police/legal difficulties

❑ Excessive use of computer/phone/gaming

❑ Use of alcohol or street drugs

❑ Witnessed domestic violence

❑ Parental divorce

❑ Family move

❑ Loss of pet

❑ Loss of friendship or romantic relationship

❑ Parental abandonment

❑ Death of family member/friend

❑ Any other problems?

Details (age, brief description) for any problems checked above:

_____

_____

_____

Patient's prebirth and delivery history:

Was pregnancy planned?	
Was delivery at full term?	
Problems or illnesses during pregnancy?	

Maternal substance use (including alcohol/tobacco) or toxic exposure during pregnancy?	
Difficult delivery?	
Caesarian section?	
Birth weight (pounds, ounces)? Birth length?	
Did baby have problems breathing?	
Was oxygen administered?	
Was there jaundice?	
Was blood transfused?	

At what age (months, years) did this child first:

Sit up unsupported?	
Crawl?	
Stand alone?	
Walk?	
Speak first words?	
Speak in compete sentences?	
Complete toilet training?	

Child's general health history:

- ❏ Allergies
- ❏ Asthma
- ❏ Diabetes
- ❏ Chicken pox or measles
- ❏ Heart problems
- ❏ Ear infections
- ❏ Urinary infections
- ❏ Poor bowel control
- ❏ Meningitis/encephalitis

- ❏ Head injury
- ❏ Rheumatic fever
- ❏ Strep throat
- ❏ Operations
- ❏ Recurrent headaches
- ❏ Frequent stomachaches
- ❏ Seizures
- ❏ Other illnesses or injuries

Details (age in years, treatment, outcome) for any problems checked above:

_____

_____

_____

Any current or past medications:

Medication name	Age when used	Dose	Reason for use and effectiveness

Vaccination history—write in age(s) at which each was given:

❑ DTaP (diphtheria, tetanus, pertussis)   ❑ MMR (measles, mumps, rubella)

❑ Hepatitis A   ❑ Polio

❑ Hepatitis B   ❑ Chicken pox

❑ Influenza   ❑ HPV (human papillomavirus)

❑ Meningococcus (meningitis)

Education:

Current school	
Grade	
Main teacher	
Current grades (range)	
Problems with specific subjects?	

Disciplinary issues?	
Repeat a grade?	
Special education needs, such as IEP or 504 plan?	
Number of schools attended	

Family data (please include information about any step- or half-siblings):

	Mother	Father	Stepmother	Stepfather
Name				
Street address				
City, state, zip/ post code				
Last school year completed				
Number of marriages				
Current occupation				
Children (names, ages)				
Grandparents' names				
Grandparents' locations				

Family history of illness:

Has any biological relative of the child (mother, father, brother, sister, uncle, aunt, grandparent, cousin) had symptoms of or been diagnosed with any of the following?

	Relative(s)	Brief description
Alcohol or other substance use		
Anxiety, phobias, obsessions		
Autism/Asperger's		
Behavior problem/conduct disorder/criminal behavior		
Conflict with family or others		
Depression		
Learning disorders or intellectual difficulties		
Mania/bipolar disorder		
Attention-deficit/hyperactivity disorder		
Psychosis/schizophrenia		
Seizures/epilepsy/traumatic brain injury		
Suicide or suicide attempt/ psychiatric hospitalization		
Tics/Tourette's		

Details for any problems checked above:

_____

_____

_____

Is the family currently undergoing any stresses, such as illness, death, military deployment, financial problems, multiple moves, job loss? If so, please describe:

_____

_____

_____

Are there any other circumstances that influence your parenting style with this child? Please describe:

_____

_____

_____

Index

Italics indicate definitions; **bold face** indicates Essential Features.